THE YEAR IN RESPIRATORY MEDICINE

VOLUME 4

EDITED BY

**R FERGUSSON, A HILL,
N HIRANI, P REID, R RIHA**

Clinical Publishing
OXFORD

Clinical Publishing

an imprint of Atlas Medical Publishing Ltd

Oxford Centre for Innovation
Mill Street, Oxford OX2 0JX, UK

Tel: +44 1865 811116
Fax: +44 1865 251550
E mail: info@clinicalpublishing.co.uk
Web: www.clinicalpublishing.co.uk

Distributed in USA and Canada by:

Clinical Publishing
30 Amberwood Parkway
Ashland, OH 44805, USA

Tel: 800-247-6553
         (toll free within US and Canada)
Fax: 419-281-6883
Email: order@bookmasters.com

Distributed in UK and Rest of World by:

Marston Book Services Ltd
PO Box 269
Abingdon
Oxon OX14 4YN, UK

Tel: +44 1235 465500
Fax: +44 1235 465555
Email: trade.orders@marston.co.uk

© Atlas Medical Publishing Ltd 2009

First published 2009

A catalogue record for this book is available from the British Library

ISBN-13 978 1 84692 014 1
e-book ISBN 978 1 84692 577 1
ISSN 1477-8114

**The publisher makes no representation, express or implied, that the dosages in
this book are correct. Readers must therefore always check the product information
and clinical procedures with the most up-to-date published product information and
data sheets provided by the manufacturers and the most recent codes of conduct
and safety regulations. The authors and the publisher do not accept any liability for
any errors in the text or for the misuse or misapplication of material in this work**

Typeset by Hope Services (Abingdon) Ltd, Abingdon, Oxon, UK
Printed by Marston Book Services Ltd, Abingdon, Oxon, UK

Contents

Part IV

Obstructive sleep apnoea/hypopnoea syndrome

Part V

Interstitial lung disease

Editors/contributors

Ron Fergusson, MD, FRCPE
Consultant Physician, Respiratory Medicine Unit, Western General Hospital, Edinburgh, UK

Adam Hill, MBChB, MD, FRCPE
Consultant Physician, Department of Respiratory Medicine, Royal Infirmary of Edinburgh, Edinburgh, UK

Nik Hirani, PhD, MRCP
Senior Clinical Lecturer and Honorary Consultant, Department of Respiratory Medicine, Royal Infirmary of Edinburgh, Edinburgh, UK

Anne Jones
Department of Sleep Medicine, Edinburgh Royal Infirmary, Edinburgh, UK

Maeve Murray, MBChB, MRCP
Clinical Research Fellow, University of Edinburgh, Edinburgh, UK

Peter Reid, MD, FRCP(Edin)
Consultant Respiratory Physician and Honorary Senior Lecturer, Lothian University Hospital Trust, Western General Hospital, Edinburgh, UK

Renata Riha, MD, FRACP, FRCPE
Department of Sleep Medicine, Edinburgh Royal Infirmary, Edinburgh, UK

John Simpson, PhD, FRCPE
Senior Clinical Lecturer and Honorary Consultant in Respiratory Medicine, MRC Centre for Inflammation Research, University of Edinburgh, Edinburgh, UK

Part I

Obstructive airway disease

1

Asthma

PETER REID

Introduction

Asthma is a chronic complex inflammatory disorder of the airways characterized by increased airway hyper-reactivity (AHR) and variable airflow obstruction. Its importance is underpinned by the recognition that an estimated 300 million people worldwide suffer from asthma and an estimated additional 100 million persons may be expected to develop the disease by 2025.

Given the magnitude of the potential impact of asthma, one of the key challenges for clinicians and scientists is the possibility of identifying the individuals at highest risk of developing the disease and then intervening in such a manner as to prevent its emergence. This area continues to attract significant interest and more papers have been published this year, with particular interest in intervention with corticosteroids. Once asthma has developed, management involves a number of different healthcare professionals working together with the patient. Lifestyle factors are invariably important, although many patients require pharmacological intervention. Inhaled corticosteroids (ICS) are the most effective anti-inflammatory therapy and are recommended for most patients with symptomatic, persistent disease. Their pre-eminent position is underpinned by clinical studies reporting prompt and effective reductions in asthma symptom scores, improvements in lung function, attenuation of AHR, a reduced incidence of hospitalization and the prevention of death. Nevertheless, important questions have remained unanswered. This year investigators have explored whether in mild asthma it is important to administer inhaled steroids as regular therapy or whether intermittent dosing guided by symptoms is sufficient. We have also seen more information on the relationship between dose and response, and there is some further information on new inhaled steroids.

For those patients whose disease remains inadequately controlled by the use of ICS alone, the addition of long-acting β_2-agonists (LABAs) has been consistently demonstrated to provide additional control, particularly with regard to important end-points such as exacerbations of asthma. This year, further information becomes available as to which dosing level we should choose for add-on therapy with a LABA. The important question of whether the combination of ICS and LABA has any additional anti-inflammatory effect is explored further, and more information has become available on the often neglected area of stepping-down therapy. An interesting study has also been published exploring the strategy of using combination inhalers for both maintenance and relief. Leukotriene receptor antagonists remain the second choice for add-on therapy but appear to be beneficial in certain patients. This year we have more information regarding the responsiveness of patients to leukotriene receptor antagonists. Further data are also available on the efficacy of omalizumab in patients with severe asthma, and the novel technique of bronchial thermoplasty, which uses radiofrequency energy to reduce the mass of airway smooth muscle, has been explored in a small number of patients.

Most guideline statements encourage practitioners to develop education and self-management programmes. These programmes have developed with the aim of increasing patients' knowledge and supplying and reinforcing the skill base necessary for the patient (or their carers) to govern changes in their own therapy, the premise being that knowledge leads to improved day-to-day self-management behaviour. However, it remains unclear whether programmes such as these have a role in patients with more severe asthma who have a history of near-fatal attacks.

Preventing the emergence of asthma

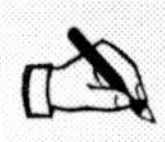

The Canadian Childhood Asthma Primary Prevention Study: outcomes at 7 years of age

Chan-Yeung M, Ferguson A, Watson W, *et al. J Allergy Clin Immunol* 2005; **116**: 49–55

BACKGROUND. **The Canadian Childhood Asthma Primary Prevention Study is a prospective, randomized, controlled trial designed to determine the effectiveness of a multifaceted intervention programme in the primary prevention of asthma in high-risk infants, implemented before birth and in the first year of life.**

INTERPRETATION. A multifaceted intervention designed to reduce exposure to allergens and environmental tobacco smoke and to encourage breastfeeding reduced the prevalence of paediatric allergist-diagnosed asthma in children aged 7.

Comment

The authors of this study identified high-risk infants (those with at least one first-degree relative with asthma or two first-degree relatives with other classic immunoglobulin (Ig) E-mediated allergic diseases) and randomly assigned them either to a control group who received the usual care recommended by their primary care physicians, or an active group who received a multifaceted intervention to minimize exposure to house dust mite (encasement of the infant's and parents' bedding, instructions to wash bedding weekly and chemical treatments of carpets and upholstered furniture), exposure to pets (parents were instructed to remove cats and dogs from the home, or, if this was not possible, to keep any pets outside the home or away from the infant's bedroom) and counselling on smoking cessation and smoke-free homes. Day care was discouraged until after the first year of life and mothers were advised to breastfeed for at least 4 months of the first year. When breastfeeding was not possible, partially hydrolysed whey formula was supplied for supplementation until 12 months of age. Assessment at age 7 included a nurse-led questionnaire on symptoms, examination by a paediatric allergist, determination of AHR by methacholine challenge and allergy skin tests.

The main finding of this study was that the proportion of children recognized by a physician to suffer from asthma was significantly lower in the intervention group (14.9%) than in the control group (23.0%; adjusted risk ratio [RR] 0.44; 95% confidence interval [CI] 0.25–0.79). Interestingly, however, the two groups did not differ with regard to two other atopic diseases: allergic rhinitis and atopic dermatitis. The prevalence and relative risks of reported symptoms in the last 12 months were lower in the intervention group compared with the control group; however, in the same group the prevalence of emergency room visits for wheeze or asthma was higher, and (with regard to the mechanism) it was interesting that there was no effect on the prevalence of AHR or sensitization to common allergens in the intervention group. Looking at a subgroup of patients defined by the presence of AHR and reported wheeze in the last 12 months (derived from a questionnaire interview conducted independently by research nurses) the prevalence of asthma in the intervention group was significantly reduced, by 61%.

The dissociation between reduction in diagnosed asthma and the prevalence of AHR is potentially confusing. Excluding explanation by incorrect diagnoses or bias, the authors argued that AHR (and atopy) may be separate but related factors that contribute to the clinical manifestation of airway disease, and they hypothesized that, for example, if their intervention had reduced the degree of airway inflammation, this may have affected the likelihood that AHR would translate into clinical symptoms. Further assessments are planned when these children reach 11–12 years.

Long-term inhaled corticosteroids in preschool children at high risk for asthma

Guilbert TW, Morgan WJ, Zeiger RS, *et al. New Engl J Med* 2006; **354**: 1985–97

BACKGROUND. Focusing therapy in subjects at high risk of developing asthma is an attractive goal as it represents a window of opportunity to either abrogate or modify the disease. Therefore, the authors designed the Prevention of Early Asthma in Kids (PEAK) study to test whether regular treatment with ICS would prevent the development of asthma in pre-school children. The primary outcome measure was the number of episode-free days during the third treatment-free observation year.

INTERPRETATION. The use of regular ICS for 2 years in pre-school children at high risk of developing asthma did not prevent the development of asthma symptoms or affect lung function during a third, treatment-free year.

Comment

The PEAK study randomly assigned 285 subjects at high risk of developing persistent asthma during their pre-school years (identified by an asthma predictive index) to either inhaled fluticasone propionate (88 µg twice daily) or placebo for 2 years. During the third year of the study, medication was discontinued and the primary outcome measure was the number of episode-free days during that year. During the treatment period, the authors found that subjects taking inhaled fluticasone reported a greater proportion of episode-free days, a lower rate of exacerbations and a reduced requirement for supplementary medications compared with placebo. However, following discontinuation of regular therapy during the third year there was no important difference between groups with regard to the proportion of episode-free days. Treatment with ICS was associated with reduced growth during the treatment year but there was evidence of catch-up during the treatment-free year.

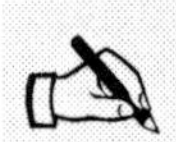

Intermittent inhaled corticosteroids in infants with episodic wheezing

Bisgaard H, Hermansen MN, Loland L, Halkjaer LB, Buchvald F. *New Engl J Med* 2006; **354**: 1998–2005

BACKGROUND. In order to test whether early intervention with ICS would affect the development of asthma in children with recurrent wheezing episodes, the authors designed the Prevention of Asthma in Childhood (PAC) study as a double-blind, randomized, controlled trial to investigate the effects of intermittent ICS therapy in a cohort of infants whose mothers had received a diagnosis of asthma. They monitored the progression of asthmatic symptoms from birth through the first 3 years of life and used symptom-free days as the primary outcome measure.

INTERPRETATION. Intermittent ICS therapy had no effect on the progression from episodic to persistent wheezing and no short-term benefit during episodes of wheezing in the first 3 years of life.

Comment

Prior observations suggest that the antecedent of impaired lung function in later childhood and adult life observed in patients with persistent wheezing and asthma is an uncontrolled airway inflammatory reaction. Thus, the authors argue that early intervention with anti-inflammatory therapy could affect the natural history favourably. The authors drew their population from a prospective, longitudinal, birth-cohort study: the Copenhagen Prospective Study on Asthma in Childhood

(COPSAC). Infants were recruited following the report of a 3-day episode of wheezing and randomized to either 400 µg/day budesonide or placebo, which was commenced after 3 days of symptoms. As with the study of the use of inhaled fluticasone propionate in wheezy infants discussed below, the results of the study were largely negative. The proportion of symptom-free days did not differ between the two groups and there were no differences with regard to persistent wheezing or the duration of acute episodes. Height and bone mineral density were unaffected. Any study on this age group is beset by the difficulties inherent in recognizing asthma; however, although such difficulties will continue to challenge clinicians and investigators alike, it would seem that treatment with ICS would be unlikely to alter the natural history of asthma.

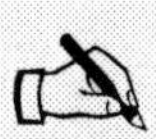

Secondary prevention of asthma by the use of inhaled fluticasone propionate in wheezy infants (IFWIN): double-blind, randomised, controlled study

Murray CS, Woodcock A, Langley SJ, Morris J, Custovic A. *Lancet* 2006; **368**: 754–62

BACKGROUND. The aim of this study was to investigate whether the introduction of ICS at the earliest identifiable point in the natural history of asthma could prevent subsequent loss of lung function and worsening of asthma in later childhood.

INTERPRETATION. The introduction of early inhaled anti-inflammatory therapy has no effect on the natural history of asthma or wheeze in later childhood and does not prevent loss of lung function.

Comment

This study shared a similar hypothesis and aims to the PAC study (see above). They tested this hypothesis by designing a randomized, double-blind, controlled study of inhaled fluticasone propionate 100 µg twice daily in young children. They identified their participants from a high-risk birth cohort consisting of children having one atopic parent and children who had had an episode of wheeze confirmed by the family doctor. Children were enrolled in the study if they had either two episodes of confirmed wheeze lasting more than 24 h or one prolonged physician-confirmed wheezy episode lasting more than 1 month. The dose of the study drug was reduced every 3 months until the minimum treatment dose was obtained, but if wheeze persisted at 3 months open-label fluticasone propionate 100 µg twice daily was commenced in addition to the study drug. The children were then followed up until the age of 5 years, when the parent or guardian was asked to complete a standard interviewer-administered respiratory questionnaire and specific airway resistance was measured.

Two-thirds of the children were younger than 2 years, most were followed up for more than 3 years and dropouts were few. However, as with previous studies, the outcome was negative. The authors reported no difference in the proportions of children with current wheeze, physician-diagnosed asthma or use of asthma medication, declining lung function or AHR between those on active treatment and those receiving placebo.

Treatment options for asthma

Inhaled corticosteroids

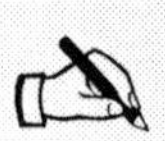

Daily versus as-needed corticosteroids for mild persistent asthma

Boushey HA, Sorkness CA, King TS, *et al*. *N Engl J Med* 2005; **352**: 1519–28

BACKGROUND. Prompted by observations that patients with asthma infrequently renew prescriptions for controller medications, the authors asked whether this may reflect over-treatment and whether intermittent therapy may therefore be an acceptable strategy in patients with mild persistent asthma. They enrolled 225 patients with mild persistent asthma in a randomized, double-blind, parallel-group trial to investigate the efficacy of short-course corticosteroid treatment guided by a symptom-based action plan alone or in addition to daily treatment with either inhaled budesonide or oral zafirlukast over a 1-year treatment period. The primary outcome measure was morning peak expiratory flow (PEF). Other outcome measures included the pre- and post-bronchodilator forced expiratory volume in 1 (FEV_1), frequency of exacerbations, second degree of asthma control, number of symptom-free days and quality of life.

INTERPRETATION. Further studies are required to determine whether this approach can be recommended.

Comment

The premise of this study was based on the observation that in real life many patients do not adhere to therapy as prescribed and adopt an as-required approach to the management of their asthma. The authors suggest that this may be because many patients do not perceive the need for daily therapy and adopt their own symptom-based action plan. The aim of this study was to determine whether, when following a symptom-based action plan, intermittent corticosteroid therapy would perform as well as either regular inhaled budesonide or oral zafirlukast. Patients were aged 18–65 and were included in the study if they fulfilled the criteria for mild persistent asthma over a 4-week run-in period. Once entered, participants were assigned to one of three parallel treatment groups, which comprised intermittent therapy with either a symptom-based action plan alone, regular inhaled budesonide or regular oral zafirlukast.

With regard to the primary outcome measure, PEF, there was no significant difference among the three groups. As might be expected in patients with mild asthma, the absolute number of exacerbations was low; however, there was no significant difference between the groups with regard to the number of patients who had one or more exacerbations. Embedded within the study is a recurring message that regular therapy with ICS is associated with important benefits. The authors reported that regular treatment with budesonide was accompanied by significantly greater improvements in the asthma control score, improved lung function (as measured by the pre-bronchodilator FEV_1), AHR, sputum eosinophilia and exhaled nitric oxide. Compared with the intermittent treatment, treatment with zafirlukast did not produce a significantly greater improvement in any outcome. The authors are careful in the interpretation of their results, suggesting that their findings must be considered preliminary and indicating only that symptom-driven intermittent treatment may be possible. Longer and larger studies will be needed before an intermittent approach to prescribing ICS can be recommended.

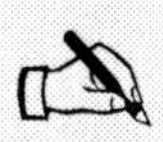

Once-daily ciclesonide improves lung function and is well tolerated by patients with mild-to-moderate persistent asthma

Pearlman DS, Berger WE, Kerwin E, LaForce C, Kundu S, Banjerji D. *J Allergy Clin Immunol* 2005; **116**: 1206–12

BACKGROUND. The authors designed this study to assess the efficacy and safety of ciclesonide administered once daily in the morning in patients with mild to moderate asthma.

INTERPRETATION. Ciclesonide 80–320 µg once daily in the morning improved lung function and symptoms in patients with mild to moderate persistent asthma. Treatment was well tolerated, with a low incidence of local side effects and no significant effect on the hypothalamic–pituitary–adrenal axis.

Comment

Ciclesonide is a prodrug that, after inhalation, undergoes metabolism by endogenous lung esterases to its active metabolite, desisobutyryl-ciclesonide (des-CIC). The molecule displays high receptor affinity and forms reversible conjugates with lipids in the lung (a possible explanation for the extended residency time within the lung). Systemic bioavailability is typically less than 1%, suggesting that the side-effect profile should be favourable.

In this study the authors analysed data from two identical 12-week multicentre, randomized, double-blind, placebo-controlled, parallel-group studies that included just over 1000 adult patients with mild to moderate asthma. Patients were administered ciclesonide once daily in the morning at one of three doses: 80, 160 and 320 µg. Outcome measures included lung function, asthma symptom scores and safety assessments. All ciclesonide groups showed a modest but significant improvement in FEV_1 from baseline to week 12 compared with the placebo group

(80 μg, 0.12 l; 160 μg, 0.13 l; 320 μg, 0.14 l). Patients taking ciclesonide also showed improvements in FEV_1 percentage predicted, morning and evening PEF, 24-h asthma symptom scores, daily rescue medication use, and night-time awakenings when compared with placebo. The drug was well tolerated and the incidence of oropharyngeal adverse events was no different from placebo. Consistent with the low oral bioavailability, the authors did not find any significant suppression of hypothalamic–pituitary–adrenal axis function (by 24-h urinary cortisol or peak serum cortisol level following cosyntropin stimulation) with any dose of ciclesonide.

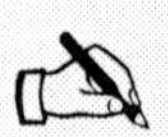

Efficacy of low and high dose inhaled corticosteroid in smokers versus non-smokers with mild asthma

Tomlinson JEM, McMahon AD, Chauduri R, Thompson JM, Wood SF, Thomson NC. *Thorax* 2005; **60**: 282–7

BACKGROUND. Inhaled corticosteroids are the most efficacious anti-inflammatory therapy for patients with persistent asthma; however, most clinical trials exclude cigarette smokers. This group from Glasgow, UK, had previously shown that the efficacy of ICS is reduced in current cigarette smokers. Exploring this further, the authors designed a randomized, double-blind, parallel-group study comparing the efficacy of 400 or 2000 μg of inhaled beclomethasone daily in smokers and non-smokers.

INTERPRETATION. Smokers with mild persistent asthma show a relative corticosteroid resistance that can be overcome by using higher doses.

Comment

The authors recruited 95 patients with persistent asthma from both primary and secondary care clinics in Glasgow. The primary end-point was the change in morning PEF. After 12 weeks of treatment the authors were able to show that the morning PEF improved in the non-smoking group but showed no improvement in the smoking group. In patients receiving 400 μg daily of inhaled beclomethasone there was a large difference in the morning PEF (mean difference –25; 95% CI –45 to –4; adjusted $P = 0.019$) and smokers reported more exacerbations of asthma than non-smokers (6 vs 1). In non-smoking patients receiving 2000 μg daily of inhaled beclomethasone an improvement in morning PEF was seen, as expected; however, smoking patients also showed a small improvement in PEF, and there was no difference in exacerbation rates between the two groups, suggesting that the insensitivity to corticosteroids could be overcome by using larger doses. No differences in compliance were found between non-smokers and smokers.

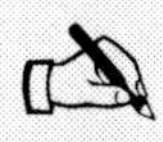

Monitoring exhaled nitric oxide to guide inhaled steroid dosage in asthma

Smith AD, Cowan JO, Brassett KP, Herbison GP, Taylor DR. *N Engl J Med* 2005; **352**: 263–73

BACKGROUND. Current guideline statements recommend that the dose of ICS should be titrated according to asthma control, as judged by reported symptoms and lung function. The authors of this study designed a prospective, randomized, single-blind, placebo-controlled trial to test whether the use of an algorithm based on the fraction of exhaled nitric oxide (FE_{NO}) had the potential to guide dose adjustment of ICS therapy and improve asthma control.

INTERPRETATION. Measurements of FE_{NO} may be used to facilitate dose adjustments of ICS in adult patients with chronic persistent asthma.

Comment

The authors recruited 110 patients (mean age 44.8 years, 63% women) from primary care who had chronic asthma and were receiving regular ICS. During the first phase of the study a considerable amount of effort was put into optimizing the dose of fluticasone (the ICS chosen for the study) so that patients commenced the second phase of the study from a stable baseline. After this first phase, subjects were randomly assigned to one of two management groups: a control group and a nitric oxide group. In the control group treatment decisions were made in response to reported symptoms, bronchodilator use and lung function (according to current Global Initiative for Asthma [GINA] guidelines) and in the nitric oxide group treatment decisions were based solely on FE_{NO}.

The main finding from the study was that participants in the FE_{NO} arm ended up requiring a lower maintenance dose of ICS (370 µg fluticasone/day) than those whose treatment decisions were based on symptoms, bronchodilator use and lung function (641 µg fluticasone/day) without any important difference in other markers of control, including the cumulative total number of exacerbations, time to first exacerbation, or the numbers of patients with one or more exacerbations. Although the authors observed a reduction of just over 45% in the number of exacerbations per patient per year, this was not deemed clinically significant. It is also noteworthy that no significant differences were observed with regard to a range of symptoms or the magnitude of airway inflammation, as measured by the percentage of eosinophils in induced sputum.

One significant problem with the study is that, rather than concentrating on increasing doses of inhaled fluticasone, current guidelines suggest that most clinicians would opt to introduce a LABA rather than increase ICS when asthma control is suboptimal; however, this would have required a much larger study and may have confounded the primary end-point. It may also be recognized that designing a study in which three parameters may effect a treatment change in one arm but only one parameter does so in the other arm will favour more treatment changes to be made in the arm of the study with the greater number of parameters.

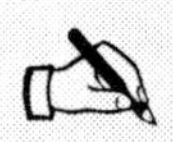

Titrating steroids in exhaled nitric oxide in children with asthma: a randomized controlled trial

Pijnenburg MW, Bakker EM, Hop WC, De Jongste J. *Am J Respir Crit Care Med* 2005; **172**: 831–6

BACKGROUND. The authors of this study explore a similar idea to that of Smith and colleagues (see above), investigating the utility of adjusting the dose of ICS on the basis of exhaled nitric oxide measurements in children. They postulated that titration of the ICS dose with reference to both FE_{NO} and symptoms would result in the administration of lower doses of inhaled steroid and better asthma control compared with titration of the steroid dose according to symptom scores alone.

INTERPRETATION. The use of FE_{NO} to guide the dose of ICS in children with allergic asthma achieves reduction in AHR without increasing the dose of steroids compared with treatment adjustments based on symptoms alone.

Comment

This study shares a similar premise to that conducted by Smith and colleagues but focuses on children with atopic asthma. Pijnenburg and colleagues studied 85 children aged between 6 and 18 years with atopic asthma and randomly allocated them to one of two groups stratified for baseline FE_{NO} ($\geq$30 or <30 p.p.b.) and dose of ICS ($\geq$400 or <400 µg budesonide or equivalent daily dose). The study ran over 12 months and patients were assessed at 3-monthly intervals. In one group (FE_{NO} group), ICS doses were adjusted in accordance with an agreed algorithm based on both the FE_{NO} and symptoms, and in the other group (symptom group) dose adjustments were based on symptoms alone. Although the authors had speculated that incorporating FE_{NO} would result in the administration of lower doses of ICS, this did not prove to be the case: in both groups there was no significant difference between the dose of steroids used; however, the degree of AHR improved significantly more in the FE_{NO} group than in the symptom group (2.5 vs 1.1 doubling doses; $P = 0.04$). As AHR is a major determinant of asthma prognosis and is associated with reduced growth of airway calibre in childhood and an accelerated decline of lung function in adulthood, the authors speculated that the FE_{NO} strategy may have the potential to improve the long-term outcome of childhood asthma. Clearly, this would need to be endorsed by adequately designed studies. Although there was no difference in FE_{NO} between the two groups at the start of the study, the FE_{NO} increased in the symptom group (32% higher): in the symptom group there was a significant increase in FE_{NO}, from 30.8 to 36.7 p.p.b. ($P = 0.035$).

Inhaled corticosteroids and long-acting β_2-agonists

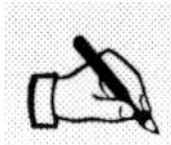

Moderate dose inhaled corticosteroid plus salmeterol versus higher doses of inhaled corticosteroids in symptomatic asthma

Masoli M, Weatherall M, Holt S, Beasley R. *Thorax* 2005; **60**: 730–4.

BACKGROUND. The recently published British Thoracic Society guidelines endorse the addition of a LABA drug as first-line add-on therapy at step 3 in patients not controlled on ICS alone. However, such advice is based on studies including dose ranges from 200 to 800 µg/day of beclomethasone dipropionate or equivalent. It remains unclear at what dose of ICS within this range clinicians should consider introducing concomitant LABA treatment. The authors of this study compared the clinical benefit of adding salmeterol in patients not controlled on moderate doses of ICS (200 µg/day fluticasone or equivalent) with increasing the dose of ICS at least twofold.

INTERPRETATION. In patients symptomatic on ICS at a dose of 200 µg fluticasone or equivalent, the addition of salmeterol is superior to increasing the dose of ICS at least twofold for all major clinical outcome measures. The results of this meta-analysis suggest that salmeterol should be considered when asthmatics remain symptomatic despite moderate doses of ICS such as fluticasone 200 µg/day or equivalent.

Comment

When asthma remains poorly controlled on ICS therapy, the British Thoracic Society guidelines recommend the addition of a LABA as the first choice. However, this advice encompasses a fourfold dose range of ICS (200–800 µg/day beclomethasone dipropionate or equivalent). Recent information on dose– response curves though suggests that the maximum effect of ICS is achieved at much lower doses than previously thought. In an attempt to compare the benefits of the two medications, the authors of this study compared the clinical benefit of adding salmeterol in patients not controlled on moderate doses of ICS (200 µg/day fluticasone or equivalent) with the benefit of increasing the dose of ICS at least twofold. Data were obtained from twelve studies with just over 4500 subjects with moderate to severe asthma. The primary outcome measures were the number of subjects withdrawn because of asthma and the number of subjects with at least one moderate or severe exacerbation. Secondary outcome measures included morning and evening PEF, FEV_1, night awakenings, and daytime and nighttime α_2-agonist use.

With regard to the primary outcomes of the study, the authors reported that there was a significant reduction in the number of subjects withdrawn because of asthma in the low-dose ICS/salmeterol group (59/2036) compared with the high-dose ICS treatment (86/1992) (odds ratio [OR] 1.58; 95% CI 1.12–2.24). More subjects in the low-dose ICS/salmeterol group reported one or more moderate or severe exacerbations of asthma (184/2312) compared with high-dose ICS treatment (243/2264): OR 1.35 (95% CI 1.10–1.66). Secondary outcomes were also better in the ICS/salmeterol group.

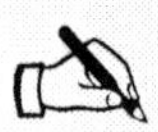

Effect of budesonide in combination with formoterol for reliever therapy in asthma exacerbations: a randomised controlled, double-blind study

Rabe KF, Atienza T, Magyar P, Larsson P, Jorup C, Lalloo UG. *Lancet* 2006; **368**: 744–53

BACKGROUND. Turning again to the question of the dose of ICS at which a LABA should be initiated, the authors of this study designed a double-blind, parallel-group study to assess whether patients with moderate to severe persistent asthma who remained symptomatic despite regular budesonide/formoterol combination maintenance therapy would benefit from additional budesonide/formoterol administered as reliever therapy.

INTERPRETATION. In patients with moderate to severe asthma who remain symptomatic despite regular combination therapy with budesonide/formoterol, the use of as-needed budesonide/formoterol reduces the risk of severe exacerbations compared with as-needed formoterol or as-needed terbutaline.

Comment

The rapid onset of action of formoterol provides a rationale for its use as a reliever as well as a controller medication and its use as such has been shown to reduce the number of asthma exacerbations compared with terbutaline in symptomatic patients despite regular budesonide treatment. In order to determine whether patients using formoterol/budesonide combination would also benefit, the authors enrolled around 3400 patients from 289 centres in 20 countries. To be eligible for entry, patients had to have symptomatic moderate to severe persistent asthma despite the regular use of combination therapy. Enrolled patients were assigned to one of three alternative reliever strategies: budesonide/formoterol, formoterol or terbutaline.

The main finding was that the time to first severe exacerbation (the primary outcome measure in this study, which was defined as an event resulting in hospitalization, emergency room treatment or both, or the need for oral steroids for ≥ 3 days) was significantly longer in patients using as-needed budesonide/formoterol versus formoterol ($P = 0.0048$, log-rank test) and with as-needed formoterol versus terbutaline ($P = 0.0051$). The rate of severe exacerbations was also reduced when taking as-needed combination therapy compared with formoterol. The authors reported a greater number of asthma control days in all treatment groups and all treatments were well tolerated.

This is an interesting study raising the potential for a new paradigm in asthma management. Concerns that such a strategy would result in patients administering excessive amounts of ICS were not realized. However, as alluded to in the accompanying editorial by Professor Pedersen from Denmark, a study should be designed comparing this strategy to an increase in the daily dose of combination therapy.

Adding salmeterol to an inhaled corticosteroid: long term effects on bronchial inflammation in asthma

Koopmans JG, Lutter R, Jansen HM, van der Zee JS. *Thorax* 2006; **61**: 306–12

BACKGROUND. Although the addition of a LABA to an ICS consistently improves clinical outcomes, it is not known whether there is any additional anti-inflammatory effect. The authors of this study designed a randomized controlled trial to run over 1 year in which the primary outcomes included sputum eosinophil and eosinophilic cationic protein concentration and secondary outcomes included neutrophil-associated sputum parameters and a marker of respiratory membrane permeability.

INTERPRETATION. The authors did not observe any sustained anti-inflammatory effect; however, they noted an improvement in the size selectivity of plasma protein permeation across the respiratory membrane.

Comment

Clinical studies have consistently demonstrated that the addition of a LABA to an ICS results in consistent improvements in a range of clinical outcomes, including symptom control and the exacerbation rate. However, to date no convincing effect has been shown on the underlying inflammatory asthmatic process. In this study the authors enrolled 54 patients with mild to moderate persistent allergic asthma, who were randomized to receive either fluticasone 250 μg twice daily or fluticasone/salmeterol 250/50 μg twice daily. Compared with subjects receiving fluticasone alone, those randomized to fluticasone/salmeterol demonstrated improved lung function, improved symptom scores, a reduced requirement for rescue medication and improved bronchial hyper-reactivity; however, using induced sputum to assess a range of eosinophil and neutrophil markers of inflammation, they were unable to demonstrate any convincing sustained anti-inflammatory effect. The one positive finding was that subjects receiving the combination therapy displayed a significantly reduced ratio of α_2-macroglobulin to albumin compared with those receiving fluticasone alone. This may suggest that the permeability of the respiratory membrane is improved by the addition of salmeterol.

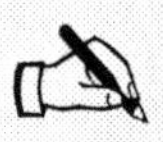

Asthma control can be maintained when fluticasone propionate/salmeterol in a single inhaler is stepped down

Bateman E, Jacques L, Goldfrad C, Atienza T, Mihaescu T, Duggan M. *J Allergy Clin Immunol* 2006; **117**: 563–70

BACKGROUND. Current international asthma guidelines recommend that once asthma control has been achieved and maintained for 3–6 months, treatment should be reviewed and dose reduction of controller medication should be attempted, with careful monitoring to ensure that control is not lost. This advice is largely based on clinical experience, and few studies have examined the options and most favourable conditions for stepping down treatment. The authors of this paper designed a prospective, double-blind, controlled study in which, using a very similar definition of asthma control to that used in the Gaining Optimal Asthma ControL (GOAL) study, they compared the effects on features of asthma of reducing either the inhaled LABA or the ICS component once control had been attained with fluticasone propionate/salmeterol in previously steroid-naive patients with chronic asthma.

INTERPRETATION. Treatment with a lower dose of ICS and a LABA is a more effective treatment option than treatment with a higher dose of ICS alone.

Comment

In order to assess two options for stepping down asthma therapy, the authors selected patients who achieved well-controlled status on fluticasone propionate/salmeterol 250/50 µg twice daily after 12 weeks of treatment. These patients were then randomized to either fluticasone propionate/salmeterol 100/50 µg twice daily or fluticasone propionate 250 µg twice daily. As might be expected, improvements in baseline lung function were obtained during the 12-week open-label part of the study; however, during the double-blind treatment period the mean morning PEF was maintained only in the group receiving fluticasone propionate/salmeterol 100/50 µg twice daily. In contrast, mean morning PEF decreased in patients treated with fluticasone propionate 250 µg twice daily. For each week of the double-blind treatment period, the proportion of patients with asthma assessed as well controlled or totally controlled was slightly lower than that seen during the last week of open-label treatment but the proportion controlled each week with fluticasone propionate/salmeterol 100/50 µg remained higher than with fluticasone propionate 250 µg.

Inhaled corticosteroids and leukotriene receptor antagonists

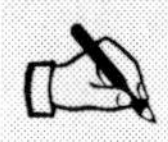

Characterization of within-subject responses to fluticasone and montelukast in childhood asthma

Szefler SJ, Phillips BR, Martinez FD, *et al*. *J Allergy Clin Immunol* 2005; **115**: 233–42

BACKGROUND. The recognition that a considerable amount of interindividual variability exists in the response to ICS and the response to leukotriene receptor antagonists suggests that more information is needed to allow the clinician to tailor therapy for individual patients. This study, conducted under the auspices of the Childhood Asthma Research and Education Network of the National Heart, Lung and Blood Institute, was designed to examine the variability of response to ICS and leukotriene receptor antagonists in children with the aim of identifying indicators that would allow prediction of a successful response to either medication.

INTERPRETATION. Significantly more children show a clinically meaningful FEV_1 response to an ICS than a leukotriene receptor antagonist.

Comment

The authors recruited 144 children with mild to moderate asthma aged between 6 and 17 years, and randomized them to one of two crossover sequences, including 8 weeks of fluticasone propionate (100 µg twice daily) and 8 weeks of the leukotriene receptor antagonist montelukast (using either a 5 or 10 mg dose depending on the age of the child). The trial ran over 18 weeks and 126 children (out of 144) completed the study. Defining response as an improvement in FEV_1 of 7.5% or greater, 17% of the 126 participants responded to both medications, 23% responded to fluticasone alone and 5% to montelukast alone. Interestingly, 55% did not respond to either medication. A favourable response to fluticasone appeared to be predicted by the presence of higher levels of exhaled nitric oxide, total eosinophil count, serum IgE, serum eosinophilic cationic protein and lower levels of AHR and lung function. A favourable response to montelukast appeared to be associated with a younger age and shorter disease duration. A greater differential response to fluticasone over montelukast was associated with greater bronchodilator response, exhaled nitric oxide level and eosinophilic cationic protein level, and a lower methacholine PC_{20} (20% fall in FEV, in response to methacholine challenge) and pulmonary function values. The 55% of patients who failed to demonstrate a significant response to either agent despite reporting symptoms tended to have better lung function and less evidence of allergic inflammation.

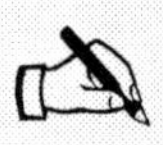

Response profiles of fluticasone and montelukast in mild-to-moderate persistent childhood asthma

Zeiger RS, Szefler SJ, Phillips BR, *et al*. *J Allergy Clin Immunol* 2005; **117**: 45–52

BACKGROUND. Recognizing the need for evidence on outcome from the use of either ICS and leukotriene receptor antagonists in children, the authors interrogated data from a multicentre, double-masked, two-sequence, 16-week crossover trial in order to determine intraindividual and interindividual response profiles and predictors of response.

INTERPRETATION. Inhaled corticosteroids have a superior clinical, pulmonary and anti-inflammatory profile in children with mild to moderate asthma compared with leukotriene receptor antagonists.

Comment

Inhaled corticosteroids should be preferred to leukotriene receptor antagonists in adults with asthma; however, fewer data are available to make a similar definitive statement in children. In this study the authors drew on a clinical trial being coordinated by The National Heart, Lung, and Blood Institute Childhood Asthma Research and Education Network in children with mild to moderate persistent asthma. One hundred and twenty-seven (out of 144) children aged between 6 and 17 years completed a randomized trial in which they were assigned to one of two crossover treatment periods (separated by a 4-week washout period) involving 8 weeks on either inhaled fluticasone propionate 100 µg twice daily or montelukast (a daily dose of 5 or 10 mg depending on the age of the child).

Consistent with the known efficacies of the two agents, the investigators reported improvements in most clinical outcomes in both limbs of the study; however, fluticasone was significantly better than montelukast with regard to the number of asthma control days, the asthma control questionnaire score, use of reliever medication, lung function and exhaled nitric oxide. They also noted that exhaled nitric oxide provided an indication of the likely number of asthma control days and could prove a useful predictor of the response to ICS.

Omalizumab

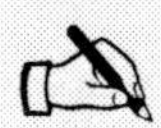

Benefits of omalizumab as add-on therapy in patients with severe persistent asthma who are inadequately controlled despite best available therapy (GINA 2002 step 4 treatment): INNOVATE

Humbert M, Beasley R, Ayres J, *et al*. *Allergy* 2005; **60**: 309–16

BACKGROUND. A subgroup analysis of previous studies using omalizumab had suggested that this drug would prove beneficial to patients with severe persistent asthma. Here the authors conducted a randomized, placebo-controlled, double-blind study over a 28-week period to establish the efficacy, safety and tolerability of omalizumab in patients whose asthma remained poorly controlled despite GINA step 4 interventions, including high-dose ICS plus LABA and additional controller medication if required.

INTERPRETATION. Omalizumab significantly reduced exacerbation rates in patients with asthma whose disease remained uncontrolled despite GINA step 4 interventions. Benefits were also seen with regard to quality of life, symptom control and lung function.

Comment

Patients with severe persistent asthma are fortunately a minority but constitute an important subgroup of patients who continue to experience symptoms and frequent exacerbations. They make a significant contribution to asthma-related health expenditure; indeed, more than half the patients enrolled by Humbert *et al*. had required emergency room assessment in the year before the study, more than one-third had required admission to hospital and 10% had been admitted to an intensive care unit.

In this study the authors enrolled 482 patients with severe persistent asthma (requiring regular treatment with >1000 µg/day beclomethasone dipropionate or equivalent and LABA [GINA step 4]) with reduced lung function (mean FEV_1 = 61% predicted) and an allergic phenotype (positive skin prick test to at least one perennial aeroallergen to which they were likely to be exposed during the study, and a total IgE level of ≥30 to ≤700 IU/ml). They also had to have reported at least two exacerbations requiring systemic corticosteroids or one severe exacerbation in the past 12 months. The primary efficacy variable was the rate of clinically significant asthma exacerbation (defined as a worsening of asthma symptoms requiring treatment with systemic corticosteroids) during the 28-week treatment phase. The primary intention-to-treat (PITT) population (a total of 419 patients) was, on advice from the European Union Committee on Proprietary Medicinal Compounds (CPMP), deemed to be the patient population randomized after implementation of the protocol amendment (CPMP) and reflected the updated GINA guidelines.

After adjustment (PITT population), the clinically significant asthma exacerbation rate was 26% lower in patients receiving omalizumab than in those receiving placebo (0.68 compared with 0.91); this difference was statistically significant. The number needed to treat for 1 year to save one clinically significant exacerbation was 2.2. Omalizumab halved the rates of severe asthma exacerbations (0.24 vs 0.48; $P = 0.002$) and emergency visits (0.24 vs 0.43; $P = 0.038$), and the number needed to treat to save one severe exacerbation was also 2.2. Omalizumab also significantly improved asthma-related quality of life, morning PEF and asthma symptom scores. The study also provided reassuring safety data in that the incidence of adverse events was similar between treatment groups and the total incidence of injection site reactions was 5.3% with omalizumab. This study provides evidence that omalizumab may be a useful add-on therapy in patients whose asthma remains poorly controlled despite GINA step 4 strategies.

Smoking cessation

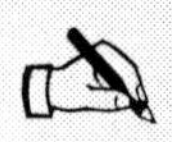

Effects of smoking cessation on lung function and airway inflammation in smokers with asthma

Chaudhuri R, Livingston E, McMahon AD, *et al. Am J Respir Crit Care Med* 2006; **174**: 127–33

BACKGROUND. Around one-fifth of patients with asthma smoke and probably as a consequence of this experience more symptoms, are more likely to present to hospital, experience an accelerated decline in lung function, and have relative corticosteroid resistance. To date, there has been very little published work exploring the effects of stopping smoking in patients with asthma. The authors of this study examined the short-term effects of smoking cessation on lung function, airway inflammation and corticosteroid responsiveness in patients with asthma who smoke.

INTERPRETATION. Smoking cessation is followed by a rapid and considerable improvement in lung function and a fall in sputum neutrophil counts.

Comment

This study is from the same group in Glasgow, UK, whose paper is discussed earlier in this chapter (Tomlinson *et al.*, 2005) In this prospective controlled study, the team enrolled 32 smoking asthmatics who were willing to consider stopping. They underwent a baseline assessment that included measurement of lung function, measurement of inflammatory cells in induced sputum, assessment of the cutaneous vasoconstrictor response to topical beclomethasone, airway responsiveness to oral prednisolone, and a peripheral blood lymphocyte proliferation assay. Assessments were repeated 1, 3 and 6 weeks into the study.

They recruited 32 subjects, of whom 11 wished to continue smoking and 21 decided to attempt smoking cessation. Smoking cessation is challenging, and the authors found that by the end of 1 week seven had relapsed and by the end of the study a further four had started smoking again. However, for those who managed to stop smoking the benefits in terms of lung function were rapid and impressive. The mean (SD) change in FEV_1 in those quitting was 356 (278) ml at the end of week 1, 390 (311) ml at the end of week 3 and 450 (471) ml at the end of week 6. There was no change in the equivalent FEV_1 measures in the smoking control group. At week 6, compared with the smoking controls, the mean improvement in FEV_1 in those who stopped smoking was 407 ml, which represented 15.2% in FEV_1 predicted. The improvement in PEF was 93 l/min.

Consistent with other studies, the authors found that smokers had a raised sputum neutrophil count, and although the authors were able to demonstrate that the neutrophil levels declined after smoking cessation, there were no changes in the levels of sputum supernatant mediators. The improvement in FEV_1 did not appear to relate to the changes in neutrophil numbers.

Smoking cessation did not improve corticosteroid responsiveness; however, the authors speculated that this may have been because the baseline lung function improved by such a large amount that there was little room for further improvement. No differences between groups were noted in the cutaneous vasoconstrictor response or lymphocyte proliferation assay.

Pneumococcal vaccination

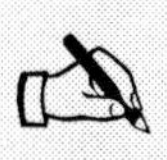

Asthma as a risk factor for invasive pneumococcal disease
Talbot TR, Hartert TV, Mitchel E, *et al. N Engl J Med* 2005; **352**: 2082–90

BACKGROUND. Pneumococcal vaccination is currently recommended for patients with chronic obstructive pulmonary disease but not asthma. The authors of this paper designed a nested case–control study using data from two large populations and then, using Tennessee's Medicaid programme, performed a cohort analysis to estimate the incidence of invasive pneumococcal disease in persons with and without asthma.

INTERPRETATION. The risk of invasive pneumococcal disease in persons with asthma is at least double that in controls, and asthma therefore represents an independent risk factor for this condition.

Comment

Data from this study was drawn from two Tennessee disease registries that form part of the Active Bacterial Core surveillance (ABCs) network for the Centres for Disease Control and Prevention (CDC), providing a study population of nearly 3 million. From this, the authors conducted a nested case–control study enrolling subjects between the ages of 2 and 49 years covered by Tennessee's Medicaid programme (TennCare). Over the period of the study the authors identified just over 600 cases of invasive pneumococcal disease (defined as isolation of *Streptococcus pneumoniae* from a normally sterile site) and just over 6000 controls. A diagnosis of asthma was based on assignation of the diagnosis from one emergency department attendance, two outpatient visits, or the prescription of asthma-related medications. High-risk asthma was defined as asthma requiring admission to hospital or an emergency department. Following adjustment for other recognized risk factors, persons with asthma had more than twice the risk of pneumococcal disease (adjusted OR 2.4; 95% CI 1.9–3.1) compared with controls. The observed increased risk remained after adjustment for the use of long-term (<120 days per year) oral corticosteroids. The authors argue that the strength of this finding suggests that persons with asthma should be considered for pneumococcal vaccination.

Peak flow monitoring

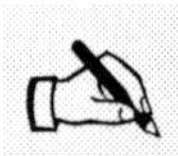

A randomized clinical trial of peak flow versus symptom monitoring in older adults with asthma

Buist AS, Vollmer WM, Wilson SR, Frazier A, Hayward AD. *Am J Respir Crit Care Med* 2006; **174**: 1077–87

BACKGROUND. Guideline statements endorse the use of patient education and self-management, including the use of peak flow readings for asthma, particularly in adults with moderate to severe asthma and a history of exacerbations. However, only a minority of patients keep a peak flow meter and an even smaller number use one regularly. In studies endorsing the use of peak flow readings it can be difficult to separate the usefulness of the peak flow readings from that conferred by other aspects of the intervention. The authors of this study designed a randomized, controlled trial to determine whether the use of peak flow readings in addition to symptom monitoring would be superior to symptom monitoring alone as a management tool in older adults with moderate to severe asthma.

INTERPRETATION. When used as part of a comprehensive asthma management programme, peak flow monitoring had no advantage over symptom monitoring in older adults with moderate to severe asthma.

Comment

In this study the authors identified nearly 300 patients aged between 50 and 92 years from a large managed care organization. Participants were randomly assigned to either symptom monitoring or peak flow monitoring interventions. The interventions were delivered through the use of four 90-min small group classes during which a personalized asthma action plan was developed and inhaler technique checked. The primary outcome measures were healthcare utilization and asthma-specific quality of life. The secondary outcome measure was lung function. No significant differences were found between the groups with regard to the primary or secondary outcome measures. Although it is often suggested that patients do not comply with long-term peak flow monitoring, the authors found that most patients randomized to peak flow monitoring persisted throughout the study, confirming that lapses in this arm did not contribute to the lack of difference between groups.

The Coping with Asthma Study: a randomised controlled trial of a home-based, nurse-led pschoeducational intervention for adults at risk of adverse asthma outcomes

Smith JR, Mildenhall S, Noble MJ, *et al. Thorax* 2005: **60**; 1003–11

BACKGROUND. Management strategies in asthma encourage the use of self-management asthma programmes. However, it is unclear at present whether the evidence of effectiveness of these programmes can be extrapolated to patients who present with fatal and near-fatal asthma. The authors designed what they felt was a pragmatic randomized controlled trial to assess effectiveness as it would be as part of normal care in a home-based programme delivered by a respiratory nurse specialist (intervention) compared with usual care (control). By necessity, the study was unblinded since additional liaison with health professionals involved in the care of study patients often formed part of the intervention.

INTERPRETATION. The effectiveness of a home-based, nurse-led psychological intervention is limited in adult asthma patients at risk of adverse outcomes.

Comment

Although self-management asthma programmes are effective in general asthma populations, patients who present with fatal or near-fatal attacks are subject to a complex interplay of clinical and psychosocial factors that are likely to reduce the effectiveness of these programmes. In particular, the recognition that these patients display a high prevalence of psychosocial factors lends support to the proposition that a home-based psychoeducational intervention may influence their presentation; however, it is uncertain whether any such intervention would be more likely to be effective, given the greater capacity for benefit, or less effective, given the impact of the psychosocial barriers to education and behaviour change.

The authors identified patients with severe asthma (British Thoracic Society step 4 or 5) that they felt to be at risk of severe events (history of non-attendance at clinics, lack of adherence to treatment, and clinical judgement) from adult asthma clinics at five hospitals in Norfolk and Suffolk, UK, and ten general practices in Norfolk. Patients were randomized to either a control arm, in which they continued with their routine asthma care as provided by primary and secondary health services, or the intervention arm, in which they received 6 months of home visits (plus supplementary telephone calls) by a specialist nurse delivering a psycho-educational programme.

Unfortunately, the results of the study were largely negative. After 6 months there were no important or significant differences between the usual care and intervention groups in mean symptom control, physical functioning or mental health scores. Although the authors did report small apparent benefits of the intervention on asthma-specific quality of life for up to 12 months and short-term effects on generic health status, the interpretation of the benefit or magnitude of these was difficult.

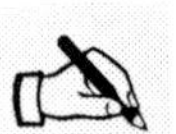

Bronchial thermoplasty for asthma

Cox G, Miller JD, McWilliams A, Fitzgerald JM, Lam S. *Am J Respir Crit Care Med* 2006; **173**: 965–9

BACKGROUND. Bronchial thermoplasty delivers energy to the airway wall at radio frequency, which has been shown to reduce the contractility of airway smooth muscle. It therefore has the potential to reduce AHR and improve asthma control. The object of this study was to examine the safety of the technique in patients with mild to moderate asthma and observe the impact on lung function and AHR.

INTERPRETATION. Bronchial thermoplasty is well tolerated and produces sustained improvements in AHR for at least 2 years.

Comment

Bronchial thermoplasty delivers radio frequency energy to the airway in a controlled manner at an intensity sufficient to heat the tissue to around 65°C, which avoids tissue destruction and scarring but reduces the mass of airway smooth muscle. The technique targets the airways distal to the mainstem bronchi down to an airway diameter of 3 mm. In this non-randomized, prospective study the investigators applied the technique to 16 subjects with asthma of mild to moderate severity. The work was performed at two sites; at one site the technique was performed with the patient under general anaesthesia and at the other the patient was under local anaesthesia with conscious sedation. The airways treated were those that were beyond the lobar bronchi but accessible to the bronchoscope, and larger than 3 mm in diameter. The authors reported that typically one treatment session was needed to treat the airways in each lower lobe and a further session to treat the upper lobes. Treatment sessions were at least 3 weeks apart.

A total of 49 bronchoscopic procedures were performed and all treatments were completed in 30 min or less. Apart from transient acute blanching of the airway wall, no sustained changes were reported with regard to the shape size or structure of the airways. Increased cough, dyspnoea, wheeze and bronchospasm represented the most frequently reported adverse events and the majority of side effects were deemed to be mild (130/155). A small number of moderate adverse events were noted (25/155); there were no serious adverse events. An improvement in AHR was observed in all 16 subjects, the mean PC_{20} increasing by 2.37 ± 1.72 ($P < 0.001$), 2.77 ± 1.53 ($P < 0.007$) and 2.64 ± 1.52 doublings ($P < 0.001$) at 12 weeks, 1 year and 2 years after the procedure respectively. Subjects also reported significant improvements over baseline in symptom-free days and both morning and evening peak flow. In terms of long-term safety, the investigators observed no deterioration in spirometry or change in CT scan appearances after 2 years.

As the authors acknowledge, the study was designed to evaluate feasibility and safety, not efficacy; however, the results give confidence to suggest that further studies should proceed.

Acute asthma

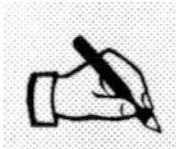

Comparison of inhaled fluticasone with intravenous hydrocortisone in the treatment of adult acute asthma
Rodrigo GJ. *Am J Respir Crit Care Med* 2005; **171**: 1231–6

BACKGROUND. The prescription of systemic corticosteroids is endorsed as a key component of the management of acute exacerbations of asthma but ICS are generally considered to be ineffective. However, several studies have suggested there may be some merit in exploring whether this traditional view should continue to be held. The author of this study designed a double-blind randomized trial to investigate the effect of high and repeated doses of fluticasone propionate with standard treatment in adult patients with acute severe asthma.

INTERPRETATION. The sequential delivery of high doses of fluticasone produces therapeutic effects as soon as 90 min after commencing treatment.

Comment

The authors recruited 106 patients presenting to the Emergency Department of the Hospital Central de las Fuerzas Armadas in Montevideo, Uruguay, with acute severe asthma. Fluticasone was administered by metered-dose inhaler (MDI) using a spacer (Volumatic) in a dose of two puffs at 10-min intervals for 3 h, giving a total dose of 3000 µg/h. Patients randomized to the systemic steroid arm received 500 mg of intravenous hydrocortisone at the beginning of treatment. All patients received four puffs of albuterol and ipratropium bromide (2400 µg of albuterol and 504 µg of ipratropium) per hour.

Patients randomized to fluticasone displayed an overall 30.5% (95% CI 6.3–54.7%) greater improvement in PEF than those receiving hydrocortisone. Notably, the improvement in patients receiving fluticasone was rapid, resulting in better peak flows at 120, 150 and 180 min. Fluticasone-treated patients also achieved discharge criteria at a faster rate than those receiving fluticasone. The fluticasone effect appeared to be greater in those with the poorest lung function. The authors speculated that the beneficial effects are probably a non-genomic steroid effect and may be attributed to enhanced noradrenergic neurotransmission in the airway vasculature promoting vasoconstriction and possibly mucosal decongestion.

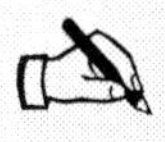

The effect of telithromycin in acute exacerbations of asthma

Johnston SL, Blasi F, Black PN, Martin RJ, Farrell DJ, Nieman RB. *New Engl J Med* 2006; **354**: 1589–600

BACKGROUND. The Telithromycin, Chlamydophila, and Asthma Trial (TELICAST) was designed to determine whether a 10-day course of telithromycin improved symptoms and peak flow in patients with an acute exacerbation of asthma compared with placebo. The primary end-point was a change in symptom score and morning PEF.

INTERPRETATION. The authors concluded that telithromycin may be of benefit in patients with acute exacerbations of asthma.

Comment

Ketolides are a new class of antibiotics that are structurally related to macrolides and have a bactericidal effect against *Chlamydophila pneumoniae* and *Mycoplasma pneumoniae*; however, in addition they are known to possess immunomodulatory effects. The authors enrolled 278 patients within 24 h of an acute exacerbation of asthma and randomly assigned participants to receive either telithromycin (800 mg daily for 10 days) or placebo in addition to their usual care. As current guidelines do not endorse the prescription of antibiotics as routine for the management of asthma, the authors specifically aimed to recruit patients with no clinically obvious need for an antibiotic and therefore excluded those deemed to have overt infection. They chose two primary end-points: change from baseline over the treatment period in symptoms and the morning PEF at home.

Of the two primary outcome measures, only asthma symptoms showed a significant improvement, the telithromycin group showing a mean decrease in symptom score of 1.3 points compared with 1.0 point in the placebo group (mean difference −0.3 point; 95% CI 0.5 to −0.1; $P = 0.004$), which was equivalent to a 40.4% reduction in symptoms compared with 26.5%. PEF did not differ significantly between the groups.

The presence of *C. pneumoniae* or *M. pneumoniae* was sought by performing serological analysis, polymerase chain reaction and culture. Somewhat surprisingly, around 60% of patients met at least one of the criteria for infection with *C. pneumoniae*, *M. pneumoniae* or both; however, it is unclear from this study whether the mechanism of apparent benefit relates to antibacterial or immunomodulatory activity. The authors allude to the need for further studies and highlight concern that recent reports have emphasized rapidly aggressive hepatotoxicity associated with telithromycin.

Conclusion

The field of asthma research continues to generate important and challenging research. The goal of preventing the emergence of asthma remains tantalizing and elusive. There are hints that multifaceted programmes such as that adopted by the Canadian Childhood Asthma Primary Prevention Study may have some benefit; however, it does appear clear that using ICS is not appropriate. ICS remain the mainstay of prophylactic anti-inflammatory therapy and once again are shown to be more efficacious than leukotriene receptor antagonists; however, although we may accept that many patients may use such therapies on an *ad hoc* basis, strategies recommending this approach cannot be endorsed. Cigarette smoking is a major contributor to relative corticosteroid resistance, alerting clinicians to the need for the prescription of higher doses in smoking asthmatics. Conversely, stopping smoking confers benefits for lung function and airway inflammation. Although asthma is fundamentally an inflammatory disease and ICS are administered for the purposes of controlling inflammation, until recently we have only been able to infer the airway inflammatory response by assessing reported symptoms and lung function. The development of techniques to measure airway inflammation, specifically the fraction of expired nitric oxide, may provide a useful tool to guide decision-making, particularly in children, although it is likely that more studies will be needed, especially in adults, before day-to-day confidence emerges. The LABAs have made an extremely important contribution to the management of asthma and have become established as the most efficacious add-on therapy, although the precise mechanisms remain elusive. However, not only can they allow asthma control to be improved, but they also facilitate step-down therapy without loss of control. The importance of smoking cessation notwithstanding, the development of new therapies for selected patients with asthma remains an important goal. Studies with omalizumab suggest that it has potential in selected atopic asthmatics and this year we have evidence that the drug has potential in patients with the severest spectrum of the disease. The development of bronchial thermoplasty also appears to offer promise to selected patients and future studies will undoubtedly be awaited with interest. Finally, as ever challenging, the development of techniques to help patients accept responsibility for the management of this illness remains an important goal and requires input from a variety of health professionals, including, in certain situations, specialist psychologists.

2

Chronic obstructive pulmonary disease

PETER REID

Introduction

Chronic obstructive pulmonary disease (COPD) continues to make a substantial impact on world health and an increasing number of papers draw attention to the escalating burden of COPD in both developing and developed countries. Although cigarette smoking remains the most important aetiological agent for most patients, occupational factors are a contributing factor in around 20% of cases, and in worldwide terms the impact of the widespread use of biomass fuels is an important aetiological factor in some of the poorest countries.

The most common presenting complaint is that of breathlessness or exercise limitation, but the totality of COPD involves a complex pathophysiological abnormality with both pulmonary and extrapulmonary features. Papers published this year provide more information on the mechanical consequences of COPD in the lung and the importance of the systemic nature of the disease. Although it is defined in terms of the irreversible nature of the airflow obstruction and is thus perceived in a somewhat nihilistic manner by some clinicians, significant improvements can be made in exercise capacity, quality of life, exacerbation frequency and severity. This year we see further information published on the use of short- and long-acting α_2-agonists in relation to their ability to act quickly and improve many of these outcomes.

Inhaled steroids are currently recommended in the management in patients with forced expiratory volume in 1 second (FEV_1) less than 50% predicted who report two or more exacerbations in the last year. This year published studies focus on the impact of withdrawing inhaled steroids from therapy after a period of stability. Although we know that inhaled steroids make little impact on the rate of decline in lung function, much interest focuses on whether they can affect mortality. Several papers continue to analyse data acquired as part of other studies in order to answer this question.

Combination therapy has been shown to improve symptoms and quality of life and to reduce the frequency of exacerbations; this year some new information has been published on the potential anti-inflammatory action of the combination. New drug treatments being evaluated include phosphodiesterase type 4 inhibitors, anti-tumour necrosis factor (TNF) agents, and antioxidants. Lung volume reduction surgery confers benefit in terms of lung function, exercise tolerance and quality of life in carefully selected individuals but many patients are deemed at too high a surgical risk for the procedure. Interest is emerging in the use of less invasive methods, such as the placement of endobronchial valves. Equally important is the investigation of treatments that are widely used but lacking in evidence; this year investigators have questioned the use of intravenous aminophylline for exacerbations and short-burst oxygen for improving patient well-being.

Pulmonary rehabilitation is often poorly provided for but should be an integral component of the management of the majority of patients with COPD. However, we continue to struggle to understand why not all patients improve and debate continues over which exercise protocols are optimal. Several papers this year have attempted to shed further light on this area.

As COPD progresses patients become more susceptible to exacerbations. As the consequences of these can be severe, including respiratory failure and death, striving to understand modifiable risk factors and improve the management of the exacerbation are key goals in COPD research. This year important papers have been published relating to the role of bacteria and viruses and the nature of the associated inflammatory response. The possibility that hyperglycaemia may be a modifiable risk factor is raised and the potential role of anti-pneumococcal vaccination in preventing community-acquired pneumonia is also explored. COPD carries a significant mortality and this year authors have examined the role of the lungs and the systemic features (including the inflammatory response) in predicting death.

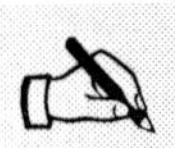

Developing COPD: a 25 year follow up study of the general population

Løkke A, Lange P, Scharling H, Fabricus P, Vestbo J. *Thorax* 2006; **61**: 935–9

BACKGROUND. Most data on the risk of developing COPD are drawn from relatively short studies. In this study the authors aimed to determine the absolute risk of developing COPD from a general population study.

INTERPRETATION. The longer people smoke the greater their risk of developing COPD.

Comment

The authors drew on data obtained as part of the Copenhagen City Heart Study, which is a large longitudinal epidemiological study enrolling members of the general population of the inner city of Copenhagen, Denmark. The authors were able to draw on data from over 8000 participants aged between 30 and 60 years who provided information on smoking and in whom spirometry was performed. Only subjects with normal lung function were included and patients with asthma were excluded. The development of COPD was assessed through spirometric examinations over a 25-year follow-up period. The authors used the staging criteria suggested by the American Thoracic Society and the European Respiratory Society:

Stage 1: FEV_1/forced vital capacity (FVC) <70% and FEV_1 >80% predicted
Stage 2: FEV_1/FVC <70% and 50% >FEV_1 <80% predicted
Stage 3: FEV_1/FVC <70% and 30% >FEV_1 >50% predicted
Stage 4: FEV_1/FVC <70% and FEV_1 <30% predicted.

Twenty-five years of spirometric data were available on just over 2000 participants and this group were analysed according to smoking status defined as: never smoker; ex-smoker; smoker with early smoking cessation; smoker with late smoking cessation; continuous smoker. Although the authors were unable to calculate the total number of years of smoking or the amount of tobacco smoked by any given individual they were able to show clearly that the risk of developing COPD was greatest in continuous smokers: for a continuous smoker compared with a never smoker the odds ratio (OR) for developing clinically significant COPD was 6.3 (95% confidence interval [CI] 4.2–9.5). Indeed, just over 35% of continuous smokers developed COPD and in a quarter of these the disease was clinically significant, being at least stage 2. The study also affirmed the importance of stopping smoking early. None of the early quitters developed severe COPD even after 25 years but the risks of developing the condition were similar in late quitters and continuous smokers.

Breathlessness, exercise limitation, diaphragmatic dysfunction and pulmonary hypertension

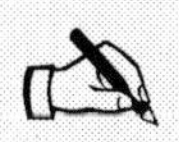

Patterns of dynamic hyperinflation during exercise and recovery in patients with severe chronic obstructive pulmonary disease

Vogiatzis I, Georgiadou O, Golemati S, *et al. Thorax* 2005; **60**: 723–9

BACKGROUND. Although hyperinflation is recognized to contribute to breathlessness and exercise limitation in COPD, the phenomenon does not seem to occur in all patients and some patients with COPD report exercise-related breathlessness despite little or no apparent hyperinflation. The authors of this study used techniques that provide information on chest wall volumes during exercise in an attempt to delineate all dynamically modified operational lung volumes during exercise in patients who progressively hyperinflate during exercise and in those who do not.

INTERPRETATION. The development of early and late hyperinflation early in response to exercise represents two distinct responses in patients with severe COPD.

Comment

The authors employed a technique known as optoelectronic plethysmography, which is capable of measuring changes in volumes of the entire chest wall (Vcw) and its rib cage and abdominal chest wall compartments on a breath-by-breath basis. It is also able to measure breath-by-breath variations in end-inspiratory and end-expiratory Vcw and volume variations of the different chest wall compartments. Studying 20 patients with severe COPD, the authors were able to show that two main patterns of change in EEVcw (the change in Vcw at the end of expiration) could be observed: twelve patients displayed a progressive, significant increase in EEVcw during exercise (so-called early hyperinflaters) and eight patients showed a relatively stable EEVcw until reaching 66% peak workload, following which EEVcw increased significantly (so-called late hyperinflaters).

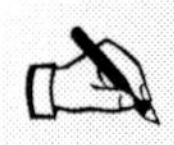

Diaphragm dysfunction in chronic obstructive pulmonary disease

Ottenheijm CA, Heunks LM, Sieck GC, *et al. Am J Respir Crit Care Med* 2005; **172**: 200–5

BACKGROUND. The diaphragm is the most important inspiratory muscle and changes in the composition of the muscle fibres of the diaphragm have been reported in patients with severe COPD; however, as no conclusive studies had been published on the direct contractile properties of the diaphragm, the authors decided to investigate this further. Using single fibres from patients with and without COPD, they assessed contractile function and myosin heavy chain content.

INTERPRETATION. Abnormalities in the force-generating ability of diaphragmatic muscle can be found in early-stage COPD.

Comment

Taking advantage of the availability of patients undergoing thoracotomy for lung cancer, the authors obtained skinned muscle biopsies from eight patients with COPD (six men) and five patients without COPD. Samples were divided to be analysed for single-fibre contractile properties and ubiquitin-conjugation analysis. With respect to the ability of the fibres to contract, the authors found that patients with COPD showed reduced force generation per unit cross-sectional area, which was probably a consequence of reduced myosin heavy-chain content in the muscle fibres. They also showed decreased Ca^{2+} sensitivity of force generation and slower cross-bridge cycling kinetics, observations that suggest the muscle is likely to perform suboptimally when contracting. Increased ubiquitin-conjugated proteins were also found, which suggested that the muscle of patients with COPD underwent accelerated muscle degradation compared with controls.

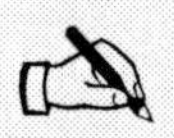

Characteristics of physical activities in daily life in chronic obstructive pulmonary disease

Pitta F, Troosters T, Spruit MA, Probst VS, Decramer M, Gosselink R. *Am J Respir Crit Care Med* 2005; **171**: 972–7

BACKGROUND. The impact of exercise-related dyspnoea in patients with COPD may lead to further deconditioning and muscle weakness; however, to date there have been no comparisons of the physical activities undertaken by healthy subjects compared with patients with COPD. The authors of this study quantified physical activities of daily life in patients with COPD compared with age- and sex-matched controls. They also sought to determine whether time spent in physical activity relates to any parameter of lung function.

INTERPRETATION. Patients with chronic obstructive pulmonary disease show a marked reduction in physical activity. Functional exercise capacity is the strongest correlate of physical activities in daily life.

Comment

The authors enrolled 62 patients (46 men) with COPD with a range of severity from mild to very severe (GOLD [Global Initiative for Chronic Obstructive Lung Disease] classes 1–IV) and compared them with 26 healthy age- and sex-matched retired control subjects. All participants were fitted with a triaxial accelerometer (a small, lightweight box that can be worn on the waist linked to a leg sensor that records the time spent walking, cycling, standing, sitting or lying, in addition to movement intensity during walking). They also measured pulmonary function, peripheral muscle force and maximal exercise capacity, and performed a 6-min walking test. The authors found that most patients with COPD have markedly reduced physical activity, with significant reductions in time spent walking (44 ± 26 vs 81 ± 26 min/day) and time spent standing (191 ± 99 vs 295 ± 109 min/day) compared with control subjects. Walking speeds were significantly slower than those of normal subjects. Patients with COPD also spent more time sitting and lying than controls. The 6-min walking test appears to be the best marker of physical activity ($r = 0.76$; $P < 0.0001$).

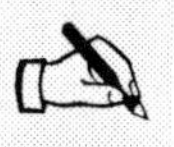

Association between markers of emphysema and more severe chronic obstructive pulmonary disease

Boschetto P, Quintavalle S, Zeni E, *et al. Thorax* 2006; **61**: 1037–42

BACKGROUND. The authors investigated whether there are differences in severity of COPD between patients with and without evidence of emphysema on high-resolution computed tomography (HRCT) scanning.

INTERPRETATION. Patients with COPD who have HRCT evidence of emphysema have greater impairment of lung function and more airway inflammation than COPD patients with no emphysema.

Comment

These authors have previously observed that patients with emphysema confirmed by quantitative HRCT scanning tend to have more severe airflow limitation. Using the inspiratory capacity to total lung capacity ratio (IC/TLC) as an indicator of respiratory severity and the BODE index (a composite score derived from body mass index, the degree of airflow obstruction, the degree of dyspnoea, and exercise capacity) as a measure of systemic disease severity, the authors set out to determine the relationship between the extent of emphysema and severity of COPD. They also obtained induced sputum for analysis of a variety of cell and molecular markers implicated in the pathogenesis of COPD. The logistical complexities of these studies are such that they tend to be quite small, and the final study population comprised 26 subjects with COPD and eight healthy non-smoking controls; however, each subject underwent HRCT scanning, pulmonary function tests and total cell counts in induced sputum, and induced sputum was assayed for neutrophil elastase, matrix metalloproteinase 9 (MMP-9) and tissue inhibitor of metalloproteinase 1 (TIMP-1). Desmosine (a marker of elastin degradation) was measured in the urine, plasma and sputum.

COPD patients with HRCT-confirmed emphysema (as defined by greater than 15% of lung area showing attenuation values lower than −950 Hounsfield units) had both a higher BODE index and a lower IC/TLC ratio than subjects without emphysema and controls. Patients with HRCT emphysema also had a lower FEV_1, FEV_1/FVC and carbon monoxide transfer coefficient, higher numbers of sputum eosinophils, a higher MMP-9 level and higher MMP-9/TIMP-1 ratio than patients without emphysema. Interestingly, it was the number of sputum eosinophils that correlated positively with the HRCT score of emphysema. The study has two important limitations. Firstly, it is a cross-sectional study, thereby making tempting speculations on causality redundant; secondly, the small numbers involved urge caution when interpreting the data.

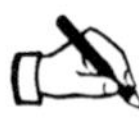

Exacerbations and time spent outdoors in chronic obstructive pulmonary disease

Donaldson GC, Wilkinson TM, Hurst JR, Perera WR, Wedzicha JA. *Am J Respir Crit Care Med* 2005; **171**: 446–52

BACKGROUND. The authors investigated whether exacerbations would affect time spent outside the house, and they therefore used time spent outside the house as an outcome measure.

INTERPRETATION. Time spent out of doors may be a relatively simple but relevant outcome measure for patients with COPD.

Comment

This is an interesting study employing a novel but important clinical end-point. One hundred and forty-seven patients with COPD ranging from moderate to very severe were recruited from the East London COPD Study and data were collected with daily diary cards on a range of respiratory symptoms and time spent out of doors. Patients completed the St George's Respiratory Questionnaire on a yearly basis. Time spent outdoors was shown to decrease by 0.16 h/day per year. The decline was faster in patients who reported frequent exacerbations. During the baseline period patients reported staying in all day on 2.1 days per week, whereas over the post-exacerbation period of 1–35 days they spent 2.5 days per week at home. The St George's Respiratory Questionnaire total, activity and impact scores were independently associated with time outdoors. Patients who experienced frequent exacerbations of COPD showed a progressive reduction in the amount of time they spent outside the home and were more likely to become housebound.

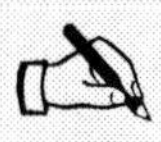

Airway inflammation and bronchial bacterial colonisation in chronic obstructive pulmonary disease

Sethi S, Maloney J, Grove L, Wrona C, Berenson CS. *Am J Respir Crit Care Med* 2006; **173**: 991–8

BACKGROUND. Although tobacco smoke remains the most significant aetiological agent in the development of COPD and induces a pulmonary inflammatory response, it is well documented that inflammation may persist after cessation of smoking. Chronic bacterial colonization may represent one potential explanation for the persistence of this inflammatory response. To test this hypothesis the authors compared airway inflammation in bronchoalveolar lavage (BAL) fluid obtained from ex-smokers with COPD, ex-smokers without COPD and non-smoking control subjects, and determined the contribution of bacterial colonization to inflammation.

INTERPRETATION. Bacterial colonization is associated with persistent neutrophilic inflammation in ex-smokers with COPD.

Comment

The authors enrolled three groups: 26 ex-smokers with stable COPD (predominantly mild to moderate); 20 ex-smokers with no evidence of COPD; and 15 healthy non-smokers. All subjects underwent BAL, from which information was gained on quantitative bacterial culture, cell counts, chemokines, cytokines, proteinase/antiproteinase, and endothelin levels. *Haemophilus* sp., *Streptococcus pneumoniae, Moraxella catarrhalis, Staphylococcus aureus, Pseudomonas aeruginosa* and Gram-negative enteric bacteria were regarded as potentially pathogenic bacteria (PPB) and a threshold concentration of 100 (10^2) colony-forming units (c.f.u.)/ml was used to define significant growth. PPB bacteria were recovered at $\geq$100 c.f.u./ml in just over one-third of patients with COPD, no ex-smokers and 7% of non-smokers.

The authors were able to demonstrate an association between PPB and neutrophilic airway inflammation in the peripheral bronchial tree in patients with COPD. They also demonstrated elevated levels of interleukin (IL) 8, the principal chemokine associated with neutrophilic infiltration, and elevated levels of MMP 9 and neutrophil elastase (bound to α_1-antitrypsin), which may support the concept of proteinase-mediated destruction. Thus they speculated whether the links between bacterial colonization and inflammation may begin to explain the susceptibility of some smokers to COPD and also contribute to the continued deterioration seen in some patients with established COPD despite smoking cessation.

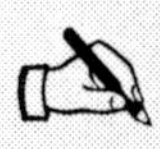

Severe pulmonary hypertension and chronic obstructive pulmonary disease

Chaouat A, Bugnet AS, Kadaoui N, *et al. Am J Respir Crit Care Med* 2005; **172**: 189–94

BACKGROUND. COPD is a recognized common cause of pulmonary hypertension; however, when patients are stable it is unusual for the pulmonary artery mean pressure (Ppa) to exceed 20–35 mmHg. The aim of this study was to characterize a small group of patients with severe pulmonary hypertension attributable to COPD.

INTERPRETATION. Severe pulmonary hypertension is uncommon in COPD and when detected another cause should be sought.

Comment

The most important message in this paper is that significant pulmonary hypertension in patients with COPD is rare. Only 27 out of nearly 1000 patients had a Ppa $\geq$40 mmHg, and in just over half of these another cause was found. In only eleven patients was the pulmonary hypertension attributable to COPD. All eleven were men, were heavy smokers, had moderate to severe airway obstruction, and suffered severe exertional dyspnoea. They were all hypoxaemic and most were hypercapnic. Gas transfer, measured in nine patients, was extremely low and the HRCT consistently showed emphysema. The authors felt that such severe pulmonary hypertension could not be explained solely on the basis of the usual mechanisms for pulmonary hypertension operative in COPD and speculated that it may represent abnormal vascular remodelling.

Cigarette smoking and endobronchial inflammation

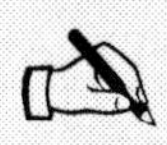

Relation between duration of smoking cessation and bronchial inflammation in COPD

Lapperre TS, Postma DS, Gosman MME, *et al. Thorax* 2006; **61**: 115–21

BACKGROUND. Stopping smoking remains the only intervention that affects the accelerated decline in lung function associated with COPD. Patients who cease smoking also experience a reduction in respiratory symptoms and an improvement in bronchial hyper-reactivity. However, it is unclear whether smoking cessation is followed by any improvement in airway inflammation. The authors of this large cross-sectional study postulated that the bronchial inflammation in patients with established COPD would differ between those who were active smokers and those who had stopped smoking, and that any differences would be influenced by the duration of smoking cessation.

INTERPRETATION. The numbers of bronchial T lymphocytes and plasma cells found in bronchial biopsies change after smoking cessation, longer periods of smoking cessation being associated with a decrease in CD8 T cells and an increase in plasma cells.

Comment

In addition to the long-term benefits of smoking cessation for lung function, quitting is usually followed by an improvement in respiratory symptoms and bronchial hyper-reactivity; the greatest improvements occur within the first year. In order to investigate their hypothesis (stated above), the authors examined data from 114 patients with COPD currently participating in the Groningen Leiden Universities and Corticosteroids in Obstructive Lung Disease (GLUCOLD) study and investigated the number of inflammatory cells in bronchial biopsies taken from current and ex-smokers. In this study population the authors found that ex-smokers had more CD3-positive, CD4-positive and plasma cells than current smokers, but the numbers of neutrophils, macrophages, eosinophils, mast cells and CD8-positive cells were no different. Short-term smoking cessation (<3.5 years) was associated with higher numbers of CD4-positive and CD8-positive T lymphocytes, whereas long-term smoking (≥3.5 years) was associated with higher numbers of plasma cells and a lower CD8/CD3 ratio, suggesting that the numbers of bronchial T lymphocytes and plasma cells in these patients were related to current smoking status and the duration of smoking cessation.

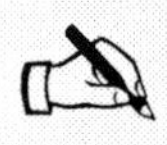

Effect of 1-year smoking cessation on airway inflammation in COPD and asymptomatic smokers

Willemse BWM, ten Hacken NHT, Rutgers B, Lesman-Leegte IGAT, Postma DS, Timens W. *Eur Respir J* 2006; **26**: 835–45

BACKGROUND. The purpose of this study was to investigate the effects of smoking cessation on subjects with COPD and asymptomatic smokers with normal lung function.

INTERPRETATION. Patients with COPD show persistence of inflammation 1 year after smoking cessation.

Comment

All participants were aged between 45 and 75 years, smoked more than ten cigarettes per day and had smoked at least 10 pack-years. The 28 patients with COPD comprised 13 patients with mild disease, eight with moderate disease and seven with severe disease. Asymptomatic smokers were identified as individuals with no history of chronic respiratory symptoms and no evidence of airflow obstruction, although they were recognized to constitute an at-risk group. Smoking cessation was delivered though an intensive group-orientated 3-month course. Urinary cotinine levels were used to confirm smoking cessation. Airway inflammation was assessed by induced sputum and bronchial biopsy at baseline with follow-up studies at 2, 6 and 12 months for induced sputum and 12 months for bronchial biopsies.

Twelve subjects with COPD achieved smoking cessation, which was followed by a slight improvement in the post-bronchodilator FEV_1 at 1 year. Smoking cessation was also accompanied by changes in airway inflammation, as assessed by assay of induced sputum (increased number of neutrophils, number of lymphocytes, IL-8 and eosinophilic cationic protein levels) but not by bronchial biopsy. Sixteen of the asymptomatic smokers managed to quit and in this group induced sputum showed decreases in the number and percentage of macrophages, percentage of eosinophils, and IL-8 levels; the percentage (not absolute number) of neutrophils increased significantly in asymptomatic smokers. In biopsy samples, quitting smoking was associated with a significant reduction in mast cells and an increase in B cells; CD3-positive cells tended to increase.

Pharmacotherapy for COPD

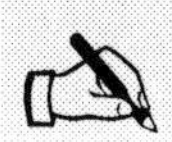

Effect of salbutamol on lung function and chest wall volumes at rest and during exercise in COPD

Aliverti A, Rodger K, Dellacà RL, *et al. Thorax* 2005; **60**: 916–24

BACKGROUND. The authors of this study had previously shown two different breathing strategies adopted by patients with COPD: euvolumic patients, who reduce end-expiratory chest wall volume during exercise; and hyperinflators, who, mainly by changing the abdominal compartment, allow chest wall volume to rise. Little is known about how bronchodilators affect the breathing strategy adopted during exercise and whether this relates to subsequent exercise performance. The authors hypothesized that bronchodilator treatment would reduce chest wall volume at rest and during exercise and predicted that those who increased their end-expiratory abdominal compartment volume during exercise would be able to exercise for longer after taking the drug.

INTERPRETATION. Patients with lesser degrees of hyperinflation at rest had less effect from salbutamol on exercise performance despite improvements in forced expiratory flow.

Comment

Bronchodilators are widely prescribed for patients with COPD in order to improve breathlessness and exercise performance; however, it is apparent that not all patients benefit equally. The reasons for lack of effectiveness in some patients but not others remain unclear. The authors of this study suggested that the patients who were likely to gain the most benefit would be those who could increase their end-expiratory abdominal compartmental volume during exercise. In a double-blind, randomized, crossover trial they examined the effect of 5 mg of nebulized salbutamol or saline on exercise endurance using a cycle ergometer in 18 patients with moderate to severe COPD. They used optoelectronic plethysmography to record chest wall volume; they also measured breathing patterns, metabolic variables and dyspnoea intensity.

The administration of salbutamol resulted in improvements in FEV_1, FVC and inspiratory capacity, and reduced functional residual capacity (FRC) and residual volume. The change in FRC at rest was mostly due to improved compliance of the abdominal compartment. However, although the authors noted improvements in both lung and chest wall mechanics, there was no significant difference in exercise duration or end-of-exercise symptoms in the patients. Separating the group into improvers and non-improvers showed that improvers were older, had more severe airflow obstruction, higher resting lung volumes and worse exercise performance after placebo than non-improvers. They also noted that a significant fall in chest wall volume was associated with an improvement in exercise endurance even though the patients then displayed progressive hyperinflation.

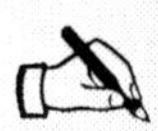

Addition of salmeterol to existing treatment in patients with COPD: a 12 month study

Stockley RA, Chopra N, Rice L, on behalf of the SMS40026 Investigator Group. *Thorax* 2006; **61**: 122–8

BACKGROUND. Recognizing that previous studies investigating the role of long-acting β_2-agonists (LABAs) such as salmeterol and formoterol have been relatively short and conducted in homogeneous patient groups, the authors investigated the effect of salmeterol on the rate of moderate to severe exacerbations over 1 year in a real-life setting. The primary end-point in the study was the number of exacerbations in the intention-to-treat (ITT) population, with secondary end-points of mild exacerbations, lung function, diary card parameters and health status.

INTERPRETATION. Salmeterol improves the clinical state of patients with COPD and reduces exacerbations.

Comment

As exacerbations are a significant event in the course of COPD, the authors designed their study to focus on the impact of the addition of salmeterol on the number of exacerbations experienced. They specifically enrolled patients ($n = 634$) with poorly reversible airflow obstruction and introduced salmeterol ($n = 316$) or placebo ($n = 318$) in addition to their current treatment. Exacerbations were defined as mild if the worsening symptoms could be managed with increased use of salbutamol alone, moderate if they required treatment with antibiotics and/or oral corticosteroids or an increase in ICS dose, and severe if they required admission to hospital. To provide information on the degree of hyperinflation, inspiratory capacity was measured in addition to other lung function tests, breathlessness and exercise capacity, symptoms and change in health status.

After randomization, 56 patients (18%) in the salmeterol group and 75 (24%) in the placebo group were withdrawn, mainly because of adverse events; 233 patients were judged to be protocol violators before unblinding treatment allocation and were omitted to form the per protocol population (PPP) group. Although the difference did not reach statistical significance, the median number of moderate/severe COPD exacerbations over 12 months in the ITT population was 21% lower in the salmeterol group than in the placebo group. However, there were significantly fewer moderate or severe exacerbations on salmeterol than on placebo, with a mean rate of reduction of 30%. Compared with placebo, regular treatment with salmeterol led to significant improvements in lung function, with increases in the inspiratory capacity becoming evident from as early as 4 weeks after treatment began and being sustained over the 12-month period. Salmeterol use was also associated with improvements in the Medical Research Council (MRC) breathlessness score and the distance achieved on a shuttle-walk test. The perception of breathlessness measured using the Borg scale before and after the shuttle walk was not significantly different between the groups. The authors were also able to demonstrate significant improvements in health status as measured by the St George's Respiratory Questionnaire.

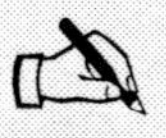

Tiotropium for stable chronic obstructive pulmonary disease: a meta-analysis

Barr RG, Bourbeau J, Camargo CA, Ram FSF. *Thorax* 2006; **61**: 854–62

BACKGROUND. Tiotropium bromide is a long-acting anticholinergic agent licensed for use in COPD. The authors of this study performed a systematic review of nine randomized, controlled trials with the aim of evaluating the efficacy of tiotropium with regard to clinical events, health-related quality of life, symptoms, lung function and adverse events compared with placebo.

INTERPRETATION. Tiotropium reduces the number of exacerbations and related hospitalizations due to COPD and improves quality of life and symptom scores.

Comment

The authors hand-searched 20 respiratory journals looking for randomized controlled trials of at least 12 weeks' duration that compared tiotropium with placebo, ipratropium bromide, or a long-acting β_2-agonist. Nine trials containing data on 8000 patients were included. The main findings were that, compared with ipratropium bromide and placebo, tiotropium reduced the odds of reporting an exacerbation (OR 0.73; 95% confidence interval [CI] 0.66–0.81) and related hospitalization (OR 0.68; 95% CI 0.54–0.84). The prescription of tiotropium was also accompanied by improvements in symptoms scores, quality of life, and lung function. Although there was no difference between the impact on exacerbations and hospitalizations when compared with the prescription of a long-acting β_2-agonist, the effects on lung function (at the time-point measured in this study) were greater with tiotropium. No benefits were reported with regard to mortality.

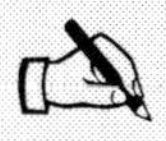

Stable COPD: predicting benefit from high-dose inhaled corticosteroid treatment

Leigh R, Pizzichine MMM, Morris MM, Maltais F, Hargreave FE, Pizzichini E. *Eur Respir J* 2006; **27**: 964–71

BACKGROUND. Given the heterogeneity of COPD, the authors of this paper argued that it may be possible to identify a subgroup of patients with COPD who showed benefit from inhaled corticosteroids and suggested that this was most likely to be seen in patients with significant sputum eosinophilia.

INTERPRETATION. The presence of sputum eosinophilia ≥3% predicts improvement in dyspnoea and lung function in response to high-dose inhaled corticosteroid.

Comment

Previous studies have shown that the presence of sputum eosinophilia predicts short-term clinical benefit from oral prednisolone. The authors of this study suggested that the same finding may assist with the identification of a subgroup of patients with COPD who would derive benefit from high-dose inhaled corticosteroids. They enrolled 44 consecutive patients with moderate to severe clinically stable COPD who, following baseline assessment (including induced sputum cell count) were given inhaled placebo for 4 weeks and then budesonide 1600 μg/day (both drugs being administered twice daily via a Pulmicort Turbuhaler®) for a further 4 weeks. Although the treatments were administered in a single-blind fashion, the results of the cell counts from induced sputum samples were kept double-blind. Sputum eosinophilia ≥3% was found in nearly 40% of participants and, consistent with their hypothesis, the authors found that the presence of eosinophilia ≥3% was associated with clinical improvement. Specifically, they found that sputum eosinophilia was associated with a clinically significant improvement in the dyspnoea domain of the disease-specific chronic respiratory questionnaire and a small but statistically significant improvement in post-bronchodilator spirometry. Those without significant sputum eosinophilia did not show any evidence of benefit.

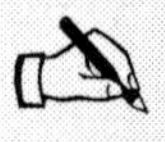

Inhaled corticosteroids in chronic obstructive pulmonary disease: results from two observational designs free of immortal time bias

Kiri VA, Pride NB, Soriano JB, Vestbo J. *Am J Respir Crit Care Med* 2005; **172**: 460–4

BACKGROUND. Previous studies suggesting that inhaled corticosteroids protect against death from COPD may have been flawed by the concept of immortal time bias, which refers to the period of time in a cohort study during which the subject cannot incur the designated outcome, in this case death. In the case of corticosteroids the designers of some studies may have underestimated the duration of person-time without inhaled corticosteroid treatment, resulting in overestimation of the benefit of treatment. The authors of this study used the UK General Practice Research Database (GPRD) to investigate the effect of inhaled corticosteroids on the risk of rehospitalization or death in just over 4500 patients with COPD within 1 year from their first hospitalization. The authors employed two different designs that were free from immortal time bias.

INTERPRETATION. The observed benefit from inhaled corticosteroids for rehospitalization and death cannot be attributed to immortal time bias.

Comment

The authors retrospectively identified all patients with newly diagnosed COPD who were aged ≥50 years between 1990 and 1999 and defined their study cohort as those who were admitted to hospital for the first time with a COPD-related diagnosis. The authors employed two different designs that were free from immortal time bias to investigate the effect of inhaled corticosteroids on rehospitalization or death. In design 1 (propensity score-matched cohort design), they used only patients whose treatment status was defined on the same day of discharge to obtain a matched cohort based on propensity scores (the conditional probability of assignment to a particular treatment given a set of observed patient-level characteristics). In design 2 (nested case–control design), they identified those members of the cohort who experienced death or rehospitalization and then matched each case with four non-cases by random sampling from the cohort risk sets without regard to treatment status. Using the propensity score-based design, the authors reported that inhaled corticosteroids were associated with a significant risk reduction (hazard ratio [HR] 0.69; 95% CI 0.52–0.93). Similar results were observed following analysis of the nested case–control design (HR 0.71; 95% CI 0.56–0.90). The authors accepted that the use of an observational database allowed potential errors to arise from other factors, such as group imbalance from unmeasured factors, and therefore would not satisfy the need for a properly designed and powered efficacy study.

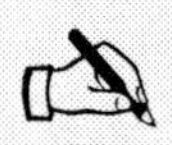

Inhaled corticosteroids and mortality in chronic obstructive pulmonary disease

Sin DD, Wu L, Anderson JA, Anthonisen NR, *et al. Thorax* 2005; **60**: 992–7

BACKGROUND. Little information is available about whether inhaled corticosteroids affect mortality from COPD. In this paper the authors pooled individual patient data from seven large randomized controlled trials, evaluating the effect of inhaled steroids in patients with stable COPD in whom the drugs were administered for at least 1 year.

INTERPRETATION. Treatment with inhaled corticosteroids seemed to be associated with a 27% reduction in all-cause mortality.

Comment

Inhaled steroids do not alter the accelerated decline in FEV_1 nor do they have a major impact on airway inflammation. Nevertheless, fairly consistent observations suggest that they can reduce the frequency of exacerbations and improve health status. The aim of this analysis was to determine whether they might affect mortality. By pooling individual patient data from seven large randomized, controlled trials it was possible to analyse data from just over 5000 individuals, 70% of whom were men and 70% current smokers.

Overall, 201 (4%) died during the trial period: 64% of deaths were from cardio-respiratory causes and 21% were due to cancer. Deaths tended to occur in those who were older and had lower post-bronchodilator FEV_1 ($PDFEV_1$) at the time of randomization. Males were more likely to die than females. The authors found that inhaled corticosteroids reduced all-cause mortality by around 25% relative to placebo (adjusted HR 0.73; 95% CI 0.55–0.96). The greatest effects were noted in women, former smokers, and in those whose baseline $PDFEV_1$ was below 60%.

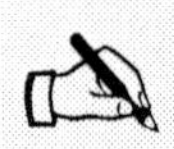

Early onset of effect of salmeterol and fluticasone propionate in chronic obstructive pulmonary disease

Vestbo J, Pauwels R, Anderson JA, Jones P, Calverly P, on the behalf of the TRISTAN study group. *Thorax* 2005; **60**: 301–4

BACKGROUND. Although long-acting β_2-agonists and inhaled corticosteroids are known to convey benefits reasonably quickly in patients with asthma, little is known about their speed of onset in patients with COPD. The authors of this study examined data acquired as part of the TRISTAN (Trial of Inhaled Steroids and Long-acting β_2 Agonists) study to determine the time of onset of action of the individual drugs in respect of lung function and breathlessness.

INTERPRETATION. The effects of salmeterol and fluticasone propionate, alone or in combination, on peak expiratory flow and breathlessness are seen within days and most of the obtainable effect is reached within 2 weeks.

Comment

The TRISTAN study was designed to compare the efficacy of a salmeterol/fluticasone propionate combination (50/500 µg twice daily) with salmeterol (50 µg twice daily), fluticasone propionate alone (500 µg twice daily) and placebo. Just under 2000 patients were recruited and around 1500 received treatment. Examining the data from this study, the authors found that the administration of both drugs resulted in prompt improvements in peak expiratory flow compared with placebo; significant differences appeared for both salmeterol and salmeterol/fluticasone propionate from day 1 and for fluticasone propionate alone on day 2. After 2 weeks the differences for salmeterol, fluticasone and salmeterol/fluticasone were 16 (95% CI 11–21), 11 (6–16) and 27 (22–33) l/min respectively. Similar differences were then maintained over the following year of the study period. Positive benefits in breathlessness were also detected quickly, those receiving salmeterol reporting a significant improvement compared with those receiving placebo from day 1. At 2 weeks the odds ratio for an improvement in breathlessness compared with placebo was 1.57 (95% CI 1.17–2.12) for salmeterol, 1.28 (0.95–1.72) for fluticasone and 2.19 (1.60–2.98) for combination therapy. A similar timescale for improvements in FEV_1 was noted but the change at 2 weeks did not necessarily reflect sustained improvement.

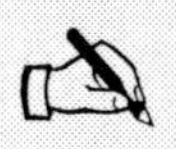

Withdrawal of fluticasone propionate from combined salmeterol/fluticasone treatment in patients with COPD causes immediate and sustained disease deterioration: a randomised controlled trial

Wouters EFM, Postma DS, Fokkens B, *et al. Thorax* 2005; **60**: 480–7

BACKGROUND. Inhaled corticosteroids are known to be beneficial in patients with moderately severe COPD who experience frequent exacerbations. Long-acting β_2-agonists improve lung function and provide symptomatic relief of breathlessness and improved exercise tolerance. The combination of an inhaled corticosteroid and a long-acting β_2-agonist is known to result in greater improvements in lung function and symptom control than the prescription of a long-acting β_2-agonist alone in patients with moderate to severe COPD. The aim of this study was to determine whether the withdrawal of the inhaled corticosteroid component of the combination therapy after 1 year would result in any deterioration of disease.

INTERPRETATION. Withdrawal of fluticasone from fluticasone/salmeterol therapy results in an increased number of mild exacerbations, a deterioration in lung function and an increase in symptoms.

Comment

The COSMIC (COPD and Seretide: a Multi-Center Intervention and Characterization) study was designed as a multicentre, randomized, double-blind, parallel-group study in which all patients received combined salmeterol 50 μg and fluticasone 500 μg (Seretide 50/500) twice daily during a 3 month run-in period following which participants were then randomized to either salmeterol/fluticasone or salmeterol alone. In total, 49 participating centres in the Netherlands enrolled 497 patients; 373 were randomized and 293 completed the study.

The investigators found that withdrawal of fluticasone resulted in a sustained decrease in FEV_1, FEV_1/FVC ratio, peak expiratory flow and MEF_{50} (maximal expiratory flow at 50% of FVC), whereas the same parameters stayed stable in patients remaining on combination therapy. Withdrawal of fluticasone was also associated with an increase in the number of exacerbations, most of which were mild, but there was no difference between either the number of exacerbations or the time to first moderate-to-severe exacerbation. The investigators questioned whether this reflected the fact that they had powered the study on lung function rather than exacerbations or whether it was a result of using medications rather than a diary card to detect exacerbations. Withdrawal of fluticasone was also associated with an increase in dyspnoea, the percentage of disturbed nights, a decrease in the number of rescue medication-free days and a worsening of quality of life.

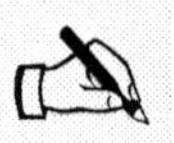

Anti-inflammatory effects of salmeterol/fluticasone propionate in chronic obstructive lung disease

Barnes NC, Qiu Y-S, Pavord I, *et al. Am J Respir Crit Care Med* 2006; **173**: 736–43

BACKGROUND. The pulmonary inflammatory response in patients with COPD is distinct from that in the lungs of asthmatic patients and appears to be relatively resistant to therapeutic intervention. The authors of this study performed a randomized, double-blind, placebo-controlled, parallel-group, multicentre trial designed to determine whether the combination of a long-acting β_2-agonist and inhaled steroid would reduce inflammation in the airway of patients with COPD. The primary end-points were biopsy for CD8-positive and CD68-positive cells and sputum neutrophils.

INTERPRETATION. The combination of inhaled salmeterol/fluticasone propionate appears to influence the numbers of anti-inflammatory cells in the airways of patients with COPD.

Comment

The inflammatory response in the airway of patients with COPD is distinct from asthma. In COPD the airways show increased numbers of CD8-positive cells. The bronchial subepithelium and alveoli show an increase in CD68-positive cells (monocytes and macrophages) and the small airways an excess of B lymphocytes. Increases in a variety of inflammatory cells in different compartments have been linked with an accelerated decline in lung function, suggesting that affecting the inflammatory response could have the potential to impact on the natural history of the disease. In this study the investigators performed induced sputum assays and undertook endobronchial biopsies in 140 current and former smokers with moderate to severe COPD. Participants were then randomized to a 13-week double-blind study to either placebo ($n = 73$) or salmeterol/fluticasone 50/500 µg ($n = 67$) twice daily. Further induced sputum samples were taken at 8 and 13 weeks and endobronchial biopsies repeated at 12 weeks.

As with previous studies, the patients treated with salmeterol/fluticasone propionate showed increases in mean prebronchodilator FEV_1 at each visit and these were significantly greater than in patients on placebo. With regard to their main hypothesis, the investigators found that, compared with placebo, combination therapy reduced the number of CD8-positive cells by 36% in the endobronchial biopsy specimens. CD68-positive cells increased in the placebo group but did not change in patients taking combination therapy. The number of biopsy CD45-positive and CD4-positive cells and cells expressing genes for TNF-α and interferon γ were also reduced compared with placebo in patients taking combination therapy. Examining induced sputum, the authors found that the number of neutrophils declined throughout the study compared with placebo and, when expressed as a percentage reduction from baseline, achieved significance. A reduction in the total number of sputum eosinophils was also noted, favouring combination therapy. The authors accept that the study would have been more informative had the design included a separate limb for each individual drug; however, this would have increased the number of patients required considerably. How much of the effect can be attributed to salmeterol alone remains unanswered.

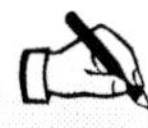

Short-burst oxygen therapy for COPD patients: a 6-month randomised controlled study

Eaton T, Fergusson W, Kolbe J, Lewis CA, West T. *Eur Respir J* 2006; **27**: 697–704

BACKGROUND. Although the prescription of oxygen for intermittent use before or after exertion is widespread, there is very little evidence to endorse its use. The authors of this study designed a randomized, double-blind, placebo-controlled, parallel-group study to determine whether short-burst oxygen therapy was of benefit. The primary outcome measures included health-related quality of life and healthcare utilization.

INTERPRETATION. The use of short-burst oxygen therapy did not improve health-related quality of life or the requirement for subsequent use of healthcare resources following hospitalization with an exacerbation of COPD.

Comment

The patients in this study were recruited from a cohort of patients admitted to hospital with an exacerbation of COPD; baseline disease was moderate to severe in severity, all patients reported symptomatic breathlessness, and had a resting arterial partial pressure of oxygen greater than 8 kPa on air at discharge. Nearly 80 patients were identified and randomized to receive cylinder oxygen, cylinder air or placebo. Those provided with a cylinder received instructions on how to use the gas when encountering distressing or limiting breathlessness. The study ran for 6 months. The main findings were negative with regard to the primary outcome measures, and add to previous literature showing that oxygen administered as such has no real benefit in terms of dyspnoea or recovery time. The costs associated with the widespread prescription of short-burst oxygen therapy could be redirected towards more useful endeavours.

New treatments for COPD

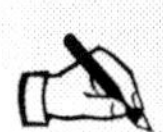

Roflumilast – an oral anti-inflammatory treatment for chronic obstructive pulmonary disease: a randomised controlled trial

Rabe KF, Bateman ED, O'Donnell D, Witte S, Bredenbröker D, Bethke TD.
Lancet 2005; **366**: 563–71

BACKGROUND. *In vitro* and *in vivo* studies suggest that phosphodiesterase type 4 inhibitors may prove beneficial in the management of COPD by providing both bronchodilation and anti-inflammatory effects. The authors of this paper report on a large clinical Phase III multicentre, double-blind, randomized, placebo-controlled trial which was designed to assess whether once daily administration of the phosphodiesterase type 4 inhibitor roflumilast had a clinically meaningful effect on lung function and health-related quality of life in patients with moderate to severe COPD. Primary outcomes were post-bronchodilator FEV_1 and health-related quality of life.

INTERPRETATION. The improved lung function and reduced exacerbation rate seen with roflumilast suggest that further studies with this drug are warranted.

Comment

The regulation of airway smooth muscle relaxation is mediated in part through the naturally occurring second messenger cyclic nucleotides adenosine 3′,5′-monophosphate (cAMP) and guanosine 3′,5′-monophosphate (cGMP), and increased intracellular concentrations of these two cyclic nucleotides lead to airway smooth muscle (ASM) relaxation and bronchodilation. Furthermore, many of the key inflammatory cells implicated in COPD appear to be regulated by the same second messengers. As both cAMP and cGMP are inactivated by hydrolysis of the 3′-phosphodiester bond, the inhibition of this process offers the potential to combine beneficial bronchodilator and anti-inflammatory effects in one medication.

The authors recruited just over 1150 patients with COPD, who were randomly assigned to treatment with roflumilast 250 µg/day, roflumilast 500 µg/day or placebo. Medications were administered orally over a treatment period of 24 weeks. Analysis was by intention to treat. With regard to the primary outcome measures, the authors found that at the end of the treatment period the post-bronchodilator FEV_1 significantly improved with roflumilast 250 µg/day (by 74 ml [SD 18]) and roflumilast 500 µg/day (by 97 ml [18]) compared with placebo. They observed improvements in health-related quality of life with both treatment doses compared with placebo; however, these were not significant. The mean numbers of exacerbations per patient were 1.13 (SD 2.37), 1.03 (2.33) and 0.75 (1.89) with placebo, roflumilast 250 µg/day and roflumilast 500 µg/day respectively. Gastrointestinal side effects occurred early during the study and were generally mild to moderate and self-limiting. Only 1% of patients assigned to roflumilast 250 µg/day and 4% of patients assigned to roflumilast 500 µg/day discontinued treatment because of diarrhoea or nausea. No cardiac side effects were reported.

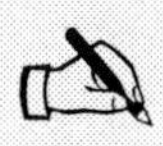

Effects of N-acetylcysteine on outcomes in chronic obstructive pulmonary disease (Bronchitis Randomised on NAC Cost-Utility Study, BRONCUS: a randomised placebo-controlled trial

Decramer M, Rutten-van Mölken M, Dekhuijzen PNR, *et al. Lancet* 2005; **365**: 1552–60

BACKGROUND. Given that increased oxidative stress appears to be important in the pathogenesis of COPD, the authors of this study postulated that antioxidant therapy represented a logical therapeutic target. They therefore designed the Bronchitis Randomized on N-acetylcysteine Cost–Utility Study (BRONCUS) as a randomized, controlled trial to test the effects of N-acetylcysteine on the rate of lung function decline and exacerbations in patients with COPD.

INTERPRETATION. N-acetylcysteine at a dose of 600 mg/day did not affect the rate of decline in lung function or the rate of exacerbations in patients with COPD.

Comment

The study was designed as a Phase III trial employing a dose of 600 mg per day of N-acetylcysteine with the primary end-points of yearly decline in lung function and exacerbation rate. Fifty centres recruited just over 500 patients and followed them for 3 years. The results were almost uniformly negative, the authors failing to show any benefit in terms of yearly decline in lung function, rate of exacerbations or health status. They performed a subgroup analysis that suggested that the drug may influence exacerbation rates in patients who were not taking inhaled corticosteroids. Considering whether the dose was too low, but noting that it was well tolerated, they suggested that further studies should employ higher doses.

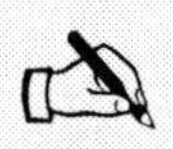

First study of infliximab treatment in patients with chronic obstructive pulmonary disease

van der Vaart H, Koeter GH, Postma DS, Kauffman HF, ten Hacken NH. *Am J Respir Crit Care Med* 2005; **172**: 465–9

BACKGROUND. A variety of observations suggest that TNF-α plays a key role in the pathogenesis of COPD. The authors of this study therefore planned to investigate the effects of a monoclonal antibody to TNF in this condition. They designed a randomized, double-blind, placebo-controlled, proof-of-principle Phase II study to evaluate whether short-term therapy with infliximab (chimeric monoclonal anti-TNF antibody) modifies airway inflammation.

INTERPRETATION. The use of infliximab was not associated with any improvement in any of the clinical or inflammatory end-points.

Comment

Infliximab is a chimeric monoclonal antibody that binds with high affinity and specificity to human soluble and membrane-bound TNF-β; therapy with this agent has been shown to improve clinical and inflammatory parameters in patients with Crohn's disease and rheumatoid arthritis. However, in this study of 22 patients with mild to moderate COPD (current smokers) there were no appreciable effects on inflammatory (percentage of sputum neutrophils, IL-8 or IL-6, exhaled nitric oxide) or clinical markers (respiratory symptoms, lung function, airway hyper-reactivity, quality of life or resting energy expenditure). The authors speculated as to whether the selection of a more severe patient group may have allowed small improvements to become more apparent or whether the inclusion of current smokers may have offset any benefit. It is also possible that the dose of infliximab was too low; however, the dosage was similar to that used in patients with inflammatory bowel disease and rheumatoid arthritis. Importantly, no serious adverse events were reported.

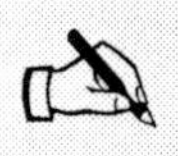

Effect of bronchoscopic lung volume reduction on dynamic hyperinflation and exercise in emphysema

Hopkinson NS, Toma TP, Hansell DM, *et al. Am J Respir Crit Care Med* 2005; **171**: 453–60

BACKGROUND. It is widely appreciated that exercise limitation in COPD results from the development of dynamic hyperinflation restricting tidal breathing. It has been shown that bronchodilators and lung volume reduction surgery produce reductions in dynamic hyperinflation. Bronchoscopic lung volume reduction involves obstructing the airways leading to the most hyperinflated areas of lung with one-way valves that allow expiration but not inspiration, thereby reducing lung volume through collapse of the area of lung supplied by that bronchus. The authors' aim was to investigate the effect of endobronchial valves on the exercise capacity of patients with emphysema and relate this to effects of exercise physiology.

INTERPRETATION. Reduction in dynamic hyperinflation and improvement in exercise tolerance follow the placement of endobronchial valves.

Comment

The study was performed on 19 patients with a mean (SD) FEV_1 of 28.4 (11.9) as a percentage of predicted. Measurements were performed before and 4 weeks after the placement of one-way endobronchial valves in endobronchial segments deemed to be leading to the most hyperinflated parts of the lung. Overall exercise capacity improved, with a 39% improvement in mean cycle endurance time; this was associated with a reduction in end-expiratory lung volume at peak exercise. The authors also observed that functional residual capacity decreased and diffusing capacity rose. Using stepwise logistic regression analysis, they demonstrated that a model containing changes in transfer factor and resting inspiratory capacity explained 81% of the variation in change in exercise time ($P < 0.0001$). In a sub-group of patients in whom invasive measurements were performed, improvement in exercise capacity was associated with a reduction in lung compliance and isotime oesophageal pressure–time product.

Exercise and pulmonary rehabilitation

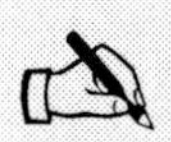

Rehabilitation decreases exercise-induced oxidative stress in chronic obstructive pulmonary disease

Mercken EM, Hageman GJ, Scols AM, Akkermans MA, Bast A, Wouters EF.
Am J Respir Crit Care Med 2005; **172**: 994–1001

BACKGROUND. An excess of oxidants relative to antioxidants is believed to underpin some of the pathophysiology of COPD. As exercise has been shown to increase systemic oxidative stress, the authors were keen to find out whether the increased exercise associated with pulmonary rehabilitation would lead to an increase in oxidative stress and potentially adversely affect the outcome of COPD.

INTERPRETATION. Patients with COPD have increased pulmonary and systemic oxidative stress both at rest and after exercise; however, pulmonary rehabilitation increases exercise capacity and is associated with reduced oxidative stress.

Comment

The authors studied eleven patients with moderate to severe COPD and a similar number of age- and sex-matched healthy controls. Oxidative stress was analysed in the peripheral blood using a variety of techniques. They used a comet assay (single-cell gel electrophoresis) designed to analyse reactive oxygen species (ROS)-induced DNA damage in peripheral blood mononuclear cells and measured the amount of malondialdehyde (MDA) in both the plasma and urine. Plasma uric acid was used to provide a marker of xanthine oxidase activity. Pulmonary oxidative stress was assessed by analysing the concentration of H_2O_2 in exhaled breath condensate. Measurements were made before and after 8 weeks of pulmonary rehabilitation.

As might be expected, compared with the healthy subjects, patients with COPD showed evidence of oxidative damage at rest but further increases followed exercise. Following the 8-week pulmonary rehabilitation programme, despite increased exercise capacity the increase in ROS-induced DNA damage was significantly lower after exercise at submaximal intensity. The reason for the improvement remains uncertain; however, the authors speculate that exercise may lead to improvement in oxidative metabolism or an increase in the capacity of endogenous antioxidative systems.

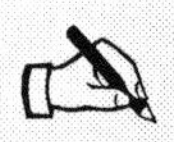

Predictors of success and failure in pulmonary rehabilitation

Garrod R, Marshall J, Barley E, Jones PW. *Eur Respir J* 2006; **27**: 964–71

BACKGROUND. The majority of patients, but not all, appear to benefit from pulmonary rehabilitation. Although a variety of hypotheses have been put forward to explain this, methods for identifying positive or negative outcomes from rehabilitation remain unclear. The aim of this study was to investigate whether any features could be identified as associated with short- and long-term outcomes following pulmonary rehabilitation.

INTERPRETATION. Predictors of response versus non-response remain elusive. The presence of depression predicts dropout from programmes.

Comment

The authors studied a population of 74 patients (mean age 68 ± 10 years; 41 males). Ten patients were current smokers, 62 were ex-smokers and two patients had never smoked. Patients were stratified according to the MRC dyspnoea score, with nine patients MRC grade 1, twelve grade 2, ten grade 3, 19 grade 4 and 24 grade 5. The mean attendance rate was just over 70%. Assessments included quadriceps torque, 6-min walking distance, a measure of depression, and health-related quality of life.

Of the 74 patients, 51 completed the study and nearly 80% showed a clinically significant improvement in either 6-min walking distance (24 patients) or health-related quality of life (32 patients). Interestingly, improvements were seen in patients with MRC grade 1 and 2 dyspnoea, supporting the inclusion of patients with mild impairment in rehabilitation schemes. Clinical improvement in walking distance did not predict improved health status. None of the baseline variables allowed prediction of response versus non-response. Patients suffering from depression were more likely to drop out of the programme.

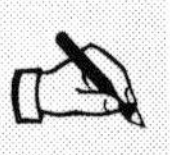

How should COPD patients exercise during respiratory rehabilitation? Comparison of exercise modalities and intensities to treat skeletal muscle dysfunction

Puhan MA, Schünemann, Frey M, Scharplatz M, Bachmann LM. *Thorax* 2005; **60**: 367–75

BACKGROUND. Exercise is an important component of any rehabilitation scheme; however, uncertainty exists over the optimal exercise programme, with a variety of different protocols being adopted by several investigators. The authors of this systematic review aimed to analyse all available randomized controlled trials that included head-to-head comparisons of at least two exercise protocols.

INTERPRETATION. The use of strength exercise rather than endurance exercise should be adopted by those implementing pulmonary rehabilitation programmes. More information is needed on the relative benefits of interval versus continuous exercise programmes and high- versus low-intensity programmes.

Comment

Skeletal muscle dysfunction is well documented in advanced COPD and undoubtedly contributes to the exercise limitation experienced by these patients. Pulmonary rehabilitation has been shown to reverse this process. However, as there is no consensus on the optimal exercise protocol, a variety of different programmes are employed. The authors of this study searched six electronic databases, congress proceedings and bibliographies of included studies and identified 15 randomized, controlled trials that included head-to-head comparisons of at least two exercise protocols (different exercise modalities and intensities or combinations thereof).

The strongest conclusions of the review relate to information from four trials comparing endurance and strength exercise, which showed that strength exercise consistently yielded larger improvements in health-related quality of life than endurance exercise. Such information as there was comparing interval exercise with continuous exercise suggested that interval exercise may be as beneficial as continuous exercise programmes, but the quality of the evidence was low. Even less information was available to comment with authority on whether high-intensity training was superior to low-intensity training, and the authors recommend that more research should be directed towards answering this important question.

Managing exacerbations of COPD

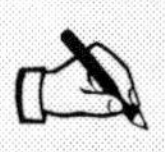

Intravenous aminophylline in patients admitted to hospital with non-acidotic exacerbations of chronic obstructive pulmonary disease: a prospective randomised controlled trial
Duffy N, Walker P, Diamantea F, Calverley PM, Davies L. *Thorax* 2005; **60**: 713–17

BACKGROUND. Despite a long history of use in the management of exacerbations of COPD, there is little evidence to validate the prescription of aminophylline in this scenario. Current guidelines suggest that aminophylline may be considered as a treatment option when response to controlled oxygen, nebulized bronchodilators (β_2-agonist and anticholinergic agent) and oral corticosteroids have been administered. As it is widely recognized that aminophylline is accompanied by potentially deleterious side effects, the authors of this study conducted a double-blind, randomized, parallel-group trial comparing intravenous aminophylline with placebo, examining the speed of spirometric recovery and length of hospital stay.

INTERPRETATION. No evidence was found for any clinically important additional effect of aminophylline treatment when used with high doses of nebulized bronchodilators and oral corticosteroids.

Comment

The authors enrolled 80 patients with known COPD presenting to a large teaching hospital in Liverpool, UK, if they complained of increased breathlessness and two or more of the following symptoms for at least 24 h: increased cough (frequency or severity); increased sputum volume or purulence; and increased wheeze. Following a loading dose, intravenous aminophylline was prescribed at a dose of 0.5 mg/kg per hour; the placebo was an equivalent volume of saline. At the 2-h time-point a small but significant improvement was reported in acid–base status and was accompanied by a fall in arterial carbon dioxide tension in patients receiving aminophylline compared with placebo; however, there was no significant or important difference between the two groups with respect to post-bronchodilator FEV_1 over the first 5 days of treatment, severity of breathlessness, post-bronchodilator FVC or length of hospital stay. Nausea was more frequently reported in patients receiving aminophylline (46 vs 22%). Therefore, when used with high doses of nebulized bronchodilators and oral corticosteroids, intravenous aminophylline adds little in terms of clinically relevant improvements and is accompanied by an increased incidence of nausea.

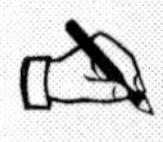

Hyperglycaemia is associated with poor outcomes in patients admitted to hospital with acute exacerbations of chronic obstructive pulmonary disease

Baker EH, Janaway CH, Philips BJ, *et al. Thorax* 2006; **61**: 284–9

BACKGROUND. Hyperglycaemia is associated with worse outcomes in patients with acute myocardial infarction, stroke and trauma. Although both diabetes mellitus and acute hyperglycaemia are common in patients with COPD, the relationship between blood glucose levels and clinical outcomes has not been fully established. This retrospective pilot study attempts to interrogate whether there is any relationship between blood glucose concentrations, length of hospital stay and mortality in patients hospitalized with acute exacerbations of COPD.

INTERPRETATION. During exacerbations of COPD, increasing blood glucose concentrations are associated with worse outcomes.

Comment

The authors retrieved data from electronic records on a total of 433 patients admitted with an acute exacerbation of COPD to St George's Hospital in London between 2001 and 2002. They included 291 subjects with a single admission and recorded the data from the first admission on 57 patients who were admitted on more than one occasion. They grouped patients according to blood glucose levels into quartiles: group 1, <6.0 mmol/l; group 2, 6.0–6.9 mmol/l; group 3, 7.0–8.9 mmol/l; and group 4, >9.0 mmol/l. When several blood glucose levels were available the highest value was used in the analysis.

Compared with group 1, the relative risk of an adverse outcome (defined as length of stay greater than 9 days) was 1.30 (95% CI 0.93–1.82) in group 2, 1.46 (95% CI 1.05–2.02) in group 3, and 1.97 (85% CI 1.33–2.92) in group 4. Following adjustment for age, sex, and previous diagnosis of diabetes mellitus, the absolute risk of an adverse outcome increased by 15% (95% CI 4–27) per 1 mmol/l increase in blood glucose. Compared with group 1, the relative risk of death was 1.22 (95% CI 0.70–2.12) for patients in group 2, 2.10 (95% CI 0.82–5.20) in group 3, and 3.42 (95% CI 1.40–8.36) for those in group 4. After adjustment, the risk of death increased by 10% (95% CI 0–22) per 1 mmol increase in blood glucose. Although the authors accepted that there were some methodological issues with the study, given the literature on myocardial infarction, this interesting paper sets the scene for a prospective study powered to determine whether tight control of blood glucose can improve the outcome of a COPD exacerbation.

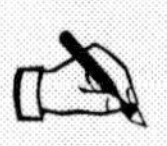

Infections and airway inflammation in chronic obstructive pulmonary disease severe exacerbations

Papi A, Bellettato CM, Braccioni F, *et al. Am J Respir Crit Care Med* 2006; **173**: 1114–21

BACKGROUND. Exacerbations of COPD are associated with enhanced airway inflammation; however, the relationship between the aetiology of the exacerbation and the inflammatory response requires further study. The aim of this study was to investigate whether the type of infection influences the inflammatory profile and the authors performed a prospective controlled study investigating viral and bacterial detection during severe COPD exacerbations when stable and when requiring hospitalization, in order to compare the relationships between aetiology, airway inflammation and exacerbation severity.

INTERPRETATION. Both viral and bacterial infections are associated with the majority of exacerbations of COPD.

Comment

In this study, 64 patients with COPD were recruited from a University Hospital Clinic in Italy and an exacerbation was defined as an increase in dyspnoea, cough or sputum expectoration (quality or quantity) that led the subject to seek medical attention. The authors found that exacerbations were associated with a decline in lung function and an increase in sputum neutrophilia. Nearly 80% of patients with a severe exacerbation of COPD who were admitted to hospital had a respiratory virus and/or bacterial infection. Patients in whom infection was identified had a more marked acute decline in lung function and experienced a longer duration of hospitalization. Sputum neutrophils were increased in all exacerbations and appeared to relate to the severity of the event, whether or not the exacerbation appeared to be triggered by viral or by bacterial infection. However, the presence of sputum eosinophilia appeared to relate to viral exacerbations.

The study contrasts with currently available evidence that antibiotics have very little impact in the management of exacerbations of COPD; however, the authors point out that these studies were performed some time ago and should be revisited. The data from this study suggest that there could be a role for antibiotic and/or antiviral therapy.

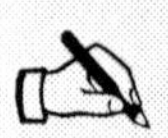

Systemic and upper and lower airway inflammation at exacerbation of chronic obstructive pulmonary disease

Hurst JR, Perera WR, Wilkinson TM, Donaldson GC, Wedzicha JA. *Am J Respir Crit Care Med* 2006; **173**: 71–8

BACKGROUND. The definition of COPD recognizes the presence of a pulmonary inflammatory response; however, it is being increasingly recognized that inflammation is also present in the upper airway and systemic compartment. The authors of this study used data from a well-defined COPD cohort in East London to investigate the inflammatory response in the lung, upper airway and systemic circulation, and related this to the occurrence of an exacerbation of the disease.

INTERPRETATION. Exacerbations of COPD are accompanied by an increased inflammatory response in the lower and upper airways and the systemic circulation. The greater the pulmonary inflammatory response, the greater the degree of systemic inflammation.

Comment

The authors examined 41 subjects from the East London COPD cohort who reported an exacerbation (the onset of two or more new or worsening symptoms on two or more consecutive days, at least one symptom of which must be major). Simultaneous samples were taken from the sputum, nasal passages and serum and analysed for pathogenic microorganisms and inflammatory indices (sputum/nasal wash leucocytes, IL-6, IL-8 and myeloperoxidase; serum IL-6 and C-reactive protein). The values were compared with those in patients with stable COPD.

The main findings from the study were that, not unexpectedly, exacerbations of COPD were associated with an increased inflammatory response compared with that seen in the stable state. They also showed that an exacerbation of COPD was associated with pan-airway inflammation and that the degree of systemic inflammation was related to the degree of inflammation present in the lungs, although not to the degree of upper airway inflammation. The presence of bacterial pathogens was associated with the greatest lower airway inflammatory response.

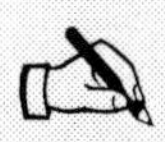

Severe acute exacerbations and mortality in patients with chronic obstructive pulmonary disease

Soler-Cataluua JJ, Martínez-García, Román-Sánchez P, Salcedo E, Navarro M, Ochando R. *Thorax* 2005; **60**: 925–31

BACKGROUND. The high mortality rate following hospital admission for an exacerbation of COPD is believed to reflect the baseline severity of the disease rather than the impact of an exacerbation *per se*. The aim of this study was to determine whether severe acute exacerbations had any direct effect on mortality.

INTERPRETATION. Severe acute exacerbations have an independent negative effect on the prognosis of patients with COPD. Mortality increases with the frequency of severe exacerbations.

Comment

Just over 300 patients with stable COPD underwent a comprehensive evaluation and were followed for 5 years. A severe acute exacerbation was defined as any sustained increase in respiratory symptoms compared with the baseline situation requiring modification of regular medication and hospital treatment. Patients were divided into three groups according to the number of exacerbations recorded: none; one or two; and three or more. Multivariate analysis of survival took into account age, comorbidity index, body mass index, FEV_1 as a percentage of predicted, FVC as a percentage of predicted, arterial partial pressure of oxygen (PaO_2)/fraction of inspired oxygen (FiO_2), $PaCO_2$, use of domiciliary oxygen and the number of acute exacerbations.

The main finding from this study was that severe exacerbations, particularly when frequent, proved one of the strongest independent adverse prognostic variables. Indeed, the adjusted mortality rate was over four times greater than that for patients reporting no exacerbations. Being older and having a higher Pa_{CO2} were also strong independent predictors of mortality.

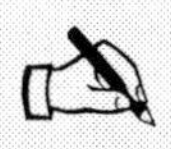

Clinical efficacy of anti-pneumococcal vaccination in patients with COPD

Alfageme I, Vazquez R, Reyes N, *et al. Thorax* 2006; **61**: 189–95

BACKGROUND. *Streptococcus pneumoniae* is one of the most important infectious disease agents and remains the most common cause of community-acquired pneumonia (CAP). The aim of this study was to evaluate the clinical efficacy of 23-serotype pneumococcal vaccine (PPV) in the prevention of pneumococcal pneumonias in immunocompetent patients with COPD.

INTERPRETATION. The 23-serotype PPV is effective in preventing radiologically proven pneumonia of pneumococcal origin in patients under 65 years and in those with severe airflow obstruction.

Comment

The potential impact of pneumococcal diseases on health around the world is significant, and although pneumococcal vaccine is known to be efficacious in preventing invasive pneumococcal disease it remains unclear whether vaccination reduces the incidence of other more common manifestations of pneumococcal disease, such as pneumonia. As patients with COPD represent a particularly vulnerable group, the authors of this study enrolled 600 patients with a diagnosis of COPD and randomized 300 to receive the 23-valent pneumococcal vaccine and the other 300 to routine clinical follow-up over 3 years.

The study reaffirms that CAP is common in patients with COPD, with 58 first episodes of community-acquired pneumonia being reported; 25 occurred in the intervention group and 33 in the non-intervention group. Examining data from the entire population, it was not possible to show any difference in survival curves between the two groups; however, when analysis was performed on patients under 65 years of age the authors noted that the efficacy of PPV was 76% and in those with severe airflow obstruction (FEV$_1$ <40% predicted) it was nearly 50%. In younger patients with severe airflow obstruction the efficacy of PPV rose even further, to 91%. *Streptococcus pneumoniae* was isolated from five patients with pneumonia in the non-intervention group and from none in the intervention group. The two groups did not differ in mortality rate, which was around 19%. Factors influencing the mortality rate among the patients were age, FEV$_1$ as a percentage of predicted, current smoking and the presence of neoplasia. The authors accept that the lack of a blind placebo comparison group was a weakness in study design, but felt that it was highly unlikely that this limitation significantly influenced the results because the vaccination status of the patient was kept in a specific encrypted database and was not stated in the patients' clinical records. The main investigator of this study was the only person with access to this database, but this investigator did not participate in the follow-up or in adjudicating the outcome events.

Prognosis in COPD

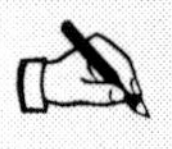

Inspiratory-to-total lung capacity ratio predicts mortality in patients with chronic obstructive pulmonary disease

Casanova C, Cote C, de Torres JP, *et al. Am J Respir Crit Care Med* 2005; **171**: 591–7

BACKGROUND. Hyperinflation is an important component of exercise limitation in patients with COPD; however, there is little information on whether it provides any information regarding survival. The investigators postulated that, because

hyperinflation is a key determinant of exercise capacity and exercise capacity is related to survival, hyperinflation may provide information on survival.

INTERPRETATION. Inspiratory capacity/total lung capacity is an independent predictor of mortality in subjects with COPD.

Comment

The authors studied just under 700 patients with COPD for just under 3 years. All patients were evaluated with pulmonary function tests, including lung volume and gas transfer. Exercise capacity was evaluated with a 6-min walk test and dyspnoea recorded according to the modified MRC dyspnoea index. Body mass index and comorbidity were recorded according to standard methods. Inspiratory capacity was measured and lung hyperinflation estimated as the ratio of inspiratory capacity to total lung capacity (IC/TLC).

Mortality was more frequent when subjects were older, had a lower body mass index, FEV_1 and IC/TLC ratio; walked less in a 6-min walking test; and had greater dyspnoea, a higher BODE index, and comorbidity. Both the FEV_1 and the BODE index have previously been shown to predict mortality in COPD patients. However, in this study the authors were able to demonstrate that the IC/TLC compared favourably with the FEV_1 and predicted mortality independently of the BODE index. Indeed, logistic regression showed that the IC/TLC was a good and independent predictor of all-cause and respiratory mortality; an IC/TLC threshold of 25% provided the best power to predict all-cause and respiratory mortality. The authors proposed that the IC/TLC could be seen as analogous to the ejection fraction in the evaluation of patients with left ventricular dysfunction.

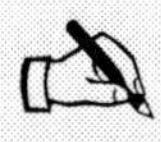

Body weight and comorbidity predict mortality in COPD patients treated with oxygen therapy

Marti S, Muñoz X, Rios J, Morell F, Ferrer J. *Eur Respir J* 2006; **27**: 689–96

BACKGROUND. The aim of this study was to determine the relationship between a number of clinical variables and all-cause mortality from COPD in patients receiving domiciliary oxygen therapy.

INTERPRETATION. This study highlights the role of body mass index in predicting both all-cause and respiratory mortality in patients with COPD on domiciliary oxygen therapy, but also emphasizes the importance of comorbid disease.

Comment

The 5-year survival of patients with COPD who meet the criteria for long-term domiciliary oxygen therapy is around 40%. The authors of this study performed a retrospective cohort study on 128 patients with COPD under the care of a teaching hospital in Barcelona. Domiciliary oxygen therapy was prescribed in accordance with the criteria agreed by the Spanish Society of Respiratory Diseases and comorbidity measured by use of the Charlson index. During a follow-up period of median length 3.2 years, just over 60% of patients died; 3-year survival was 55%. Examining all-cause mortality, the authors found that having a body mass index <25 kg/m^2, comorbid conditions, being at least 70 years of age and the presence of cor pulmonale were predictive. When restricting analysis to those with a respiratory cause for mortality, they found that the only significant predictive parameters were the body mass index and comorbidity.

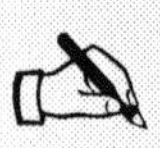

Body mass, fat-free body mass, and prognosis in patients with chronic obstructive pulmonary disease from a random population sample

Vestbo J, Prescott E, Almdal T, *et al. Am J Respir Crit Care Med* 2006; **173**: 79–83

BACKGROUND. This study was designed to examine the effect of body mass index and fat-free mass in a general population free of referral bias. They therefore drew on subjects enrolled in the Copenhagen City Heart Study (CCHS) and obtained data on just over 10 000 subjects, just over 2400 of whom had COPD.

INTERPRETATION. Patients with COPD are at risk of a low fat-free mass even when the body mass index is normal and a low fat-free mass index (FFMI, calculated as fat-free mass/height^2 [kg/m^2]) appears to carry an adverse prognostic influence. The authors suggest that fat-free mass should be considered as a component in the routine evaluation of COPD.

Comment

Body mass index is known to be an important prognostic indicator in patients with COPD, patients who display a decline in body mass index having the poorest prognosis. Recognition that body mass may be categorized as either fat mass (a metabolically inactive energy store) or fat-free mass (comprising the metabolically active organs, including the skeletal muscles) led the investigators to postulate that the most important component of the body mass index as regards prognosis would be fat-free mass, as this was most likely to reflect systemic inflammation. Fat-free mass was measured by bioelectrical impedance analysis and standardized for height as the fat-free mass index, calculated as shown above. COPD was classified according to the GOLD criteria. Patients were followed up for a mean of 7 years. The authors found that body mass index and FFMI do not necessarily go hand in hand. Even in those with a normal body mass index they found that just over one-quarter had an FFMI that fell below the lowest 10th percentile of the general population. Both body mass index and FFMI appeared to provide independent predictions of mortality, and having an FFMI in the lowest 10th percentile of the general population was associated with a hazard ratio of 1.5 (95% CI 1.2–1.8) for overall mortality and 2.4 (95% CI 1.4–4.0) for COPD-related mortality. The authors measured serum fibrinogen as a surrogate for a systemic inflammatory response and reported higher fibrinogen levels in patients with a low FFMI.

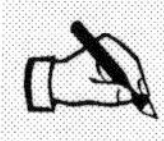

C-reactive protein and mortality in mild to moderate chronic obstructive pulmonary disease

Man SFP, Connett JE, Anthonisen NR, Wise RA, Tashkin DP, Sin DD. *Thorax* 2006; **61**: 849–53

BACKGROUND. As COPD is associated with a low-grade systemic inflammation, the authors of this study wished to determine whether a marker of systemic inflammation, in this case serum C-reactive protein (CRP), was associated with (i) an increase in all-cause and disease-specific causes of mortality, (ii) an increased risk of fatal and non-fatal cardiovascular events, and (iii) an accelerated decline in lung function as measured by the FEV_1.

INTERPRETATION. Serum CRP appears to be an independent predictor of prognosis.

Comment

The authors measured serum CRP levels in nearly 5000 patients participating in the Lung Health Study who had mild to moderate COPD, and then determined the risk of all-cause and disease-specific mortality. Mortality end-points included coronary heart disease, cardiovascular disease, lung cancer, other cancer, respiratory disease excluding lung cancer, other and unknown. After correcting for age, sex, cigarette smoking and lung function, it was found that CRP (as measured with a highly sensitive assay) was associated with all-cause, cardiovascular and cancer-specific causes of mortality. Endorsing the utility of CRP, the authors found that (even after adjustment) the risk of all-cause mortality showed a linear increase along the CRP gradient. Individuals in the highest CRP quintile showed a relative risk of all-cause mortality of 1.79 (95% CI 1.25–2.56) compared with those in the lowest CRP quintile. For cardiovascular and cancer deaths the relative risks were 1.51 (1.20–1.90) and 1.85 (1.10–3.13) respectively. CRP levels were also associated with the rate of decline in lung function. Comparing the highest and the lowest CRP quintiles, the relative risk was 4.03 (1.23–13.21) for 1-year mortality, 3.30 (1.38–7.86) for 2-year mortality, and 1.82 (1.22–2.68) for ≥5-year mortality.

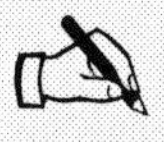

Survival of patients with chronic obstructive pulmonary disease due to biomass smoke and tobacco

Ramírez-Venegas A, Sansores RH, Pérez-Padilla R, *et al. Am J Respir Crit Care Med* 2006; **173**: 393–7

BACKGROUND. The impact of biomass fuel on the development of airflow limitation is recognized but not well characterized. The aim of this study was to describe the

clinical, functional, health-related quality of life and survival characteristics of patients with COPD exposed to biomass fuels.

INTERPRETATION. COPD associated with exposure to biomass fuels predominantly affects women but the disease displays similar characteristics to that attributable to tobacco smoking.

Comment

The impact of biomass fuels on respiratory health is of worldwide concern. The World Health Organization has estimated that indoor air pollution from such fuels is responsible for more than 1.6 million annual deaths and nearly 3% of the global burden of disease. Such exposure occurs in economically deprived countries and affects mainly women who perform their cooking in poorly ventilated homes. This study was performed in Mexico City. Over a 7-year period the authors enrolled just over 500 patients attending the COPD clinic at the National Institute of Respiratory Diseases. Comprehensive assessments were performed on all patients, including spirometry, arterial blood gases, body mass index, exercise capacity and health-related quality of life. This study analysed data on around 480 patients, comparing characteristics of COPD associated with biomass fuels with that associated with tobacco smoke. The main outcome of the study focused on survival.

Patients with COPD secondary to biomass smoke tended to be women and had less severe airflow obstruction, whereas those with COPD secondary to tobacco smoke tended to be men and had more severe airflow obstruction. Health-related quality of life and exercise capacity were similar in the two groups. Using regression analysis to analyse survival, the authors found that although age, FEV_1 as a percentage of predicted, body mass index and oxygen saturation all predicted mortality, neither sex or type of exposure appeared to have any impact.

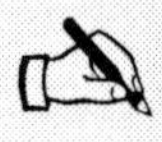

UK National COPD Audit 2003: impact of hospital resources and organisation of care on patient outcome following admission for acute COPD exacerbation

Price LC, Lowe D, Hosker HSR, Anstey K, Pearson MG, Roberts CM, on behalf of the British Thoracic Society and Royal College of Physicians Clinical Effectiveness Evaluation Unit (CEEu). *Thorax* 2006; **61**: 837–42

BACKGROUND. COPD is a common reason for admission to hospital in the UK. The authors of this study were interested in determining whether there was any relationship between resources, organization of patient care and outcome.

INTERPRETATION. Patients with exacerbations of COPD who were admitted to units with more respiratory consultants and better organized care spent less time in hospital and were less likely to die.

Comment

This study was a joint initiative between the Clinical Effectiveness and Evaluation Unit of the Royal College of Physicians and the British Thoracic Society. Just over 200 participating units in the UK collected data on 40 consecutive patients admitted with an exacerbation of COPD, completing an individual clinical proforma for each patient and an organizational questionnaire for the unit. Data on around 7500 patients were audited.

Although often treated with complacency, the mortality rate following an exacerbation of COPD requiring hospital admission is high and the authors reported inpatient mortality at just over 7% and the 90-day mortality rate at just over 15%. Interestingly, performance status was closely associated with mortality and patients with the best pre-morbid performance status showed a mortality rate of 2% whereas those with the worst status approached 40%. Nevertheless, after controlling for the case mix of the patients, resources and organization of care both affected the outcome.

The best correlate with outcome was the number of respiratory specialists per 1000 hospital beds, and those units with $\geq 4/1000$ hospital beds (a target recommended by the Royal College of Physicians) had lower mortality rates. Organizational issues (availability of local management guidelines and a composite organizational score derived from good medical practice) affected the length of stay. However, neither organizational factors nor resources appeared to have any effect on the re-admission rate, which averaged around 30%.

Conclusion

This year we have been given new insights into the consequences of COPD for pulmonary mechanics and the behaviour of respiratory muscles, which have provided deeper understanding of the mechanisms that lead to breathlessness, exercise limitation and, for some, social isolation. Similarly, we have been given further evidence that underpins the use of bronchodilators and pulmonary rehabilitation to improve breathlessness. It is widely held that pulmonary hypertension may be a feature of advanced disease; however, an important clinical message is that it is usually of only mild or moderate severity and that finding severe pulmonary hypertension should prompt a search for an alternative explanation.

The combination of a long-acting β_2-agonist with inhaled corticosteroid therapy is now employed in patients with moderate and severe COPD, and prompt improvements in breathlessness are accompanied by a change in the inflammatory cell profile in the airway. Whereas the place of long-term oxygen therapy is established, many patients who do not fulfil criteria are prescribed short-burst oxygen therapy; however, it appears there is little evidence for benefit and such prescriptions should be resisted. Pulmonary rehabilitation improves exercise tolerance and quality of life and reduces hospitalizations, and appears to be accompanied by a reduction in oxidative stress. Depressed patients appear to be at risk of dropping out and more information is needed on the merits of different exercise regimens.

The development of new drugs is challenging. Against a considerable background of experimental work, the phosphodiesterase type 4 inhibitors are beginning to emerge. Roflumilast appears to improve lung function and reduce exacerbation rates; further studies employing these drugs are awaited. However, the prospects for using N-acetylcysteine and infliximab appear less good. Whilst lung volume reduction surgery benefits very carefully selected subgroups of patients with COPD, this year we have been provided with exciting new evidence for a less invasive endoscopic method of effecting lung volume reduction surgery: more information is eagerly awaited!

The occurrence of exacerbations has important consequences for patients: deterioration in lung function, the development of respiratory failure, cor pulmonale, and the risk of death. Intravenous aminophylline is widely used; however, it appears to confer little objective benefit. On the other hand, paying attention to glycaemic control may improve the outcome of an exacerbation.

Part II

Respiratory infectious diseases

3

Tuberculosis

ADAM HILL, MAEVE MURRAY

Introduction

It is estimated by the World Health Organization (WHO) that one-third of the world's population has latent tuberculosis. Treatment of latent tuberculosis is central to the elimination of this disease. Compliance has been poor with traditional regimens and there is an ongoing search for the optimum regimen that is safe, effective, short and with limited side effects.

Latent tuberculosis

The first two papers explore the role of tuberculin skin testing using the conventional purified protein derivative and the newer interferon γ assays in peripheral blood using tuberculosis-specific antigens.

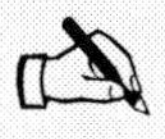

Transmission of *Mycobacterium tuberculosis* undetected by tuberculin skin testing

Anderson ST, Williams AJ, Brown JR, *et al. Am J Respir Crit Care Med* 2006; **173**: 1038–42

BACKGROUND. Investigation of tuberculosis infection has previously involved reliance on the tuberculin skin test. The cutaneous response to the intradermal administration of purified protein derivative can be variable, particularly in immunosuppressed subjects, those with previous BCG (Bacillus Calmette-Guérin) vaccination and those with overwhelming tuberculosis infection. The authors of this study compared the tuberculin skin test with a whole-blood interferon γ assay using a combination of the tuberculosis-specific antigens early secretory antigenic target (ESAT-6) and culture filtrate protein (CFP-10) during a contact-tracing investigation. There were 75 contacts in a UK school where there had been two related index cases of severe pulmonary tuberculosis. The authors also investigated the ability of the strain of tuberculosis to stimulate cytokine secretion from monocytes *in vitro*.

INTERPRETATION. The tuberculin skin test identified only two out of 75 cases (3%) of latent tuberculosis infection (both had Heaf grade 2 or Mantoux equivalent 5–14 mm, with no history of BCG vaccination) (Table 3.1). The whole-blood interferon γ release assay identified 16 out of 75 (22%) contacts with significant responses using the combination of the tuberculosis-specific antigens ESAT-6 and CFP-10. This outbreak strain of tuberculosis (in the two related index cases in this study), compared with the two reference strains of tuberculosis (H37Rv and CDC1551), induced lower levels of tumour necrosis factor α (TNF-α) and interleukin 12p40 (P <0.04), which are cytokines associated with the development of delayed-type hypersensitivity.

Comment

This study highlights that the tuberculin skin test, in comparison with whole-blood interferon γ assays, may underestimate tuberculosis infection. Transmission to healthy people can occur in the absence of skin test conversion, which may be related to the differing capacity of strains of tuberculosis to elicit delayed-type hypersensitivity reactions.

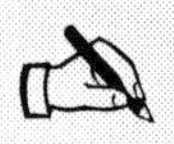

Use in routine clinical practice of two commercial blood tests for diagnosis of infection with *Mycobacterium tuberculosis*: a prospective study

Ferrara G, Losi M, D'Amico R, *et al. Lancet* 2006; **367**: 1328–34

BACKGROUND. This prospective study compared the efficacy of the tuberculin skin test, using 5 U purified protein derivative, with two recently developed interferon γ blood tests (T-SPOT.TB and Quantiferon-TB Gold tests) that are intended to improve diagnostic accuracy. The study involved 393 participants – both inpatients and outpatients – all undergoing investigation for latent or active tuberculosis, of whom 318 were investigated with all three tests.

INTERPRETATION. Twenty-four patients were eventually confirmed to have active tuberculosis. Overall agreement with the tuberculin skin test was good (T-SPOT.TB, k = 0.508; Quantiferon-TB Gold, k = 0.460) (Table 3.1). Fewer BCG-vaccinated individuals were identified as positive by the two blood assays than by the skin test (P <0.005). The overall agreement between the two blood tests was high, irrespective of BCG status (k = 0.699). Despite this, the T-SPOT.TB test had significantly fewer indeterminate results (3%) than the Quantiferon-TB Gold (11%) (P <0.001) and these indeterminate results were associated with immunosuppression. Indeterminate results were significantly more frequent with both blood tests in study participants undergoing chemotherapy for cancer, and also for patients younger than 5 for the Quantiferon-TB Gold test. Close contacts of patients with active tuberculosis were more likely to be positive with T-SPOT.TB than with Quantiferon-TB Gold (P = 0.001).

Table 3.1 Results of tuberculin skin test, T-SPOT.TB and Quantiferon Gold-TB tests in 24 patients with active tuberculosis

Test result	Tuberculin skin test ≥5 mm*	T-SPOT.TB	Quantiferon-TB Gold
Positive	14	20	17
Negative	6	4	6
Indeterminate	0	0	1

Data are number of persons.
*Tuberculin skin test was not available in four cases.
Source of data: Ferrara *et al.* (2006).

Comment

T-SPOT.TB and Quantiferon-TB Gold have higher specificity than the tuberculin skin test. Rates of indeterminate and positive results, however, differ between the blood tests, suggesting that they might provide different results in routine clinical practice. The blood assays are, however, more costly than the tuberculin skin test. The choice of diagnostic test to be used will depend on the population being tested, the purpose of testing and the resources available.

Isoniazid therapy in HIV and chronic renal failure

The next two papers are concerned with the efficacy of isoniazid in patients with human immunodeficiency virus (HIV) and chronic renal failure.

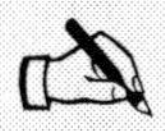

Effect of routine isoniazid preventive therapy on tuberculosis incidence among HIV-infected men in South Africa: a novel randomized incremental recruitment study

Grant AD, Charalambous S, Fielding KL, *et al. JAMA* 2005; **293**: 2719–25

BACKGROUND. HIV infection is a significant risk factor for the development of active tuberculosis. Without antiretroviral therapy there is an estimated 10% annual risk of tuberculosis. This large randomized study assessed the effect of 6 months of preventive therapy with isoniazid 300 mg/day on the incidence of tuberculosis in HIV-positive men between 1999 and 2001, before the availability of antiretroviral therapy.

INTERPRETATION. The initial study population consisted of 1655 HIV-infected men (71% at WHO disease stage 1, 7% at stage 2, 16% at stage 3 and 6% at stage 4; median age 37 years, interquartile range 33–43 years). Six hundred and seventy-nine of 702 men eligible to start primary preventive therapy with isoniazid did so. The rates of tuberculosis before and after isoniazid therapy were compared (median 11.2 months before and after enrolment). A total of 254 episodes of active tuberculosis occurred, although 39 (15%) of these were thought to have been diagnosed as a result of active screening at the study entry point and were therefore excluded from the final analysis. The risk of tuberculosis was significantly associated with age (increasing risk with increasing age; $P = 0.009$), a previous history of tuberculosis ($P = 0.004$), HIV disease stage 3 or 4 ($P = 0.001$) and a diagnosis of silicosis ($P = 0.01$).

Before study entry, the incidence of tuberculosis was 11.9 per 100 person-years and after isoniazid treatment it was 9 per 100 person-years ($P = 0.03$). In a multivariate analysis after adjustment for calendar period, age and silicosis grade, the incidence rate ratio of tuberculosis in patients who received isoniazid chemoprophylaxis was 0.62 (95% confidence interval [CI] 0.43–0.89). Excluding patients with a history of tuberculosis and hence ineligible for isoniazid preventive therapy, the incidence rate ratio of tuberculosis in patients who received isoniazid chemoprophylaxis was 0.54 (95% CI 0.35–0.83).

Comment

The routine provision of isoniazid chemoprophylaxis to HIV-infected individuals reduced the incidence of tuberculosis by 38% overall and by 46% in those with no previous history of tuberculosis. Since this study was conducted, antiretroviral therapy has been used routinely. Further studies exploring the role of chemoprophylaxis are needed in HIV patients on antiretroviral therapy.

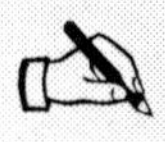

Prospective randomized control trial of isoniazid chemoprophylaxis during renal replacement therapy

Vikrant S, Agarwal SK, Gupta S, *et al. Transpl Infect Dis* 2005; **7**: 99–108

BACKGROUND. The recent guidelines of the National Institute for Clinical Excellence (NICE; UK) cite the relative risk of developing active tuberculosis in those with chronic renal failure or receiving haemodialysis to be 10–25 times greater than normal |1|. This prospective, randomized, placebo-controlled trial evaluated the efficacy of daily isoniazid 300 mg therapy given for 12 months compared with placebo in patients receiving haemodialysis and registered for renal transplantation. The primary outcome was the development of tuberculosis within a 3-year follow-up period. The development of tuberculosis was defined microbiologically, histologically or as a clinical syndrome consistent with a diagnosis of tuberculosis and documented response to antituberculous treatment (50–56% of the patients were diagnosed clinically in this study).

INTERPRETATION. The clinical outcomes for those receiving therapy are summarized in Table 3.2.

Comment

Isoniazid therapy in patients receiving haemodialysis was significantly protective against the development of active tuberculosis compared with placebo, although it remains a concern that 17% of this group still developed active tuberculosis despite chemoprophylaxis.

Table 3.2 Clinical outcomes for those receiving isoniazid therapy versus placebo

	Isoniazid group	Placebo	P-value
No. participants	54	55	
Developing active tuberculosis	16.7%	32.7%	0.04
No. developing significant hepatitis*	9 (16.7%)	6 (10.9%)	n.s.
No. with significant hepatitis attributable to viral hepatitis	7/9 (78%)	5/6 (83%)	n.s.

Data are number or percentage of persons, or number (%).
*Significant hepatitis was defined as AST/ALT more than five times the upper limit of normal, with or without elevated bilirubin.
n.s., not significant.
Source of data: Vikrant et al. (2005).

In view of the increased incidence of viral hepatitis in patients with end-stage renal failure, it would be recommended to monitor liver function tests for the duration of isoniazid treatment.

Compliance with treatment

Daily single-agent isoniazid therapy for at least 6 months (9–12 months in the USA) has been the standard treatment for latent tuberculosis infection over the past few decades. However, concerns regarding compliance, the risk of adverse effects and the increased prevalence of isoniazid-resistant tuberculosis have led to concern that such management may be a suboptimally effective strategy for tuberculosis control. The next four papers explore these issues. The first of these papers aims to identify features present at baseline that may predict poor compliance; the second compares completion rates for the traditional 6-month isoniazid regime with a 4-month rifampicin regime; the third compares completion and toxicity rates between 9 months of isoniazid and 4 months of rifampicin therapy, and the fourth assesses the safety, compliance and efficacy of two alternative regimes, both shorter than the traditional isoniazid course: once-weekly rifapentine and isoniazid for 12 weeks, and daily rifampicin and pyrazinamide for 8 weeks.

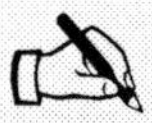

Predicting non-completion of treatment for latent tuberculous infection: a prospective survey

Shieh FK, Snyder G, Horsburgh CR, Bernardo J, Murphy C, Saukkonen JJ. *Am J Respir Crit Care Med* 2006; **174**: 717–21

BACKGROUND. In this prospective study of 217 patients, a 9-month regime of daily isoniazid therapy was prescribed and questionnaires were administered to all participants immediately before the commencement of treatment, exploring potential factors thought to influence compliance. Monthly follow-up appointments according to the tuberculosis clinic's standard protocol were issued to all participants.

INTERPRETATION. Ninety per cent of participants were born outside the USA, 82.5% in a tuberculosis-endemic country. Twenty-nine per cent of the study population completed 6 months of isoniazid therapy and 19.4% completed 9 months. Two-thirds of the patients discontinued treatment of their own accord, determined by failing to attend for review at 3 months or by their own admission. Univariate and multivariate analysis identified significant risk factors for non-completion of treatment as concern about venepuncture and an initial perceived low risk of developing active tuberculosis. These accounted for 75% of non-completers. On univariate analysis alone, not having a primary care physician and not valuing regular visits to a healthcare professional for health maintenance were also identified as factors predictive of poor compliance.

Comment

The two main predictors of non-completion of treatment were reluctance to have venepuncture and a perceived low risk of tuberculosis. These health concerns and beliefs can be discussed at the first clinic review and, importantly, may help promote the completion of treatment.

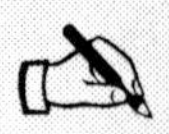

Enhancement of treatment completion for latent tuberculosis infection with 4 months of rifampicin

Lardizabal A, Passannante M, Kojakali F, Hayden C, Reichman LB. *Chest* 2006; **130**: 1712–17

BACKGROUND. This historical prospective review of 474 patients assessed treatment completion with a 9-month isoniazid regime compared with a 4-month rifampicin (rifampin) regime, but it was not a randomized controlled trial. The primary outcome of the study was treatment completion.

INTERPRETATION. The isoniazid regime was predominantly administered in the year 2000 to 194 patients. The rifampicin regime was predominantly administered in 2003 to 260 patients, except that 19 people presenting with latent tuberculosis in 2003 received an isoniazid regime. A significantly greater percentage of patients completed the rifampicin treatment course (80.5%) than the isoniazid course (53.1%) (P <0.0001). There was no significant difference in reported side effects between the isoniazid group (5.8% and the rifampicin group (3.1%)).

Comment

Patient adherence with a 4-month regime of rifampicin was significantly better than with a 9-month regime of isoniazid. Further studies exploring the efficacy of rifampicin compared with isoniazid in preventing active tuberculosis are needed. The rifampicin regime may be particularly relevant if there is a high suspicion of exposure to isoniazid-resistant tuberculosis or if poor adherence is suspected.

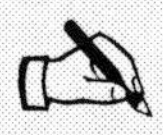

Improved adherence and less toxicity with rifampin vs isoniazid for treatment of latent tuberculosis: a retrospective study

Page KR, Sifakis F, Montes de Oca R, *et al. Arch Intern Med* 2006; **166**: 1863–70

BACKGROUND. This large retrospective case-note review compared treatment completion and adverse events of 770 patients who received the standard 9-month isoniazid regime with corresponding results for 1379 patients who received a 4-month rifampicin regime. A significantly greater percentage of the 9-month isoniazid group received directly observed therapy (5.1 vs 1.1%; *P* = 0.001). The primary outcomes of this study were treatment completion and adverse drug reactions.

INTERPRETATION. In the rifampicin group, 71.6% completed treatment compared with 52.6% in the isoniazid group (*P* <0.001). Variables affecting treatment completion were analysed. In multivariate analysis, adjusting for age, race, region of origin, treatment regimen, pre-treatment liver function tests and adverse events, the factor most strongly associated with completion was treatment regimen (rifampicin significantly better than isoniazid; adjusted odds ratio [OR] 2.88; 95% CI 2.27–3.66). Patients prescribed 4 months of rifampicin treatment were less likely to have an adverse reaction leading to permanent treatment discontinuation (1.9%) than those receiving 9 months of isoniazid treatment (4.6%) (*P* <0.001).

Hepatotoxicity (i.e. symptomatic alanine aminotransferase [ALT]/aspartate aminotransferase [AST] at least three times the upper limit of normal, or asymptomatic and ALT/AST at least five times the upper limit of normal) was significantly lower in the rifampicin group (0.08%) than in the isoniazid group (1.8%) (*P* <0.001). There was no significant difference between the two groups in the frequency of rash, gastrointestinal disturbance, thrombocytopenia or fatigue.

Comment

A 4-month treatment regime with rifampicin achieved better adherence with fewer hepatotoxic side effects than a 9-month isoniazid regime in the management of latent tuberculosis infection. Further studies exploring the efficacy of rifampicin compared with isoniazid in preventing active tuberculosis are needed. The rifampicin regime may be particularly relevant if there is a high suspicion of exposure to isoniazid-resistant tuberculosis or poor adherence is suspected.

Weekly rifapentine/isoniazid or daily rifampin/pyrazinamide for latent tuberculosis in household contacts

Schechter M, Zajdenverg R, Falco G, *et al. Am J Respir Crit Care Med* 2006; **173**: 922–6

BACKGROUND. In this study 399 household contacts of pulmonary tuberculosis with tuberculin skin test readings of ≥5 mm and with no radiographic evidence of active tuberculosis were randomly allocated to receive either once weekly rifapentine 900 mg/isoniazid 900 mg for 12 weeks (*n* = 206) or daily rifampicin 450–600 mg/pyrazinamide 750–1500 mg for 8 weeks (*n* = 193). The two groups were equally matched: about 65% in each group had a previous BCG vaccination, no study participants had any baseline hepatic or renal impairment and only one participant had HIV. The primary outcome was the development of tuberculosis within the 2-year follow-up. The expected risk of developing tuberculosis in untreated contacts is 8% over 2 years.

INTERPRETATION. Table 3.3 shows the number of participants, the percentage completing treatment, the percentage developing grade 3 or 4 hepatotoxicity and the percentage developing active pulmonary tuberculosis within 2 years. The study was terminated early because of the high rates of hepatotoxicity in the rifampicin/pyrazinamide group. There were, however, no hospitalizations or deaths due to hepatoxicity and all patients' liver function tests returned to normal after discontinuation of treatment.

Table 3.3 Development of important adverse effects and active pulmonary tuberculosis in patients receiving weekly rifapentine/isoniazid compared with those receiving rifampicin/pyrazinamide

	Rifapentine/ isoniazid	Rifampicin/ pyrazinamide	*P*-value
Total no. of participants	206	193	
Completing treatment	93%	94%	0.8
Developing grade 3 or 4 hepatotoxicity*	1%	10%	<0.001
Developing active pulmonary tuberculosis within 2-year follow-up period	1.5%	0.5%	0.7

*Grade 3 hepatotoxicity was defined as ALT/AST five to ten times normal upper limit; grade 4 hepatotoxicity was defined as ALT/AST more than ten times upper limit of normal range.
Source of data: Schechter *et al.* (2006).

Comment

The once weekly rifapentine/isoniazid regime (lasting 12 weeks) had significantly less hepatotoxicity than the daily rifampicin/pyrazinamide regime (lasting 8 weeks). The two groups had similar levels of compliance and degrees of efficacy. The study, however, gave chemoprophylaxis to household contacts 18 years or older who had a tuberculin skin response ≥5 mm. Approximately 65% had received BCG vaccination previously.

The NICE guidelines for tuberculosis would only offer chemoprophylaxis in tuberculosis contacts with previous BCG vaccination who were aged under 35 years and had a strong (≥15 mm) response [1]. Further studies are needed of the new weekly rifapentine/isoniazid regimen for 12 weeks in comparison with 6 months of daily isoniazid. Preliminary studies with this shorter regimen look promising, with high adherence rates, limited toxicity and good efficacy.

Risk factors, diagnosis and treatment of pulmonary tuberculosis

The next papers explore the risk factors for pulmonary tuberculosis and the diagnostic value of spontaneous sputum, induced sputum and bronchoalveolar lavage (BAL) in pulmonary tuberculosis. The last two papers then focus on the treatment of tuberculosis. The first of these compares therapy directly observed by healthcare workers with therapy directly observed by family members. The final paper evaluates predictors of sputum culture conversion from positive to negative in patients with multidrug-resistant tuberculosis.

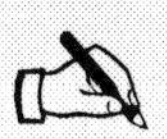

Risk factors for pulmonary tuberculosis in Russia: case–control study

Coker R, McKee M, Atun R, *et al*. *BMJ* 2006; **332**: 85–7

BACKGROUND. The incidence of tuberculosis in Russia is rising and the authors of this case–control study sought to identify potential risk factors for pulmonary tuberculosis by assessing 334 consecutively diagnosed new patients with equally matched controls. A detailed questionnaire was administered to all study participants. The primary outcome of this study was the risk factors associated with the development of tuberculosis.

INTERPRETATION. The authors identified several factors that were associated with an increased risk of developing pulmonary tuberculosis (Table 3.4).

Table 3.4 Significant risk factors for developing pulmonary tuberculosis in Russia

Variable	Univariate odds ratio (95% CI)
Few assets	16.7 (8.87–31.43)
History of imprisonment	12.5 (3.8–41.3)
History of illicit drug use	8.74 (3.06–25.01)
Unemployment	6.10 (4.32–8.61)
History of drinking raw milk	3.58 (2.58–4.97)
History of diabetes mellitus	2.66 (1.1–6.46)
History of living with a relative with tuberculosis	2.94 (1.79–4.85)

Source of data: Coker *et al*. (2006).

Table 3.5 Microscopy and culture results for spontaneous sputum, induced sputum and bronchoscopy

Time-point and collection method	No. of cases referred	No. of available specimens	No. smear positive	No. culture positive	Yield for smear: % of all positive cases detected	Yield for culture: % of culture positive
Initial spontaneous	101	83	7	13	54%	39%
Initial induced	101	91	6	12	46%	36%
Early morning spontaneous	101	84	8	16	62%	49%
Early morning induced	101	91	8	17	62%	52%
Bronchoscopy	92	87	4	15	n.a.	63%

n.a., not applicable
Source of data: Schoch *et al.* (2007)

Comment

This study confirms several established risk factors that may be influencing the increased rate of tuberculosis in Russia. In the study population, exposure to raw milk and unemployment were thought to be the most important contributors to the burden of tuberculosis. The study did not, however, explore immuno-suppression, which is a major risk factor for tuberculosis; the immunosuppression produced by HIV is key to the increased rates of tuberculosis seen internationally (similarly, other immunosuppressing agents, such as corticosteroids, immuno-suppressant therapy, chemotherapy and TNF-α blockers, were not explored in this study).

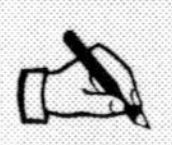

Diagnostic yield of sputum, induced sputum, and bronchoscopy after radiologic tuberculosis screening

Schoch OD, Rieder P, Tueller C, *et al. Am J Respir Crit Care Med* 2007; **175**: 80–6

BACKGROUND. Active tuberculosis screening and case-finding, particularly at points of immigration, is a crucial measure in the control of infection. Following chest radiographs highly suggestive of active tuberculosis in 101 asylum-seekers, this prospective multicentre Swiss study assessed the diagnostic yield of spontaneous and induced sputum samples and bronchoscopy with lavage. An initial spontaneous sputum sample was collected, followed by an induced sample. This routine was then repeated as an early morning procedure. All cases reported from these samples as sputum smear-negative proceeded to bronchoscopy with lavage.

INTERPRETATION. The main findings are summarized in Table 3.5. Pulmonary tuberculosis was confirmed with at least one culture-positive specimen in 33 cases (33%). Two spontaneous sputum samples combined confirmed 20 cases (61%) of culture-confirmed cases. Two induced sputum samples yielded a further seven cases on culture (82%). Bronchoscopy performed in smear-negative cases yielded a further six cases (100%) on culture.

Comment

In this study, in the screening for active TB in asylum-seekers, the diagnostic yield of any single specimen was low (36–63%). The recommendation would be that in asylum-seekers who have a high radiographic suspicion of active tuberculosis, further investigation should include the collection of initial and early morning spontaneous and induced sputum samples followed by BAL in those who are smear-negative to be sent for mycobacterial culture.

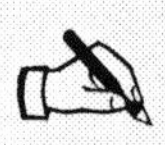

Family-member DOTS and community DOTS for tuberculosis control in Nepal: cluster-randomised controlled trial

Newell JN, Baral SC, Pande SB, Bam DS, Malla P. *Lancet* 2006; **367**: 903–9

BACKGROUND. 'Directly Observed Treatment' (DOTS) by healthcare workers is a WHO-recommended strategy for tuberculosis control but is often not feasible. In this cluster-randomized, controlled trial, the authors designed, implemented and evaluated an alternative to community healthcare worker-observed treatment: family member DOTS. Over a 12-month period, 907 patients from a total of 10 districts in Nepal with a new diagnosis of tuberculosis were allocated to receive daily community-observed treatment (five districts, *n* = 549) or daily observed treatment from a patient-nominated family member (five districts, *n* = 358). The primary outcome of this study was the success rate (cure or completed treatment).

INTERPRETATION. The success rate of treatment in the family member DOTS group (89%) was significantly higher than the WHO target of 85% (Table 3.6).

Comment

Both healthcare worker community DOTS and family DOTS can achieve WHO targets for treatment success in the management of tuberculosis. Family member DOTS may be applicable to areas of the world where healthcare worker DOTS is not feasible.

Table 3.6 Treatment completion rates for those receiving family Directly Observed Treatment Short Course (DOTS) compared with community DOTS

	Community DOTS	Family DOTS
Completion	465 (85%)	319 (89%)
Non-completion	22 (4)	14 (4)
Death	47 (9)	18 (5)

Data are number of persons (%).
Source of data: Newell *et al.* (2006)

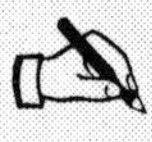

Time to sputum culture conversion in multidrug-resistant tuberculosis: predictors and relationship to treatment outcome

Holtz TH, Sternberg M, Kammerer S, *et al. Ann Intern Med* 2006; **144**: 650–9

BACKGROUND. Multidrug-resistant tuberculosis (MDRTB) (defined as tuberculosis resistant to at least rifampicin and isoniazid) is becoming increasingly common internationally. The efficacy of individualized tuberculosis treatment regimes is

typically assessed by conversion of positive to negative growth in sputum cultures for *Mycobacterium tuberculosis*. This was a retrospective cohort study of 167 patients in Latvia receiving therapy for MDRTB. The aim of this study was to evaluate the time to conversion of sputum cultures to negative growth, predictors of conversion and treatment outcome.

INTERPRETATION. One hundred and twenty-nine (77%) patients achieved sputum conversion in a median time of 60 days. Patients who were cured or completed treatment took a median of 48 days to conversion compared with 169 days in those with a poor outcome, defined as death, default or failure (P <0.001). In a multivariate analysis, factors associated with a prolonged time to sputum culture conversion were previous treatment for MDRTB, a high mycobacterial load, the presence of bilateral cavitation on the chest radiograph, and the number of drugs resistant at treatment initiation (Table 3.7).

Table 3.7 Multivariate accelerated failure time model estimates of percentage difference in time to initial sputum culture conversion in 166 patients with multidrug-resistant tuberculosis*

Characteristic	Initial conversion time	
	Difference in initial conversion time (95% CI), †	*P*-value
Previously treated for multidrug-resistant TB	169 (49 to 384)	0.001
Previously treated for TB	31 (−18 to 105)	0.23
Never treated for TB	Referent	
Colony count of initial culture		
3+ or 4+	49 (5 to 111)	0.027
1+ or 2+	Referent	
Chest radiography at treatment initiation		
Bilateral cavitations	47 (2 to 113)	0.042
No bilateral cavitations	Referent	
Number of drugs resistant to at treatment initiation	16 (3 to 30)	0.014

* One patient had a missing colony count; culture done on BACTEC (Becton, Dickinson and Company, Franklin Lakes, New Jersey). TB, tuberculosis.
† For continuous variables, such as drug resistance at treatment initiation, this value represents the percentage difference in time to conversion for a 1-unit increment in the explanatory variable. For categorical variables, it represents the percentage difference in time to conversion in the presence (versus absence) of the explanatory variable. Positive values imply longer time to conversion, and negative values imply shorter time.
Source: Holtz *et al.* (2006).

Comment

This study highlighted important pre-treatment factors predictive of delayed sputum conversion in MDRTB. The time taken to sputum conversion was also a strong predictor of treatment outcome.

Conclusion

Anderson *et al.* (2006) highlight that the tuberculin skin test, in comparison with whole-blood interferon γ assays, may underestimate tuberculosis infection. Transmission to healthy people can occur in the absence of skin test conversion, which may be related to the differing capacity of strains of tuberculosis to elicit delayed-type hypersensitivity reactions. The interferon γ assays T-SPOT.TB and Quantiferon-TB Gold have higher specificity than the tuberculin skin test. However, Ferrara *et al.* (2006) found that rates of indeterminate and positive results differ between the blood tests, suggesting that they might provide different results in routine clinical practice. The assays are also more costly compared with the tuberculin skin test. The choice of diagnostic test to be used will depend on the population being tested, the purpose of testing and available resources.

The routine provision of isoniazid chemoprophylaxis to HIV-infected individuals described by Grant *et al.* (2005) reduced the incidence of tuberculosis by 38% overall and by 46% in those with no previous history of tuberculosis. Since this study was conducted, antiretroviral therapy has been used routinely. Further studies exploring the role of chemoprophylaxis are needed in HIV patients on antiretroviral therapy.

Vikrant *et al.* (2005) showed that isoniazid therapy in patients receiving haemodialysis was significantly protective against the development of active tuberculosis compared with placebo, although it remains a concern that 17% in this group still developed active tuberculosis despite chemoprophylaxis. In view of the increased incidence of viral hepatitis in patients with end-stage renal failure, it would be recommended to monitor the liver function tests for the duration of isoniazid treatment.

The two main predictors of non-completion of treatment with isoniazid chemoprophylaxis for tuberculosis were reluctance to have venepuncture and a perceived low risk of tuberculosis, as reported by Shieh *et al.* (2006). These health concerns and beliefs can be discussed at the first clinic review and, importantly, this may help promote the completion of treatment. Lardizabal *et al.* (2006) demonstrated that patient adherence with a 4-month regime of rifampicin for tuberculosis chemoprophylaxis was significantly better than with a 9-month isoniazid regime. Page *et al.* (2006) also demonstrated that a 4-month treatment regime with rifampicin achieved better adherence with fewer hepatotoxic side effects than a 9-month isoniazid regime in the management of latent tuberculosis infection. Further studies exploring the efficacy of rifampicin compared with isoniazid in preventing active tuberculosis are needed. The rifampicin regime may be particularly relevant if there is a high suspicion of exposure to isoniazid-resistant tuberculosis or if poor adherence is suspected.

In addition, Schechter *et al.* (2006) reported that a once-weekly rifapentine/isoniazid regime (for 12 weeks) had significantly less hepatotoxicity than a daily rifampicin/pyrazinamide regime (for 8 weeks) for tuberculosis chemoprophylaxis. The two groups had similar levels of compliance and degrees of efficacy. Further studies are needed of the new weekly rifapentine/isoniazid regimen for 12 weeks in comparison with 6 months of daily isoniazid; preliminary studies with this shorter regimen look promising, with high adherence rates, limited toxicity and good efficacy.

Coker *et al.* (2006) confirmed several established risk factors that may also be influencing the increased rate of tuberculosis in Russia. In this study, exposure to raw milk and unemployment were thought to be the most important contributors to the burden of tuberculosis in the population studied. The study did not, however, explore a major risk factor—immunosuppression; the immunosuppression produced by HIV is key to the increased rates of tuberculosis seen internationally (similarly, other immunosuppressing agents, such as corticosteroids, immunosuppressant therapy, chemotherapy and TNF-α blockers, were not explored in this study).

In the study by Schoch *et al.* (2007) the diagnostic yield of any single specimen for the diagnosis of pulmonary tuberculosis was low (36–63%). The recommendation would be that in patients in whom the radiographic suspicion of active tuberculosis is high, further investigation should include collection of initial and early morning spontaneous and induced sputum specimens, followed by bronchoalveolar lavage in those with a negative smear.

Both healthcare worker community DOTS and family DOTS can achieve WHO targets for treatment success in tuberculosis management, as shown by Newell *et al.* (2006). This may be applicable to other areas of the world where healthcare worker DOTS is not feasible.

Finally, Holtz *et al.* (2006) highlighted important pre-treatment factors predictive of delayed sputum conversion in multidrug-resistant tuberculosis, including previous treatment for multidrug-resistant tuberculosis, high mycobacterial loads, the presence of bilateral cavitation and the number of drugs against which there was resistance at the initiation of treatment. The time taken for sputum sample cultures to convert to negative growth was also a strong predictor of treatment outcome, with a poorer prognosis for those that took a longer time for sputum conversion.

References

1.   National Collaborating Centre for Chronic Conditions. Tuberculosis: clinical diagnosis and management of tuberculosis, and measures for its prevention and control. London: Royal College of Physicians, 2006.

4

Community-acquired pneumonia

ADAM HILL, MAEVE MURRAY

Introduction

Community-acquired pneumonia is common and affects five to eleven persons per 1000 in the adult population. The incidence rises with age, with rates of 34 per 1000 population at age 75 and above. Community-acquired pneumonia scores are validated criteria that are used to assess disease severity at presentation and often predict morbidity and mortality. Several scores exist and are used internationally.

Assessment

The following four papers review the most commonly used scores currently in practice, exploring and comparing their roles in predicting defined clinical end-points – including mortality, the need for intensive care management – and whether they can be safely used to determine whether patients require to be hospitalized for management.

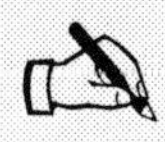

CRB-65 predicts death from community-acquired pneumonia
Bauer TT, Ewig S, Marre R, Suttorp N, Welte T; The CAPNETZ Study Group.
J Intern Med 2006; **260**: 93–101

BACKGROUND. This study aimed to validate the CURB, CRB and CRB-65 scores as mortality indicators, analysing data gathered prospectively from 1343 patients (208 outpatients and 1135 inpatients) with community-acquired pneumonia presenting to several centres in Germany over a 12-month period. The primary aim of the study was to establish whether the severity assessment scores CURB, CRB or CRB-65 could predict 30-day mortality. The scores are defined as follows:

CURB = confusion; blood urea nitrogen >7 mmol/l; respiratory rate >30 breaths/min; diastolic blood pressure ≤60 mmHg or systolic blood pressure <90 mmHg. One point for each feature present (range 0–4).

CRB = confusion; respiratory rate >30 breaths/min; diastolic blood pressure ≤60 mmHg or systolic blood pressure <90 mmHg. One point for each feature present (range 0–3).

CRB-65 = confusion; respiratory rate >30 breaths/min; diastolic blood pressure ≤60 mmHg or systolic blood pressure <90 mmHg; age ≥65 years. One point for each feature present (range 0–4).

The primary aim of the study was to establish whether the severity assessment scores CURB, CRB or CRB-65 could predict 30-day mortality.

Table 4.1 (a) Mortality at 30 days according to CURB, CRB and CRB-65 for patients with all data sets complete; (b) mortality at 30 days according to CURB, CRB and CRB-65 for patients with complete data for CRB and CRB-65.

n (%)	Outpatients (n = 208)	Hospitalized patients (n = 1135)	P-value
(a)			
CURB			
0	0/141 (0)	2/399 (0.5)	1.0
1	0/56	23/450 (3.6)	0.095
2	1/9 (11.1)	28/234 (9.0)	1.0
3	1/2 (50)	11/45 (24.4)	0.450
4	–	2/7 (28.6)	n.a.
CRB			
0	0/165 (0)	17/645 (2.6)	0.031
1	1/37 (2.6)	30/402 (7.5)	0.502
2	1/5 (20.0)	16/78 (20.5)	1.0
3	–	3/10 (30.0)	n.a.
CRB-65			
0	0/115 (0)	0/268 (0)	n.a.
1	0/80 (0)	21/524 (4.0)	0.095
2	1/10 (10.0)	31/283 (11.0)	1.0
3	1/3 (33.3)	12/53 (22.6)	0.555
4	–	2/7 (28.6)	n.a.
	Outpatients (n = 482)	**Hospitalized patients (n = 1485)**	
(b)			
CRB			
0	1/385 (0.3)	22/867 (2.0)	0.005
1	1/88 (1.1)	37/511 (7.2)	0.031
2	1/8 (12.5)	17/96 (17.7)	1.0
3	–	3/11 (27.3)	n.a.
CRB-65			
0	0/284 (0)	0/375 (2.0)	n.a.
1	1/166 (0.6)	27/686 (3.9)	0.028
2	1/29 (3.4)	37/350 (10.6)	0.338
3	1/3 (33.3)	13/66 (19.7)	0.449

n.a., not applicable.
Source: Bauer (2006).

INTERPRETATION. The 30-day mortality rate was 4.3% (0.6% for outpatients and 5.5% for hospitalized patients). The greater the number of risk factors present in each scoring system, the greater the risk of death at 30 days (Table 4.1). Overall, the CURB, CRB and CRB-65 scores provided comparable prediction of death. The CRB score, however, placed 17 inpatients in risk class 0 who subsequently died (17/66, 26% of all deaths). The CURB score placed two inpatients in risk class 0 who subsequently died (2/66, 3% of all deaths). The CRB-65 did not place any patient in risk class 0 who subsequently died.

Comment

This study provides support for the use of the severity scores CURB and CRB-65 in predicting 30-day mortality in patients presenting with community-acquired pneumonia, whether treated in the community or in hospital.

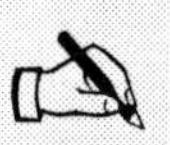

A prospective comparison of severity scores for identifying patients with severe community-acquired pneumonia: reconsidering what is meant by severe pneumonia

Buising KL, Thursky KA, Black JF, et al. Thorax 2006; **61**: 419–24

BACKGROUND. The authors compared the predictive values of the pneumonia severity index (PSI), the revised American Thoracic Society score (rATS), the British Thoracic Society (BTS) scores CURB, modified BTS severity score and CURB-65, for four specific, clinically important end-points: death; admission to the intensive care unit (ICU); need for ventilatory support with subsequent death; and need for inotropic support with subsequent death. Pneumonia severity scores were evaluated in 392 patients presenting to hospital with community-acquired pneumonia. Severe community-acquired pneumonia was defined by each scoring system as follows:

PSI: class IV and V;

CURB score: presence of two or more variables;

CURB-65 score: presence of three or more variables;

Modified BTS score: presence of at least two CURB variables or presence of one CURB variable and either aged >50 years or presence of one comorbidity with either oxygen saturation <92% on air or presence of bilateral/multilobar infiltrates on chest radiograph;

rATS: either one major criterion (mechanical ventilation or septic shock) or two minor criteria (systolic blood pressure <90 mmHg, multilobar chest radiograph changes or PaO_2/FiO_2 <250).

INTERPRETATION. There were 392 patients, of whom 9.4% died and 6.6% required ventilator and/or inotropic support. The median age of the patient population was 74 years (range 18–96 years). The positive and negative predictive values for the chosen end-points are shown in Tables 4.2 and 4.3. The authors concluded that the modified BTS severity score performed best for all four outcomes; PSI and CURB were similar; rATS identified the need for ICU admission but not for mortality; and CURB-65 predicted mortality but performed less well when the requirement for ICU admission was included.

Table 4.2 Positive predictive values for mortality, ICU admission and death and/or need for ventilatory or inotropic support using PSI, CURB, CURB-65, modified BTS score and rATS

	End-point positive predictive value (95% CI)				
	PSI classes IV and V	CURB ≥2	CURB-65 ≥3	Modified BTS score	rATS
Mortality	16 (12–22)	18 (13–25)	21 (14–28)	16 (11–22)	22 (13–33)
ICU admission	10 (6–14)	12 (7–17)	10 (6–17)	11 (7–16)	33 (22–46)
Death and/or need for ventilatory or inotropic support	22 (17–28)	26 (19–32)	27 (20–35)	24 (19–31)	45 (33–57)

Source of data: Buising *et al.* (2006).

Table 4.3 Negative predictive values for mortality, ICU admission and death and/or need for ventilatory or inotropic support using PSI, CURB, CURB-65, modified BTS score and rATS

	End-point positive predictive value (95% CI)				
	PSI classes IV and V	CURB ≥2	CURB-65 ≥3	Modified BTS score	rATS
Mortality	99 (97–100)	98 (95–99)	97 (94–99)	98 (95–100)	93 (90–96)
ICU admission	98 (94–99)	98 (95–99)	96 (92–98)	99 (97–100)	99 (98–99)
Death and/or need for ventilatory or inotropic support	97 (93–99)	96 (93–98)	94 (90–96)	98 (95–100)	93 (89–95)

Source of data: Buising *et al.* (2006).

Comment

The scores consistently have high negative predictive values. The main strength of all these severity scores is that patients with low scores have a low risk of mortality, need for ICU admission or the combined end-point of need for ventilatory support with subsequent death or need for inotropic support with subsequent death.

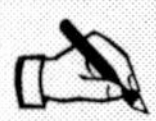

Outpatient care compared with hospitalization for community-acquired pneumonia: a randomized trial in low-risk patients

Carratala J, Fernandez-Sabe N, Ortega L, *et al. Ann Intern Med* 2005; **142**: 165–72

BACKGROUND. The aim of this study was to assess whether patients with a low PSI score could be safely and effectively managed in an outpatient setting. The PSI stratifies patients into five risk classes, with 30-day mortality ranging from 0.1% in class I to 27% in class V. The investigators randomly assigned patients with a PSI risk class of II or III to outpatient care with oral levofloxacin 500 mg/day (*n* = 103) or to hospital admission with sequential treatment with intravenous and oral levofloxacin 500 mg/day (*n* = 104), with review arranged at days 2, 7 and 30 for assessment of study parameters. The primary end-point in this study was the percentage with a successful outcome at the end of treatment (i.e. meeting all seven criteria: cure of pneumonia; no need for additional visits; no change with levofloxacin; no hospital admissions; no mortality at 30 days; no complications during treatment; no adverse drug reactions). Secondary end-points included patients' satisfaction and quality of life.

INTERPRETATION. There was no significant difference in mean length of antibiotic therapy required (10.19 days in the outpatient group vs 10 days in those hospitalized; *P* >0.2). Overall successful outcome was achieved in 83.6% of the outpatient group and 80.7% in the hospitalized group (not significantly different). This difference remained non-significant following multivariate analysis adjusting for comorbid conditions, sex, age and PSI score. No significant difference in health-related quality of life was found between the groups. However, a significantly greater percentage of the outpatient group reported more frequent satisfaction with care (91% vs 79.9%; absolute difference 12.1%; *P* = 0.03).

Comment

In patients with community-acquired pneumonia, PSI risk class II or III and no evidence of respiratory failure or any unstable comorbidities requiring hospitalization, without complicated pleural effusions, and who had adequate social support, outpatient management achieved comparable clinical outcomes and greater patient satisfaction compared with those managed as inpatients.

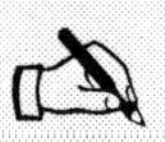

Low-risk patients admitted with community-acquired pneumonia

Marrie TJ, Huang JQ. *Am J Med* 2005; **118**: 1357–63

BACKGROUND. This was a prospective observational study of 3065 patients with community-acquired pneumonia deemed to be at low risk (PSI classes I and II), presenting to several tertiary referral centres in Canada over a 24-month period. PSI stratifies patients into low risk (PSI 1–3) and they have a low mortality (<1%). Those with a PSI 4 have 9% mortality and those with PSI 5, 27% mortality. The aim was to describe low-risk patients admitted with community-acquired pneumonia.

INTERPRETATION. Five hundred and eighty-six (19%) of these low-risk patients with community-acquired pneumonia were admitted to hospital. They were compared with 2479 treated as outpatients. Multivariate analysis revealed that the risk factors for admission were female sex, living in an inner city area, diminished pre-morbid functional status, comorbidities likely to be made worse by pneumonia (such as chronic obstructive pulmonary disease, asthma, heart disease or inflammatory bowel disease), or suffer with substance abuse or have psychiatric illness. Those requiring admission were more likely to have pre-existing comorbidities: only 11% of those with no comorbidity were admitted compared with 24.6% with one comorbidity, 45.2% with two comorbidities and 63.2% with three comorbidities. A respiratory rate of 28 or more breaths per minute and symptoms of shaking chills, breathlessness, nausea or diarrhoea were the remaining factors predicting admission. The mean length of stay was 7.4 ± 11 days and 48% stayed more than 5 days. Nineteen per cent of inpatients suffered at least one complication. None of the patients managed as outpatients required admission within the following month.

Comment

The patients included in this study were classified as having low risk according to the PSI scoring system. However, nearly one-fifth still required an admission to hospital, which lasted on average 1 week. This study therefore emphasizes that, while such scores can be used to classify risk, the patient population remains heterogeneous, and that it is critical to combine physician judgement with the severity scores.

Treatment with antibiotics

The next paper compares pathogen-directed antibiotic treatment and empirical broad-spectrum antibiotic treatment in patients with community-acquired pneumonia. The following paper compares discontinuing antibiotic therapy after 3 and 8 days in community-acquired pneumonia. The last two studies concern severe community-acquired pneumonia; the first assesses the effectiveness and safety of an early switch from intravenous to oral antibiotics and the second evaluates the added benefit of intravenous hydrocortisone.

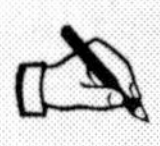

Comparison between pathogen directed antibiotic treatment and empirical broad spectrum antibiotic treatment in patients with community-acquired pneumonia: a prospective randomised study

van der Eerden MM, Vlaspolder F, de Graaff CS, *et al. Thorax* 2005; **60**: 672–8

BACKGROUND. **Antibiotic selection for the management of community-acquired pneumonia may be targeted to the suspected causative organism or an empirical strategy with broad-spectrum antibiotics may be used. This prospective study randomized a total of 262 patients, presenting to hospital between 1998 and 2000 with community-acquired pneumonia, to either empirical antibiotic treatment (intravenous erythromycin and a β-lactam/β-lactamase inhibitor; n = 128) or therapy directed to the suspected pathogen according to microbial investigation or clinical presentation (n = 134). The subjects in the targeted treatment group were significantly younger (mean age 62.0 vs 66.7 years; P = 0.03) and included significantly more patients with a lower PSI (risk classes I and II) than the empirically treated subjects (37 vs 25%; P = 0.03). The primary end-point of the study was length of hospital stay. The main secondary end-points were therapeutic failure on antibiotics,**

30-day mortality rate, duration of antibiotic therapy, resolution of fever, side effects and quality of life.

INTERPRETATION. There was no significant difference in the duration of hospital admission between the targeted treatment group and the empirically treated group (mean 14.3 and 13.2 days respectively; $P = 0.75$). The total duration of antibiotic treatment was similar for the two groups (9.9 days in the empirical group and 10.8 days in the targeted group; $P = 0.19$). There was no significant difference in 30-day mortality rate, clinical failure or resolution of fever. Significantly more adverse events after antibiotic treatment occurred in the empirically managed group (60% compared with 17% in the targeted group), although these events had no influence on the clinical outcome in terms of length of hospital stay, treatment failure or mortality.

Comment

This prospective study demonstrated that empirical antibiotic therapy for community-acquired pneumonia has clinical efficacy comparable to that of pathogen-specific antibiotic therapy.

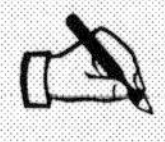

Effectiveness of discontinuing antibiotic treatment after three days versus eight days in mild to moderate-severe community-acquired pneumonia: randomised, double blind study

El Moussaoui R, de Borgie CA, van den Broek P, et al. *BMJ* 2006; **332**: 1355–62

BACKGROUND. Current international guidelines for the treatment of community-acquired pneumonia in patients admitted to hospital do not agree on the duration of antibiotic therapy, but the usual treatment is 7–14 days depending on severity. This study was a randomized, double-blind, placebo-controlled trial investigating whether discontinuing antibiotic therapy after 3 days of intravenous amoxicillin therapy was less effective in treating pneumonia than a total of 8 days of amoxicillin therapy (3 days intravenously followed by 5 days orally). Following an initial good clinical response to 3 days of intravenous amoxicillin, 121 patients were randomly assigned to receive either amoxicillin 750 mg three times daily for 5 days ($n = 64$) or placebo ($n = 57$). The primary outcome of this study was clinical success at day 10. A cure was defined as resolution or improvement of symptoms and clinical signs related to pneumonia without the need for additional or alteration of antibiotic therapy. The main secondary outcomes were bacteriological and radiological success and clinical cure at day 28. Bacteriological success was defined as the eradication or presumed eradication of the isolated pathogen. Radiological success was defined as resolved or improved chest abnormalities.

INTERPRETATION. Baseline characteristics were comparable except for the symptom severity score, which was worse in the placebo group. Fifty-nine per cent had mild pneumonia (PSI I or II) in both groups. The median age was 60 years in the 8-day therapy

Table 4.4 Clinical, bacteriological and radiological outcomes for adults with community-acquired pneumonia randomized to oral placebo or oral amoxicillin for 5 days after 3 days of amoxicillin treatment

Outcomes	Three-day treatment group	Eight-day treatment group	Difference (95% CI)
Day 10:			
Clinical cure (per protocol analysis)	50/54 (93)	56/60 (93)	0.1 (–9 to 10)
Clinical cure	50/56 (89)	56/63 (89)	0.4 (–11 to 12)
Bacteriological success	22/25 (88)	19/20 (95)	–7 (–23 to 9)
Radiological success	48/56 (86)	52/63 (83)	3 (–10 to 16)
Day 28:			
Clinical cure (per protocol analysis)	47/52 (90)	49/56 (88)	2 (–9 to 15)
Clinical cure	47/56 (84)	49/63 (78)	6 (–8 to 20)
Bacteriological success	20/25 (80)	15/20 (75)	5 (–20 to 30)
Radiological success	48/56 (86)	50/63 (79)	6 (–7 to 20)

Values are number (percentage) unless stated otherwise.
Source: El Moussaoui *et al.* (2006).

group and 54 years in the placebo group. There was comparable clinical, bacteriological and radiological success between the 8-day therapy and placebo groups at days 10 and 28 (Table 4.4).

Comment

In adult patients with mild to moderate-severe community-acquired pneumonia who show a good clinical response to 3 days of intravenous amoxicillin therapy, there is no significant additional clinical benefit gained by continuing antibiotics for a further 5 days.

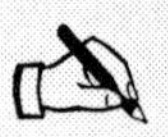

Effectiveness of early switch from intravenous to oral antibiotics in severe community-acquired pneumonia: multicentre randomised trial

Oosterheert JJ, Bonten MJ, Schneider MM, *et al. BMJ* 2006; **333**: 1193–8

BACKGROUND. Patients with severe community-acquired pneumonia who are admitted to hospital are typically initially treated aggressively with intravenous antibiotic therapy to provide optimal antimicrobial concentrations in the tissue. This open-label clinical trial of 265 patients assessed the clinical efficacy of discontinuing intravenous therapy after 72 h and completing a total of 10 days of treatment with oral antibiotics (*n* = 132, intervention group) as opposed to completing a standard regimen of 7 days of intravenous antibiotic treatment (*n* = 133, control group) in patients with

severe community-acquired pneumonia not requiring admission for intensive care. The primary outcome was clinical cure (defined as discharged in good health without signs and symptoms of pneumonia and no treatment failure during 28-day follow-up). The secondary outcome was the duration of hospital stay.

INTERPRETATION. The baseline characteristics of the patients were similar and most patients received empirical monotherapy with amoxicillin or amoxicillin and clavulanic acid ($n = 174$; 58%) or cephalosporin ($n = 59$; 20%). Similar percentages of patients in the intervention (83%) and control groups (88%) were placed in PSI class IV or V. The duration of intravenous treatment was significantly shorter in the intervention group (mean 3.6 ± 1.5 vs 7 ± 2.0 days). Total length of hospital stay was significantly reduced to 9.6 ± 5.0 days in the intervention group compared with 11.5 ± 4.9 days for patients in the control group. There was no significant difference between the groups in mortality at day 28 (intervention group 4%, control group 6%). Clinical cure was 83% in the intervention group and 85% in the control group, which again was not a significant difference.

Table 4.5 Outcomes in a multicentre randomized trial of early switching from intravenous to oral antibiotics in severe community-acquired pneumonia

	Treatment group		
Clinical outcome	Intervention ($n = 132$)	Control ($n = 133$)	Mean difference (95% CI)
Death after day 3	5 (4)	8 (6)	2% (−3% to 8%)
Clinical cure	110 (83)	113 (85)	2% (−7% to 10%)
Clinical failure:	22 (17)	20 (15)	−2% (−10% to 7%)
Clinical cure but still in hospital	9 (7)	6 (5)	−2% (−4% to 8%)
Clinical deterioration	8 (6)	6 (5)	−1% (−4% to 7%)
Death	5 (4)	8 (6)	2% (−3% to 8%)
Clinical deterioration and death	13 (10)	14 (11)	1% (−1% to 8%)
Mean (SD) length of hospital stay (days)	9.6 (5.0)	11.5 (4.9)	1.9 (0.6 to 3.2)
Mean (SD) duration of intravenous treatment (days)	3.6 (1.5)	7.0 (2.0)	3.4 (2.8 to 3.9)

Values are number of patients (percentage) unless otherwise stated.
Source: Oosterheert *et al.* (2006).

Comment

This study found that early transition from intravenous to oral antibiotic therapy in patients with severe community-acquired pneumonia not requiring ICU admission is safe and not detrimental to overall clinical outcome and can reduce the length of hospital stay.

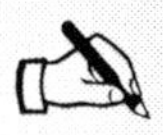

Hydrocortisone infusion for severe community-acquired pneumonia: a preliminary randomized study

Confalonieri M, Urbino R, Potena A, *et al. Am J Respir Crit Care Med* 2005;
171: 242–8

BACKGROUND. The mortality rate of patients with severe community-acquired pneumonia admitted to ICUs is high. The role of systemic steroids in life-threatening severe community-acquired pneumonia is not known. It is postulated that systemic steroids may reduce systemic inflammation, lead to earlier resolution and reduce sepsis-related complications. This randomized, double-blind, placebo-controlled trial evaluated the efficacy and safety of a 7-day hydrocortisone infusion in such a patient population. Patients meeting either two minor criteria or one major criterion of the ATS 1993 criteria for severe community-acquired pneumonia received either an initial 200 mg hydrocortisone bolus followed by a 7-day infusion of hydrocortisone at 10 mg/h (n = 23) or placebo (n = 23). The primary end-points were improvement in PaO_2:FiO_2 (PaO_2:FiO_2 >250 or an increase of ≥100 from study entry), multiple organ dysfunction syndrome score and delayed septic shock at day 8. At day 8, PaO_2:FiO_2 was assessed and multiple organ dysfunction syndrome was scored. Participants were followed to the point of death or ICU discharge or to 60 days from admission.

INTERPRETATION. The treatment group at baseline had a significantly lower PaO_2:FiO_2 (141 ± 49 vs 178 ± 58; P = 0.03), higher C-reactive protein concentration (55 [14–349] vs 29 [6–200] mg/dl; P = 0.04) and a greater chest radiograph score (P = 0.03). At day 8, compared with placebo, the treatment group had a significant improvement in PaO_2:FiO_2 and C-reactive protein concentration (Fig. 4.1). There was also a significant improvement in multiple organ dysfunction syndrome score (P = 0.003) and chest radiograph score (P <0.0001) in the treatment group. Hydrocortisone treatment appeared to be associated with a protective effect against delayed septic shock (odds ratio [OR] 0.03; CI 0.0015–0.51; P = 0.0005). The final outcome of the patients in the treatment group was significantly better in terms of mortality at 60 days (0 vs 38%; P = 0.001) and the length of hospital stay (median [interquartile range] 13 [10–53] vs 21 days [3–72]; P = 0.03).

Comment

Hydrocortisone administration initiated early in the course of severe community-acquired pneumonia that requires ICU admission may lead to earlier resolution of pneumonia, prevent sepsis-related complications and reduce mortality. The benefits of hydrocortisone therapy were considered great enough after the randomization of only 48 patients for the study to be discontinued early. This is, however, a small study and larger, multicentre trials are needed to validate the results.

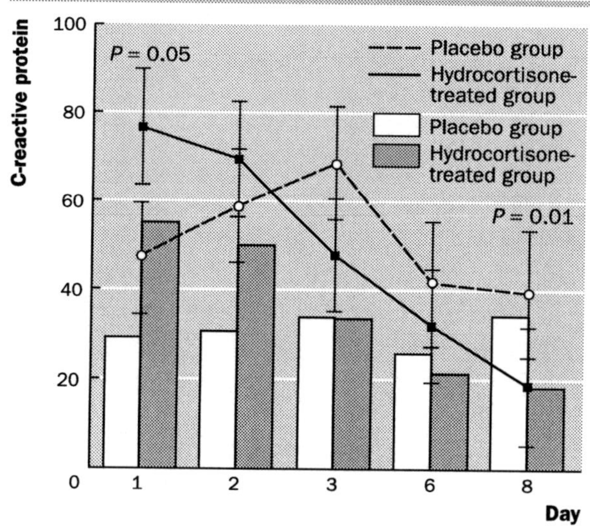

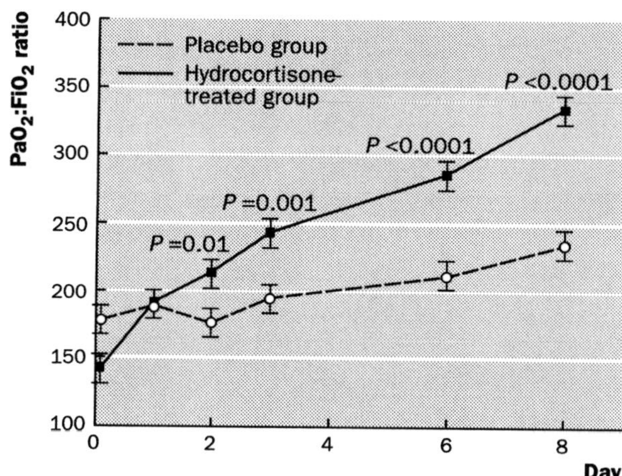

Fig. 4.1 Values over time for serum C-reactive protein (CRP) (top) and PaO_2:FiO_2 (*bottom*) in patients randomized to hydrocortisone and placebo. *Dashed lines* represent the placebo group and *solid lines* represent the hydrocortisone-treated group. The CRP graph contains two censored outliers for day 8, as shown in the line graph. Two placebo patients were censored because their day 8 CRP value was beyond 3 SD of the mean day 8 value. If the outliers were included, the difference between groups on day 8 is more significant ($P = 0.008$). The bar graph represents median values; *white bars* represent the placebo group and *grey bars* represent the hydrocortisone-treated group. *P*-values shown are median comparisons between groups. The PaO_2:FiO_2 graph contains censoring for days 6 and 8 values of the placebo patient, who exited to receive hydrocortisone therapy for septic shock. Source: Confalonieri *et al.* (2005).

Conclusion

Several studies provide support for the use of the severity scores CURB and CRB-65. Bauer *et al.* (2006) found them to be effective in predicting mortality in patients presenting with community-acquired pneumonia, whether treated in the community or in hospital; Buising *et al.* demonstrate that several severity scores (PSI, rATS, CURB, modified BTS and CURB-65) consistently have high negative predictive values. The main strength of all these severity scores is that patients with a low score have a low risk of mortality, need for ICU admission or low risk for the combined end-point of need for ventilatory support with subsequent death or need for inotropic support with subsequent death. In addition, a useful study by Carratala *et al.* showed that, in patients with community-acquired pneumonia PSI risk class II or III and no evidence of respiratory failure or any unstable comorbidities requiring hospitalization, or without complicated pleural effusions but with adequate social support, outpatient management achieved comparable clinical outcomes and greater patient satisfaction compared with inpatient management. However, in the study by Marrie *et al.* nearly one-fifth of patients classified as having a low risk according to the PSI scoring system still required an admission to hospital, lasting on average 1 week. This study therefore emphasizes that while such scores can be used to classify risk, the patient population remains heterogeneous and that it is critical to combine physician judgement with the severity scores.

The pneumococcal vaccine was not shown to reduce the incidence of pneumonia significantly, but it did reduce the risk of death from pneumonia, as reported by Vila-Corcoles *et al.* The implication from this study is that vaccination can reduce the severity of community-acquired pneumonia.

A prospective study by van der Eerden *et al.* demonstrated that empirical antibiotic therapy for community-acquired pneumonia has clinical efficacy comparable to that of pathogen-specific antibiotic therapy (as measured by the duration of hospital admission, total duration of antibiotic treatment, 30-day mortality rate, clinical failure or resolution of fever). There were significantly more adverse events after antibiotic treatment in the empirically managed group, although these events had no influence on clinical outcome in terms of length of hospital stay, treatment failure or mortality. El Moussaoui *et al.* reported that in adult patients with mild to moderate-severe community-acquired pneumonia who showed a good clinical response to 3 days of intravenous amoxicillin therapy, there was no significant additional clinical benefit gained by continuing antibiotics for a further 5 days.

Oosterheert *et al.* reported that early transition from intravenous to oral antibiotic therapy in patients with severe community-acquired pneumonia not requiring ICU admission was safe and not detrimental to the overall clinical outcome and could reduce the length of hospital stay. In the case of severe community-acquired pneumonia necessitating ICU admission, Confalonieri *et al.*

demonstrated that hydrocortisone administration initiated at an early stage may lead to earlier resolution of pneumonia, prevent sepsis-related complications and reduce mortality. However, this was a small study and larger multicentre trials are needed to validate the results.

5

Hospital-acquired infection and empyema

ADAM HILL, MAEVE MURRAY

Hospital-acquired infections

The first paper in this section assesses the risk factors for intensive care unit-acquired methicillin-resistant *Staphylococcus aureus* (MRSA) infections and the second explores whether microbial airway colonization is associated with failure of non-invasive positive pressure ventilation in patients with exacerbations of chronic obstructive pulmonary disease (COPD).

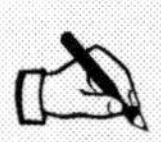

Risk factors for ICU-acquired methicillin-resistant Staphylococcus aureus infections

Oztoprak N, Cevik MA, Akinci E, *et al*. *Am J Infect Control* 2006; **34**: 1–5

BACKGROUND. MRSA is a major nosocomial pathogen, frequently and internationally responsible for severe morbidity and mortality. This prospective study followed 249 patients admitted to intensive care with the aim of identifying potential risk factors for intensive care unit-acquired MRSA infection.

INTERPRETATION. Twenty-one (8.4%) of patients developed MRSA infection. In 47% (*n* = 10) the site of infection was the bloodstream, 38% (*n* = 8) had pneumonia and in 14% (*n* = 3) the site of infection was a surgical wound site. A multivariate analysis of risk factors independently associated with MRSA infection is shown in Table 5.1.

Comment

This study identified risk factors for MRSA infection. Awareness of these may allow clinicians to be more aware of vulnerable patients and to have a lower threshold for suspecting, diagnosing and managing MRSA infection.

Table 5.1 Multivariate analysis of risk factors for intensive care unit-acquired MRSA infections

Risk factors	Odds ratio	95% confidence interval	P-value
Length of ICU stay	1.090	1.038–1.144	0.001
Presence of more than 2 patients colonized with MRSA in the same ICU at the same time	1.398	1.020–1.917	0.037
Previous antibiotic use	2.337	1.326–4.119	0.003
Central venous catheter insertion	1.822	1.095–3.033	0.021

Source: Oztoprak *et al.* (2006).

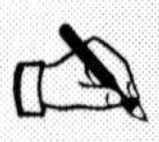

Microbial airway colonization is associated with noninvasive ventilation failure in exacerbation of chronic obstructive pulmonary disease

Ferrer M, Ioanas M, Arancibia F, Marco MA, de la Bellacasa JP, Torres A. *Crit Care Med* 2005; **33**: 2003–9

BACKGROUND. **Patients with severe exacerbations of COPD often require non-invasive positive pressure ventilation (NIV). This study assessed whether airway colonization (defined as isolation of potentially pathogenic microorganisms at concentrations $\geq 10^4$ colony-forming units (c.f.u.)/ml) affected success with NIV therapy and the acquisition of nosocomial pneumonia. It also analysed patients who required immediate invasive mechanical support at presentation.**

INTERPRETATION. In this prospective cohort study, 86 patients with severe COPD exacerbations required NIV and 51 required invasive mechanical support for respiratory failure on admission to hospital. Compared with the NIV-success group, colonization by potentially pathogenic microorganisms was greater in the NIV-failure group on admission (13 [59%] vs 14 [22%]; *P* <0.001) and at follow-up, while patients still underwent NIV (14 [93%] vs 7 [4%]; *P* <0.001) and invasive mechanical support at follow-up (20 [50%]; *P* = 0.027).

The most frequently isolated colonizing pathogens in all groups were non-fermenting Gram-negative bacteria, mainly *Pseudomonas aeruginosa*. The presence of these pathogens was significantly associated with NIV failure both on admission (odds ratio [OR] 5.6; *P* = 0.02) and at day 3 (OR 23.5; *P* <0.001). Colonization at day 3 (OR 8.8; *P* = 0.008) and inadequate antimicrobial treatment (OR 11.3; *P* = 0.001) were associated with increased hospital mortality.

Table 5.2 Colonization rates in patients receiving non-invasive positive pressure ventilation (NIV) or invasive mechanical support (IMV)

Group	Day	Patients colonized	P-value
NIV success	0	22%	<0.001
NIV failure	0	59%	
NIV success	3	14%	<0.001
NIV-dependent	3	93%	
NIV success	3	14%	0.027
IMV	3	50%	

Source of data: Ferrer *et al.* (2005).

Comment

This study provides evidence that airway colonization with non-fermenting Gram-negative bacteria in patients presenting with severe exacerbations of COPD is associated with failure of NIV therapy. The efficacy of decreasing airway colonization in preventing NIV failure needs to be assessed.

Ventilator-associated pneumonia

Ventilator-associated pneumonia (VAP) is a common problem in critically ill patients, affecting about 27% and is responsible for significant morbidity and mortality. Oropharyngeal colonization with potentially pathogenic microorganisms has a key role in the pathogenesis of VAP. The next two papers investigate the effect of gingival/dental plaque and oral antiseptic decontamination on the incidence of VAP in the intensive care patient population.

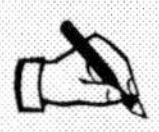

Effect of gingival and dental plaque antiseptic decontamination on nosocomial infections acquired in the intensive care unit: a double-blind placebo-controlled multicenter study

Fourrier F, Dubois D, Pronnier P, et al. *Crit Care Med* 2005; **33**: 1728–35

BACKGROUND. In this randomized, double-blind, placebo-controlled trial, 228 ventilated patients anticipated to require intensive care unit admission for ≥5 days were randomly assigned to either a daily 8-hourly application of 0.2% chlorhexidine oral gel for the duration of their admission (*n* = 114) or to an identical regimen with placebo (*n* = 114). The primary end-point was the effect on the incidence of bacteraemia, bronchitis and VAP.

INTERPRETATION. Twenty-one patients (18.4%) in the intervention group and 20 (17.5%) in the placebo group acquired bacteraemia, bronchitis or VAP. There was no significant difference between the groups in the time to develop nosocomial infection and no significant difference in the type of nosocomial infection that developed. The concordance rate between pathogens isolated from dental plaque and from the lung (by bronchoalveolar lavage or quantitative tracheal aspirate) in those who acquired infection was high: on day 8, 67% in the placebo arm and 67% in the interventional arm who had developed late-onset respiratory infection were found to have had preceding dental plaque colonization with the same bacteria. Positive dental plaque cultures taken at day 10 were significantly less frequent in the chlorhexidine group (29 vs 66%; *P* <0.05).

Comment

This study further supports the association of oropharyngeal colonization with nosocomial infection in the intensive care unit setting. Despite demonstrating good clinical efficacy of antiseptic plaque decontamination therapy in reducing oropharyngeal colonization, this study failed to demonstrate any further benefit of such treatment for the actual incidence of hospital-acquired infection.

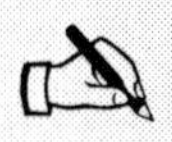

Oral decontamination with chlorhexidine reduces the incidence of ventilator-associated pneumonia

Koeman M, van der Ven AJ, Hak E, *et al. Am J Respir Crit Care Med* 2006; **173**: 1348–55

BACKGROUND. This randomized, double-blind, placebo-controlled trial allocated 385 patients requiring mechanical ventilation to receive 4-hourly applications of buccal paste containing chlorhexidine 2% (*n* = 127) or chlorhexidine 2% with colistin 2% (*n* = 128) or placebo (*n* = 130). The primary outcome was the incidence and time taken to the development of VAP. VAP was defined as the presence of new/persistent or progressive radiological changes and at least three of the following: (i) temperature >38°C or <35.5°C; (ii) leucocytosis >10 x 10^3/mm^3 or leucopenia <3 x 10^3/mm^3; (iii) purulent tracheal aspirate; and (iv) positive semiquantitative tracheal aspirate culture (≥10^5 c.f.u./ml).

INTERPRETATION. A total of 52 patients from the study population developed VAP: 23 in the placebo group, 16 in the combination group and 13 in the chlorhexidine group. The daily risk of development of VAP was significantly lower in both intervention groups compared with the placebo group (chlorhexidine, hazard ratio [HR] 0.35; 95% confidence interval [CI] 0.16–0.79; *P* = 0.012; chlorhexidine/colistin, HR 0.45; 95% CI 0.22–0.92; *P* = 0.03). Endotracheal colonization was significantly less frequent in both intervention groups compared with placebo on days 5–8 only and not in the time periods days 1–4 and 9–12 days. No differences in the duration of mechanical ventilation, length of stay in the intensive care unit or survival could be detected between the groups.

Comment

Oropharyngeal decontamination reduced the incidence and daily risk of developing VAP. It had no effect, however, on the duration of mechanical ventilation, length of stay in the intensive care unit or survival. The antiseptic agents used in this study are preferable to the use of continuous prophylactic antibiotic therapy, in which there is a risk of encouraging the emergence of resistant pathogens.

The final paper in this section evaluates the efficacy of aerosolized colistin for the treatment of nosocomial pneumonia due to multidrug-resistant Gram-negative bacteria in patients without cystic fibrosis.

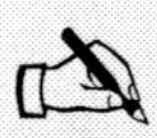

Aerosolized colistin for the treatment of nosocomial pneumonia due to multidrug-resistant Gram-negative bacteria in patients without cystic fibrosis

Michalopoulos A, Kasiakou SK, Mastora Z, Rellos K, Kapaskelis AM, Falagas ME. *Crit Care* 2005; **9**: R53–9

BACKGROUND. Nosocomial pneumonia, particularly in the intensive therapy unit setting, has a high mortality rate. The authors retrospectively assessed whether the addition of aerosolized colistin to standard intravenous antibiotic therapy was of benefit in managing Gram-negative nosocomial pneumonia.

INTERPRETATION. Out of 152 patients managed with intravenous colistin in the intensive therapy unit for multidrug-resistant Gram-negative bacterial infections, eight received adjunct treatment with aerosolized colistin. Six of the eight patients had VAP. The causative organism in seven of these patients was *Acinetobacter baumannii* and in one it was *Pseudomonas aeruginosa*. Half of the isolated pathogens were sensitive to colistin only. The daily dose of aerosolized colistin was not standardized and ranged from 1.5×10^6 to 6×10^6 IU in three or four daily divided doses. The mean duration of treatment was 10.5 days. Seven out of eight patients had concomitant therapy with intravenous colistin or other antimicrobial agents. No adverse effects (bronchoconstriction or chest tightness) occurred due to aerosolized colistin. In four patients the pneumonia was cured, three patients improved and one patient died.

Comment

This retrospective study assessed whether adding treatment with aerosolized antibiotics to treatment with intravenous antibiotics is superior to intravenous antibiotic therapy alone. Randomized controlled trials are needed to address whether adjunctive aerosolized antibiotics confer any benefit.

Empyema

The next five papers address empyema complicating bacterial pneumonia. The first two papers in this section assess the incidence and natural history of empyema and evaluate factors associated with increased hospital stay.

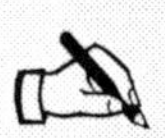

Thoracic empyema in patients with community-acquired pneumonia

Ahmed RA, Marrie TJ, Huang JQ. *Am J Med* 2006; **119**: 877–83

BACKGROUND. The aim of this study was to study the incidence and natural history of empyema in patients admitted to hospital with community-acquired pneumonia. This Canadian prospective study evaluated the outcome of 3675 patients admitted to hospital with community-acquired pneumonia. The diagnosis of empyema was based on one or more of the following: microorganisms in pleural fluid Gram stain or culture; pleural pH <7.2 with radiographic features of empyema; and frank pus in the pleural space. Patients with empyema were compared with those with community-acquired pneumonia without empyema.

INTERPRETATION. Of the 3675 patients admitted to hospital with community-acquired pneumonia only 0.7% had empyema defined by the above criteria. Compared with patients with community-acquired pneumonia without empyema, patients with empyema were younger (mean + SD age 55.2 + 19.2 vs 69.1 + 17.8 years; $P = 0.001$), had a higher incidence of illicit drug misuse (13 vs 2.4%; $P = 0.02$), were more likely to have received antibiotics previously in the community (52 vs 29%; $P = 0.02$) and were more likely to be admitted to the intensive care unit (33 vs 10%; $P = 0.002$). The only significant laboratory feature was a higher initial white cell count (18.1 ± 9.0 [empyema] vs 13.4 ± 12.2 × 10^9/l; $P = 0.001$) in patients without empyema.

Among patients with empyema, significantly higher percentages had fevers, rigors, sweats and pleurisy ($P <0.05$). The most significant pathogen identified in the empyema group was *Streptococcus milleri* (isolated in 50%). Patients with empyema had a longer hospital admission (23.5 ± 17 vs 12.4 ± 20.2 days; $P = 0.007$). Mortality was 4% in those with empyema and 10% in those with community-acquired pneumonia, but this difference was not statistically significant.

Comments

This large prospective Canadian population-based study showed a low incidence of empyema complicating community-acquired pneumonia in patients admitted to hospital. Clinical and laboratory features were non-specific and pleural fluid characteristics remain the gold standard for differentiating empyema from simple parapneumonic effusions.

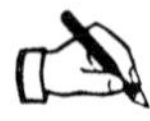

Factors influencing length of hospital stay in patients with bacterial pleural effusion

Soriano T, Alegre J, Aleman C, *et al. Respiration* 2005; **72**: 587–93

BACKGROUND. Previous published studies concerning the management of parapneumonic pleural effusions have often used length of hospital stay as an important end-point. The aim of this study was to evaluate factors that cause increased hospital stay in patients with parapneumonic effusions complicating pneumonia. This Spanish study compared 112 patients: 32 with empyema, 50 with complicated parapneumonic effusion and 30 with simple parapneumonic effusion. Empyema was defined as macroscopically purulent pleural fluid; complicated parapneumonic effusion was defined as non-purulent pleural fluid but with positive microbiology on Gram stain or culture, or pH <7.2, or glucose <40 mg/dl; simple parapneumonic effusion was defined as non-purulent pleural fluid with negative microbiology on Gram stain or culture and pH >7.2 and glucose >40 mg/dl.

INTERPRETATION.   Patients with empyema had a longer hospital stay (empyema, mean 24.6 ± 13.9 days; complicated parapneumonic effusion, 16.1 ± 8.2; simple effusion, 18.5 ± 10.3; P <0.05). Other risk factors for increased length of stay were the presence of comorbid illness and requirement for medical or surgical pleural intervention. Higher concentrations of pleural fluid neutrophil elastase and lactate dehydrogenase were both associated with a longer length of hospital stay.

Comment

This study highlighted that complications of community-acquired pneumonia such as empyema will lead to prolonged hospitalization as a result of both comorbid illness and medical/surgical intervention.

Intrapleural fibrinolytic agents

Conflicting evidence currently exists in the literature regarding the role of intrapleural fibrinolytic therapy in the management of empyema and complicated parapneumonic effusions following pneumonia in adults. The final group of papers discussed in this chapter present the most recent evidence in the debate and are summed up in the last paper, which is a meta-analysis of several recent trials exploring the therapeutic role of these drugs.

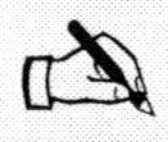

Early use of intrapleural fibrinolytics in the management of postpneumonic empyema. A prospective study

Misthos P, Sepsas E, Konstantinou M, Athanassiadi K, Skottis I, Lioulias A.
Eur J Cardiothorac Surg 2005; **28**: 599–603

BACKGROUND.   This prospective study randomly allocated 70 patients with empyema to management with closed-tube thoracostomy (28–32 French) alone and 57 equally matched patients with management with closed-tube thoracostomy (28–32 French) and three daily cycles of intrapleural streptokinase (250 000 IU). Empyema was secondary to bacterial pneumonia in this study and was defined as one or more of the following from the pleural fluid: grossly purulent pleural fluid; positive effusion Gram stain or culture for bacteria; pH <7.2; glucose <40 mg/dl; and lactate dehydrogenase >1000 IU/l.

INTERPRETATION. The streptokinase-treated group had a significantly higher percentage of patients who were successfully treated with a reduced need for surgical intervention, a reduction in length of hospital stay and reduced mortality (Table 5.3). The only adverse event with streptokinase was mild discomfort in 15.7% of patients.

Table 5.3 Outcomes for those receiving intrapleural streptokinase versus closed-tube drainage alone

	Number	Successful treatment	Need for surgical intervention	Length of hospital stay (days; mean ± SD)	Mortality rate
Streptokinase group	57	87.7%[a]	32.9%[a]	7.0 ± 1.7 days[b]	1.7%[b]
No streptokinase	70	67.1%	12.3%	15.5 ± 4 days	4.2%

[a]P <0.05; [b]P <0.001.
Source of data: Misthos *et al.* (2005).

From multiple regression analysis, the sole independent favourable factor for pleural drainage was fibrinolysis during the course of chest tube drainage, with an odds ratio of 4.29 (95% CI 1.5–12.1; $P = 0.006$).

Comment

This study supports the use of intrapleural streptokinase in the management of empyema complicating bacterial pneumonia.

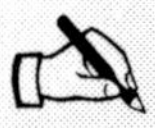

U.K. Controlled trial of intrapleural streptokinase for pleural infection

Maskell NA, Davies CW, Nunn AJ, et al. N Engl J Med 2005; **352**: 865–74.
Erratum in: N Engl J Med 2005; **352**: 2146

BACKGROUND. In this double-blind trial, 454 patients with pleural infection were randomly assigned to receive intrapleural streptokinase (250 000 IU twice daily for 3 days) or placebo. The primary end-points in this study were the number of patients who needed surgical drainage, and mortality at 3 months. Empyema was defined by the presence of purulent pleural fluid, or pH from pleural fluid <7.2 with signs of infection or proven bacterial invasion of the pleural space).

INTERPRETATION. There were 427 patients who received streptokinase or placebo (206 received streptokinase and 221 did not). Thirty-one per cent and 27% died or needed thoracic surgery in the streptokinase and placebo groups respectively ($P = 0.4$). The need for thoracic surgical intervention was not standardized in this study and was left to the discretion of the treating physician. There was no benefit with streptokinase in terms of mortality, rate of surgery, radiographic outcomes or length of hospital stay. Compared with placebo, there were more serious adverse events in the streptokinase group, such as chest pain, fever or allergy, although the difference did not reach statistical difference (7% in the streptokinase group and 3% in the placebo group; $P = 0.08$).

Comment

In this study, intrapleural streptokinase did not improve mortality, the rate of surgery or the length of hospital stay in patients with empyema.

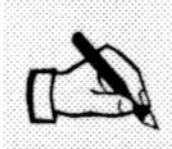

Intrapleural fibrinolytic agents for empyema and complicated parapneumonic effusions: a meta-analysis

Tokuda Y, Matsushima D, Stein GH, Miyagi S. *Chest* 2006; **129**: 783–90

BACKGROUND. This paper reports a meta-analysis of five randomized placebo-controlled trials conducted between 1980 and 2005 exploring the efficacy of intrapleural streptokinase in reducing the need for surgical intervention and mortality.

INTERPRETATION. This meta-analysis included five trials with 575 patients. The treatments used and length of treatment are shown in Table 5.4 and the outcomes are shown in Table 5.5. Compared with placebo, intrapleural fibrinolytic therapy did not significantly reduce the need for surgical intervention or mortality (27.6% in the fibrinolytic group and 32.8% in the control group; risk ratio 0.55; 95% CI 0.28–1.07). A separate analysis for either death or the need for surgical intervention failed to show significant results.

Comments

This meta-analysis concluded that intrapleural fibrinolysis of empyema and complicated parapneumonic effusion cannot be routinely recommended in all patients. It does not exclude the possibility that there is a role for intrapleural fibrinolytic therapy in selected patients, although it is beyond the scope and aim of this study to identify the potential characteristics of such patients.

Conclusion

Oztoprak *et al.* (2006) identified risk factors for MRSA infection (length of stay in intensive therapy unit, the presence of more than two patients colonized with MRSA in the same intensive care unit at the same time, previous antibiotic use and central venous catheter insertion). Awareness of these may allow clinicians to be more aware of vulnerable patients and have a lower threshold for suspecting, diagnosing and managing MRSA infection.

The study by Ferrer *et al.* provides evidence that airway colonization with non-fermenting Gram-negative bacteria in patients presenting with severe exacerbations of COPD is associated with failure of NIV therapy. The efficacy of decreasing

Table 5.4 Design of trials included in the meta-analysis

Trial, year	Patients' eligibility	Enrolled, no.		Male, %		Mean age ± SD, yr		Chest tube size, Fr	Fibrinolyties	Treatment dose per day, IU	Duration, d
		TG	CG	TG	CG	TG	CG				
Davies et al., 1997[1]	PE or CPE	12	12	75	67	62 ± 23	60 ± 23	14	Streptokinase	250 000	3
Bouros et al., 1999[2]	PE or CPE†	15	16	73	81	54‡	57§	28 to 32	Urokinase	100 000	3
Tuncozgur et al., 2001[3]	PE stage II‡	24	25	83	72	34 ± 14	33 ± 16	24 to 36	Urokinase	100 000	5
Diacon et al., 2004[4]	PE or CPE	22	22	82	68	40 ± 13	40 ± 14	24 or 28	Streptokinase	250 000	up to 7‖
MISTI, 2005[5]	PE or CPE	208	222	67	72	60 ± 18	61 ± 18	12 (12 to 20)¶	Streptokinase	500 000	3

TG, treatment group; CG, control group; PE, pleural empyema; CPE, complicated parapneumonic effusion.
† Defined by Light's classification.
‡ Staging defined by the American Thoracic Society.
§ Median values.
‖ Or until net drainage was <100 ml/d.
¶ Median (interquartile range).
Source: Tokuda et al. (2006).

Table 5.5 Outcomes of individual trials and pooled relative risks*

Trial, year	Surgery or death		Surgery		Death	
	Fibrinolysis	Placebo	Fibrinolysis	Placebo	Fibrinolysis	Placebo
Davies et al., 1997[1]	0/12 (0)	3/12 (25)	0/12 (0)	3/12 (25)	0/12 (0)	0/12 (0)
Bouros et al., 1999[2]	2/15 (13.3)	6/16 (37.5)	2/15 (13.3)	6/16 (37.5)	0/15 (0)	0/16 (0)
Tuncozgur et al., 2001[3]	7/24 (29.2)	15/25 (60)	7/24 (29.2)	15/25 (60)	0/24 (0)	0/25 (0)
Diacon et al., 2004[4]	4/22 (18.2)	11/22 (50)	3/22 (13.6)	10/22 (45.5)	1/22 (4.5)	1/22 (4.5)
MISTI, 2005[5]	64/206 (31.1)	62/221 (28.1)	32/206 (15.5)	32/221 (14.5)	32/206 (15.5)	30/221 (13.6)
Total	77/279 (27.6)	97/296 (32.8)	44/279 (15.8)	66/296 (22.3)	33/279 (11.8)	31/296 (10.5)
Pooled RR (95% CI)	0.55 (0.28–1.07)†		0.17 (0.28–1.02)†		1.14 (0.72–1.79)‡	
Q statistic (P-value)	11.4 (0.023)		8.60 (0.072)		0.01 (0.923)	

* Data are presented as no. of patients/total patients (%) unless otherwise indicated.
†Pooled estimation was performed using DerSimonian & Laird method.
‡Pooled estimation was calculated using 2 studies by Diacon et al. and MISTI.
Source: Tokuda et al. (2006).

airway colonization in preventing the failure of NIV therapy needs to be assessed. The study by Fourrier *et al.* further supports the association of oropharyngeal colonization with nosocomial infection in the intensive care unit setting. Despite demonstrating good clinical efficacy of antiseptic plaque decontamination therapy in reducing oropharyngeal colonization, this study failed to demonstrate any further benefit of such treatment on the actual incidence of hospital-acquired infection. Koeman *et al.* demonstrated that oropharyngeal decontamination reduced the incidence and daily risk of developing VAP, but that it had no effect on the duration of mechanical ventilation, length of stay in the intensive care unit or survival. The antiseptic agents used in this study are preferable to continuous prophylactic antibiotic therapy, where there is risk of encouraging the emergence of resistant pathogens. Finally, a retrospective study by Michalopoulos *et al.* assessed whether adding aerosolized antibiotics to treatment with intravenous antibiotics is superior to intravenous antibiotic therapy alone. Randomized controlled trials are needed to address whether adjunctive aerosolized antibiotics confer any benefit.

The large prospective Canadian population-based study by Ahmed *et al.* showed a low incidence of empyema complicating community-acquired pneumonia in patients admitted to hospital. Clinical and laboratory features were non-specific and pleural fluid characteristics remain the gold standard for differentiating empyema from simple parapneumonic effusions. The study by Soriano *et al.* highlights that complications of community-acquired pneumonia such as empyema will lead to prolonged hospitalization due to both comorbid illness and medical/surgical intervention. Although Maskell *et al.* show that intrapleural streptokinase did not improve mortality, the rate of surgery or the length of hospital stay in patients with empyema, the work of Misthos *et al.* supports the use of intrapleural streptokinase in the management of empyema complicating bacterial pneumonia. The meta-analysis by Tokuda *et al.* concludes that intrapleural fibrinolysis of empyema and complicated parapneumonic effusion cannot be routinely recommended in all patients. It does not exclude the possibility that there is a role for intrapleural fibrinolytic therapy in selected patients, although it was beyond the scope and aim of this study to identify potential characteristics of such patients.

References

1. Davies RJ, Traill ZC, Gleeson FV. Randomised controlled trial of intrapleural streptokinase in community acquired pleural infection. *Thorax* 1997; 52: 416–21.
2. Bouros D, Schiza S, Tzanakis N, Chalkiadakis G, Drositis J, Siafakas N. Intrapleural urokinase versus normal saline in the treatment of complicated parapneumonic

effusions and empyema: a randomized double-blind study. *Am J Respir Crit Care Med* 1999; **159**: 37–42.

3. Tuncozgur B, Ustunsoy H, Sivrikoz MC, Dikensoy O, Topal M, Elbeyli L. Intrapleural urokinase in the management of parapneumonic empyema: a randomised controlled trial. *Int J Clin Pract* 2001; **55**: 658–60.

4. Diacon AH, Theron J, Schuurmans MM, Van de Wal BW, Bolliger CT. Intrapleural streptokinase for empyema and complicated parapneumonic effusions. *Am J Respir Crit Care Med* 2004; **170**: 49–53.

5. Maskell NA, Davies CW, Nunn AJ, Hedley EL, Gleeson FV, Miller R, Gabe R, Rees GL, Peto TE, Woodhead MA, Lane DJ, Darbyshire JH, Davies RJ; First Multicenter Intrapleural Sepsis Trial (MIST1) Group. UK controlled trial of intrapleural streptokinase for pleural infection. *N Engl J Med* 2005; **352**: 865–74.

6

Bronchiectasis and chronic obstructive pulmonary disease

ADAM HILL, MAEVE MURRAY

Bronchiectasis

A vicious cycle of infection, bronchial inflammation and damage with subsequent further infection exists in bronchiectasis. The airways are frequently chronically colonized with bacteria. Nebulized antibiotics offer local and targeted therapy to the airways and indeed nebulized tobramycin is a recognized, standard and effective treatment in cystic fibrosis patients chronically colonized with *Pseudomonas aeruginosa*. However, the role of long-term antibiotics in non-cystic fibrosis bronchiectasis is not currently known. The following three papers assess the efficacy and safety of nebulized tobramycin in both acute exacerbations and as a long-term management strategy in adults with idiopathic non-cystic fibrosis bronchiectasis.

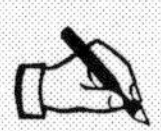

Addition of inhaled tobramycin to ciprofloxacin for acute exacerbations of Pseudomonas aeruginosa infection in adult bronchiectasis

Bilton D, Henig N, Morrissey B, Gotfried M. *Chest* 2006; **130**: 1503–10

BACKGROUND. This randomized, double-blind, placebo-controlled trial assessed whether nebulized tobramycin (300 mg twice daily) for 14 days in combination with the standard 14-day treatment regime of oral ciprofloxacin (750 mg twice daily) (*n* = 27) achieved greater clinical efficacy than 14 days of oral ciprofloxacin with a placebo in place of tobramycin (*n* = 26) in 53 patients who were chronically colonized with *P. aeruginosa* and who had acute exacerbations of non-cystic fibrosis bronchiectasis. The primary end-point was clinical outcome at day 21 (improved or resolved [cure] or whether their symptoms persisted/had worsened [failed]).

INTERPRETATION. The outcomes at day 21 are shown in Table 6.1. There was a 20% higher cure rate in the placebo/ciprofloxacin group but the difference between groups was not statistically significant. Compared with placebo/ciprofloxacin, the group receiving tobramycin/ciprofloxacin had a greater reduction in sputum densities at days

7 and 14, but not day 21. Further analysis showed that there was a higher rate of eradication of *P. aeruginosa* from sputum in the tobramycin/ciprofloxacin group (34.6% vs 18.5%) at day 21, although the difference was not statistically significant. The tobramycin/ciprofloxacin group reported more wheeze (50%) compared with placebo/ciprofloxacin (15%).

Table 6.1 Clinical assessments of test of cure (day 21) in study population*

Clinical assessment	Placebo/Cip group (*n* = 27)	TIS/Cip group (*n* = 26)
Cured	19 (70.4)	13 (50.0)
Failed	5 (18.5)	10 (38.5)
Indeterminate	2 (7.4)	2 (7.7)
Not evaluable	1 (3.7)	1 (3.8)

* Values are given as no. (%).
TIS, tobramyein inhaled solution
Source: Bilton *et al.* (2006).

Comment

The addition of inhaled tobramycin to a standard 2-week regime of oral ciprofloxacin in bronchiectasis patients chronically colonized with *P. aeruginosa* and suffering from an acute exacerbation reduced the bacterial load but had no clinical benefit compared with placebo. The authors postulated that the lack of clinical benefit might be due to the side effects of nebulized tobramycin.

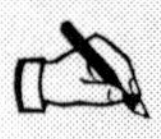

A pilot study of the safety and efficacy of tobramycin solution for inhalation in patients with severe bronchiectasis
Scheinberg P, Shore E. *Chest* 2005; **127**: 1420–6

BACKGROUND. This open-label multicentre trial aimed to assess the efficacy and safety of inhaled tobramycin by administering three treatment cycles (14 days with twice-daily inhaled tobramycin 300 mg and then 14 days without) to 41 adult patients with diffuse non-cystic fibrosis bronchiectasis, chronically colonized with *P. aeruginosa*.

INTERPRETATION. The 12-week treatment led to an improved symptom score (a composite score assessing cough severity, shortness of breath, sputum production, fatigue and wheeze; mean reduction of 1.5 units; *P* = 0.006). There was also a significant improvement in the St George's Respiratory Questionnaire score (mean reduction of 9.8 units; *P* <0.001). Twenty-two per cent of patients had eradication of *P. aeruginosa*. Two patients (about 5%) developed tobramycin resistance. However, 24% stopped treatment, mostly due to cough, wheezing and dyspnoea.

Comment

This study demonstrated that regular inhaled tobramycin treatment in non-cystic fibrosis bronchiectasis over 3 months had significant clinical benefits. There were, however, significant local adverse effects. Patients should have a tobramycin challenge before therapy and be monitored for these complications during treatment. Further longitudinal studies are needed to determine whether there are long-term benefits in terms of symptoms, exacerbation frequency and health-related quality of life.

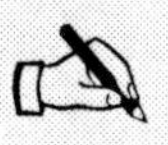

Inhaled tobramycin in non-cystic fibrosis patients with bronchiectasis and chronic bronchial infection with Pseudomonas aeruginosa

Drobnic ME, Sune P, Montoro JB, Ferrer A, Orriols R. *Ann Pharmacother* 2005; **39**: 39–44

BACKGROUND. This double-blind, placebo-controlled crossover study aimed to determine the clinical efficacy and safety of twice-daily nebulized tobramycin (300 mg) for 6 months compared with placebo in 30 patients with non-cystic fibrosis bronchiectasis and chronically colonized with *P. aeruginosa*. Patients received 300 mg aerosolized tobramycin or placebo twice daily in two cycles, each for 6 months, with a 1-month washout period. Study end-points included the effects on the number of exacerbations, hospital admissions, length of hospital stay, antibiotic use, lung function and quality of life. Tobramycin toxicity, density of *P. aeruginosa* in sputum, emergence of bacterial resistance and emergence of other opportunistic bacteria were also analysed.

INTERPRETATION. A total of 20 patients completed the study. Inhalation of tobramycin significantly reduced the number of exacerbations necessitating hospital admission (mean ± SD: tobramycin, 0.15 ± 0.37; placebo, 0.75 ± 1.16; $P = 0.038$). Inhalation of tobramycin also significantly reduced the number of days in hospital (tobramycin, 2.05 ± 5.03 days; placebo, 12.65 ± 21.8; $P < 0.05$). Nebulized tobramycin did not, however, have a significant effect on overall exacerbation frequency. No effect was observed on antibiotic usage, lung function or quality of life. A reduction in *P. aeruginosa* density in sputum was associated with tobramycin administration (Fig. 6.1). Two patients developed tobramycin-resistant *P. aeruginosa* during the treatment phase of the study, the washout month and the first 3 months of placebo therapy. Bronchospasm was the main adverse event reported, affecting three participants who subsequently withdrew from the study; one further participant required nebulized bronchodilators prior to both tobramycin and placebo administration. There was no detectable ototoxicity or nephrotoxicity.

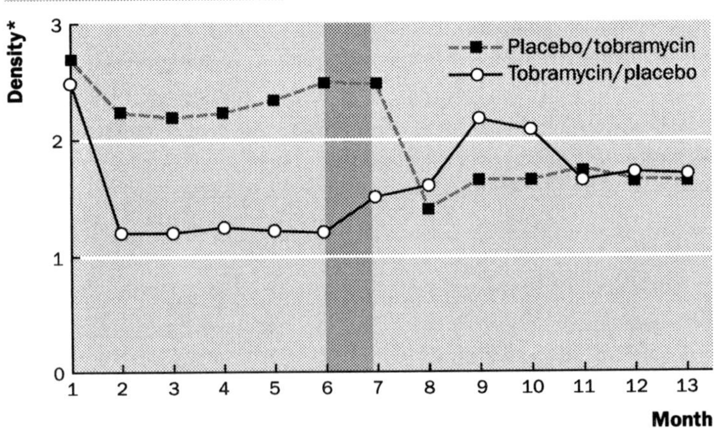

Fig. 6.1 Mean change in *Pseudomonas aeruginosa* density expressed as number of colonies growing in quantitative and/or conventional culture in the study groups. *Density was expressed as follows: no calories (0), <10 (1): between 10 and 10^6 (2); >10^6 (3). Month 6–7 corresponds to the wash out period.
Source: Drobnic *et al.* (2005).

Comment

This study shows that twice-daily administration of nebulized tobramycin in patients with non-cystic fibrosis bronchiectasis and chronically colonized with P. aeruginosa is effective in reducing bacterial density and hospital admissions for exacerbations. Further longitudinal studies are needed to determine whether there are long-term benefits in terms of symptoms, exacerbation frequency and health-related quality of life.

Chronic obstructive pulmonary disease

The next two papers evaluate the efficacy of pneumococcal vaccination in patients with chronic obstructive pulmonary disease (COPD) and whether corticosteroids affect its efficacy. The third paper in this section is a Cochrane review of the efficacy of influenza vaccination in patients with COPD.

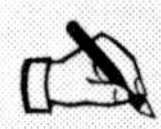

Clinical efficacy of anti-pneumococcal vaccination in patients with COPD

Alfageme I, Vazquez R, Reyes N, *et al. Thorax* 2006; **61**: 189–95

BACKGROUND. This randomized controlled trial assessed the clinical efficacy of the 23-valent pneumococcal polysaccharide vaccine in 596 patients with COPD. All

patients were followed up for 3 years. Two hundred and ninety-eight participants were vaccinated and the primary outcome was radiographically proven community-acquired pneumonia (CAP) (pneumococcal or other aetiology).

INTERPRETATION. There was no significant difference between the groups for age and COPD severity. The median (interquartile range) age was 69 (62–73) years in the vaccinated group and 68 (61–73) years in the unvaccinated group; median forced expiratory volume in 1 s (FEV_1) in the two groups was 42% (32–54%) of predicted and 43% (33–55%) of predicted respectively. Forty-four per cent and 38% of patients in the vaccinated and unvaccinated groups respectively had severe COPD, with an FEV_1 <40% of predicted. There were 58 first episodes of CAP (25 in the vaccinated group and 33 in the unvaccinated group); this difference did not reach statistical significance. For episodes of CAP requiring hospitalization, the median length of stay was 9.5 (6.5–17) days for vaccinated patients and 12 (8–20) days for the unvaccinated group, but this difference did not reach statistical significance. There was no difference in mortality rate (all causes) between the two groups, which was around 19%.

The efficacy of the vaccine in reducing radiologically proven pneumonia was shown to depend on the age of the patient and the severity of lung function impairment; there was no sign of efficacy in older patients (≥65 years) but in younger patients (<65 years) efficacy was 76% (20–93%; $P = 0.01$) and in those who also had severe airflow obstruction with FEV_1 <40% of predicted the efficacy was 91% (35–99%; $P = 0.002$).

Comment

Pneumococcal vaccination is effective in preventing community-acquired pneumonia in patients with COPD who are younger than 65 years and in those with severe airflow obstruction.

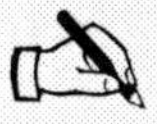

Response to pneumococcal vaccine in chronic obstructive lung disease—the effect of ongoing, systemic steroid treatment

Steentoft J, Konradsen HB, Hilskov J, Gislason G, Andersen JR. *Vaccine* 2006; **24**: 1408–12

BACKGROUND. Systemic steroid therapy may influence the response to vaccination. The aim of this study was to explore whether the response to administration of the pneumococcal vaccine was affected by ongoing treatment with systemic steroids in 49 patients with COPD (mean FEV_1 44–50% of predicted). The primary outcome was an increase in antibody level at 4 weeks and 6 months.

INTERPRETATION. The study involved randomization of 49 participants to four groups. Group 1 (13 patients) received no steroids in the preceding 3 months; they were vaccinated and then treated with steroids for 4 weeks (37.5 mg tailing to 0 mg over 4 weeks). Group 2 (nine patients) received steroids continuously before and after vaccination (dose of steroids not given in the paper). Group 3 (twelve patients) were not vaccinated (controls). Group 4 (15 patients) received no steroids in the preceding 3 months; they were treated with steroids for 4 weeks (37.5 mg tailing to 0 mg over

4 weeks) and then vaccinated. Every patient had antibodies at the start of the study. In the vaccinated groups an increase in antibody level and a later decrease was seen in 60–78% of patients, compared with 17% of the control patients (P <0.01) (Table 6.2). There were no differences in clinical variables, such as pneumonia, exacerbations and admittance to hospital, increased use of steroids or β_2-agonists, or the use of antibiotics.

Table 6.2 Antibody levels in patients after pneumococcal vaccination

Group	Number of patients with increasing and later decreasing levels	Number of patients with an increase in antibody level >1.5 (FI)	FI in antibody levels (median, range) after	
			4 weeks	6 months
1	10/13*	7/13	2.09* (0.8–10.7)	1.33 (0.6–2.3)
2	7/9*	7/9*	2.85 (0.3–14.7)	1.58 (0.3–3.3)
3	2/12	1/12	0.97 (0.7–1.2)	0.93 (0.7–1.3)
4	9/15	7/15	1.08 (0.5–5.2)	1.33 (0.5–4.2)

Fold increase (FI) in median antibody level. Group 1: no steroid 3 months before vaccination, steroid for 4 weeks after vaccination; group 2: continuous steroid treatment, before and after vaccination; group 3: control group, no vaccination, 4 weeks or continuous steroid treatment; and group 4: vaccinated after 4 weeks with steroid treatment, no steroids after that.
* P<0.05 compared to controls.
Source: Steentoft *et al.* (2006).

Comment

The authors concluded that an increase in antibody level after pneumococcal vaccination could be expected in patients with COPD despite the use of systemic steroids. This study involved only a small number of patients and larger studies are needed to address the clinical efficacy of the vaccine.

Prophylaxis

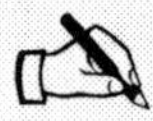

Protective effect of pneumococcal vaccine against death by pneumonia in elderly subjects

Vila-Corcoles A, Ochoa-Gondar O, Llor C, Hospital I, Rodriguez T, Gomez A. *Eur Respir J* 2005; **26**: 1086–91

BACKGROUND. Pneumococcal pneumonia causes significant morbidity and mortality in the elderly. This prospective cohort study of 11 241 individuals aged ≥65 years assessed the effectiveness of the 23-valent pneumococcal polysaccharide vaccine. The primary outcomes were the incidence of community-acquired pneumonia and mortality from the disease.

INTERPRETATION. Patients were considered vaccinated 14 days after vaccine administration. All cases were validated for a diagnosis of pneumonia by medical record review, and the presence of an infiltrate on chest radiograph was essential for diagnosis.

During 12 months of follow-up, 117 cases of community-acquired pneumonia occurred and there were 18 deaths due to pneumonia. In the multivariate analysis, pneumococcal vaccination did not significantly alter the risk of community-acquired pneumonia (hazard ratio [HR] 0.85; 95% confidence interval [CI] 0.56–1.31) or of hospitalization from community-acquired pneumonia (HR 0.81; 95% CI 0.51–1.30). Pneumococcal vaccination was, however, associated with a significant reduction in death from community-acquired pneumonia (of pneumococcal or other aetiology; HR 0.28; 95% CI 0.09–0.80; $P = 0.018$).

Comment

The pneumococcal vaccine was not shown to reduce the incidence of pneumonia significantly in this study, but did reduce the risk of death from pneumonia. The implication is that vaccination can reduce the severity of community-acquired pneumonia.

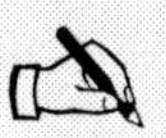

Influenza vaccine for patients with chronic obstructive pulmonary disease

Poole PJ, Chacko E, Wood-Baker RW, Cates CJ. *Cochrane Database Syst Rev* 2006; CD002733

BACKGROUND. This Cochrane review evaluated the evidence available until May 2006 for a treatment effect of the influenza vaccination in patients with COPD. It included eleven randomized, controlled trials, six of which specifically involved COPD patients. The remaining five trials included either elderly or high-risk individuals. All trials compared live or inactivated virus vaccines with placebo, either alone or with another vaccine. The outcomes evaluated were exacerbation rate, hospitalizations, mortality, lung function and adverse effects.

INTERPRETATION. A significant reduction was found in the total number of exacerbations per vaccinated patient compared with placebo (weighted mean difference –0.37, 95% confidence interval [CI] –0.64 to –0.11; $P = 0.006$) (Fig 6.2). There was a significant reduction in influenza-related respiratory infections (odds ratio [OR] 0.19; 95% CI 0.07–0.48; $P = 0.0005$). There was no significant effect of vaccination compared with placebo on hospitalizations (data were available on 88 vaccinated patients and 92 patients in the placebo group). There was no significant effect of vaccination on mortality (data were available on 88 vaccinated patients and 92 patients in the placebo group). There was no significant effect of vaccination compared with placebo on FEV_1 (data were available on 36 vaccinated patients and 19 patients in the placebo group). Influenza vaccinations were generally well tolerated but there was a significant increase in local effects, ranging from pain at the site of injection to erythema; all effects were mild and transitory.

Comment

This systematic review highlights the limited number of recent randomized controlled trials assessing the role of influenza/pneumococcal vaccination in

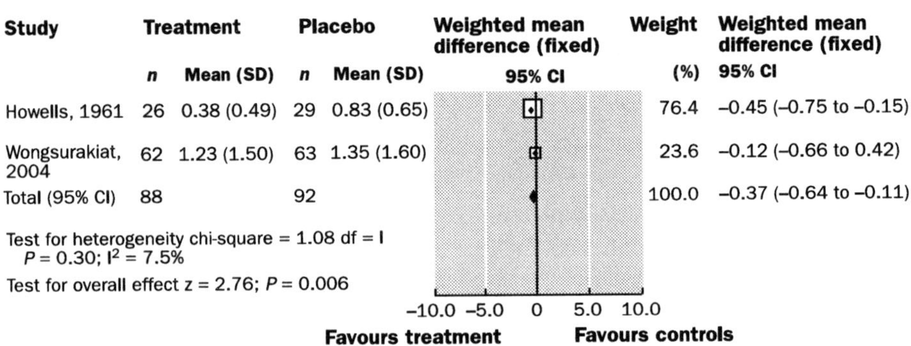

Study	Treatment		Placebo		Weighted mean difference (fixed)	Weight	Weighted mean difference (fixed)
	n	Mean (SD)	*n*	Mean (SD)	95% CI	(%)	95% CI
Howells, 1961	26	0.38 (0.49)	29	0.83 (0.65)		76.4	−0.45 (−0.75 to −0.15)
Wongsurakiat, 2004	62	1.23 (1.50)	63	1.35 (1.60)		23.6	−0.12 (−0.66 to 0.42)
Total (95% CI)	88		92			100.0	−0.37 (−0.64 to −0.11)

Test for heterogeneity chi-square = 1.08 df = I
   P = 0.30; I^2 = 7.5%

Test for overall effect z = 2.76; P = 0.006

Fig. 6.2 Comparison of influenza vaccination with placebo
Source: Poole et al. (2006).

COPD. It supports use of the vaccination as part of a wider management plan to reduce exacerbation frequency. Although associated local side effects are reported with vaccination, these are predominantly mild and transient.

The next three papers explore exacerbations and the role of antibiotics in patients with COPD. The first paper evaluates whether sputum colour is a useful marker of bacterial exacerbations. The next paper explores factors that influence short- and long-term outcomes of acute exacerbation, and the last paper studies the effect of 3 months of oral clarithromycin treatment in stable COPD.

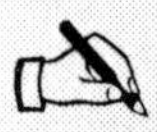

Sputum color as a marker of acute bacterial exacerbations of chronic obstructive pulmonary disease

Allegra L, Blasi F, Diano P, et al. *Respir Med* 2005; **99**: 742–7

BACKGROUND. Patients with exacerbations of COPD associated with increased sputum volume, purulence and worsening symptoms are thought to benefit from antibiotic therapy. This study analysed 795 sputum samples from a total of 315 patients with acute exacerbations of moderate to severe COPD (mean FEV$_1$ 42.5 ± 7.8% of predicted) presenting over a 5-year period. The aim was to establish if there was any association between sputum colour and the infectious aetiology of COPD exacerbations.

INTERPRETATION. Five hundred and eighty-one samples were suitable for analysis, with 145 described as mucoid and 436 as purulent. There was no bacterial growth (<10^6 colony-forming units/ml) in 22% of mucoid phlegm but only 5% of purulent phlegm (P <0.001). Isolation of Gram-positive bacteria was significantly associated with mucoid sputum (P <0.001) whereas Gram-negative bacteria (*P. aeruginosa* and Enterobacteriaceae) were more frequent with purulent sputum (P <0.001) (Fig. 6.3).

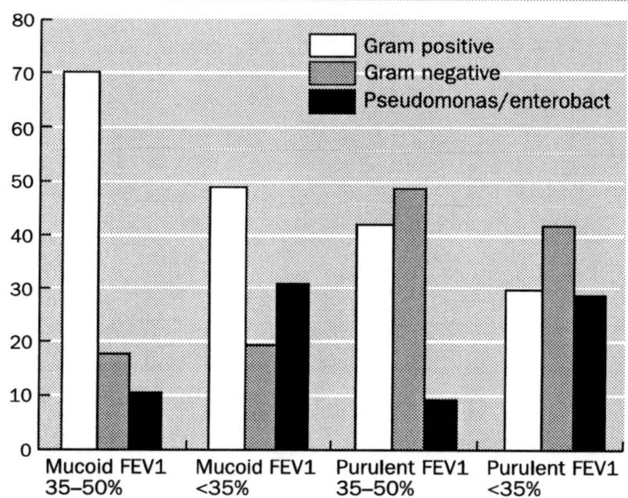

Fig. 6.3 Bacterial growth according to purulence and pulmonary function (FEV_1 % of predicted), in 581 sputum specimens (845 isolates) obtained from 335 COPD patients suffering from 795 exacerbations. Source: Allegra *et al.* (2005).

Subjects with FEV_1 <35% of predicted had Gram-negative bacteria, with *P. aeruginosa* and Enterobacteriaceae isolated more frequently.

Comment

This study demonstrated that purulent sputum is associated with bacterial growth in acute exacerbations of COPD. The greater the purulence the greater the likelihood of isolating Gram-negative bacteria, *P. aeruginosa* and Enterobacteriaceae. These organisms were more likely to be present in those with FEV_1 <35% of predicted.

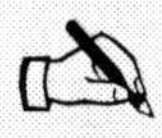

Antibiotic treatment and factors influencing short and long term outcomes of acute exacerbations of chronic bronchitis

Wilson R, Jones P, Schaberg T, *et al. Thorax* 2006; **61**: 337–42

BACKGROUND. The role of antibiotic treatment in type 1 exacerbations of chronic bronchitis has yet to be proven. This particular paper involved further analysis of the large prospective, randomized, double-blind MOSAIC (**M**oxifloxacin **O**ral tablets to **S**tandard oral antibiotic regimen given as first-line therapy in out-patients with **A**cute **I**nfective exacerbations of **C**hronic bronchitis) study |1|, which allocated 730 patients with a history of chronic bronchitis presenting with an Anthonisen type 1 acute exacerbation (defined as the presence of increased dyspnoea, sputum production and sputum purulence) to receive treatment with either moxifloxacin or one of three

standard antibiotic regimes (amoxicillin, clarithromycin, cefuroxime). The aim of this study was to identify prognostic factors of short- and long-term clinical outcomes.

INTERPRETATION. From multivariate analysis, clinical cure (complete return to the pre-exacerbation state of health 7–10 days after the end of antibiotic treatment) was positively influenced by treatment with moxifloxacin, the absence of cardiopulmonary disease, FEV_1 >50% of predicted and fewer than four exacerbations in the preceding year (Table 6.3). Multivariate analysis showed that the occurrence of a composite event (failure of study treatment, new exacerbation or further need for antibiotic treatment) was less likely if the patient was treated with moxifloxacin, aged <65, had FEV_1 ≥50% of

Table 6.3 Prognostic factors associated with the clinical cure rate 7–10 days after the end of treatment using a stepwise logistic model (intention-to-treat population)

Parameter	Odds ratio	Probability	95% confidence interval	
			Lower limit	Upper limit
Treatment (0 = comparator; 1 = moxifloxacin)	1.485	0.015	1.079	2.044
Cardiopulmonary disease (0 = no; 1 = yes)	0.585	0.016	0.378	0.903
FEV_1 (%) at enrolment (0 = ≥50; 1 = <50)	0.482	<0.001	0.349	0.666
Number of AECBs in previous year (0 = 2–3; 1 = ≥4)	0.684	0.032	0.483	0.967

There was no interaction between treatment and any of the individual factors (cardiopulmonary, P = 0.241; FEV_1, P = 0.452; number of acute exacerbations of chronic bronchitis (AECBs) in previous year, P = 0.547).
Source: Wilson *et al.* (2006).

Table 6.4 Independent prognostic factors for occurrence of the composite event using a stepwise Cox model (intention-to-treat population)

Parameter	Hazard ratio	Probability	95% confidence interval	
			Lower limit	Upper limit
Treatment (0 = comparator; 1 = moxifloxacin)	0.816	0.031	0.678	0.982
Age (0 = <65 years; 1 = ≥65 years)	1.219	0.039	1.010	1.470
FEV_1 (%) at enrolment (0 = ≥50; 1 = <50)	1.265	0.014	1.048	1.526
Number of AECBs in previous year (0 = 2–3; 1 = ≥4)	1.631	<0.001	1.338	1.988
Bronchiodilators (0 = no; 1 = yes)	1.477	0.001	1.166	1.872

There was no interaction between treatment and any of the individual factors (age, P = 0.80; FEV_1, P = 0.505; number of previous AECBs, P = 0.247; acute bronchodilators, P = 0.752).
Source: Wilson *et al.* (2006).

predicted, had fewer than four exacerbations in the preceding year and had no need for acute bronchodilator use (Table 6.4).

Comment

This study identified significant prognostic factors of short- and long-term outcomes of antibiotic treatment in acute exacerbations of chronic bronchitis. Future studies should take these into account.

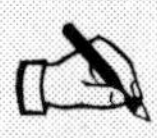

The effect of oral clarithromycin on health status and sputum bacteriology in stable COPD

Banerjee D, Khair OA, Honeybourne D. *Respir Med* 2005; **99**: 208–15

BACKGROUND. The prophylactic role of long-term antibiotic treatment in patients with clinically stable COPD is unknown. Macrolides are a popular class, with both antibacterial and anti-inflammatory properties. Sixty-seven patients with moderate to severe COPD (mean FEV_1 around 43% of predicted) were involved in this prospective, randomized, double-blind, placebo-controlled trial, which assessed the effect of 3 months of treatment with clarithromycin 500 mg once daily ($n = 31$) on health status, quantitative sputum bacteriology and exacerbation rate compared with placebo ($n = 36$).

INTERPRETATION. Compared with placebo, clarithromycin did not improve quality of life scores assessed with the St George's Respiratory Questionnaire (SGRQ) and the Short Form 36-item questionnaire (SF-36) questionnaire, except symptom domain in the SGRQ and physical domain in SF-36. Clarithromycin did not significantly change the sputum bacterial load, nor did it improve shuttle walk distance, spirometry or the C-reactive protein level. Throughout the study period there were five episodes of infective exacerbation in the clarithromycin group and two in the placebo group, but this difference was not statistically significant.

Comment

Three months of oral clarithromycin in stable, moderate to severe COPD had no impact on health status, bacterial load or exacerbation frequency. Further larger and longer-term studies are needed to address whether long-term antibiotics affect patients with COPD with recurrent exacerbations.

Conclusion

Bilton *et al.* showed that the addition of inhaled tobramycin to a standard 2-week regime of oral ciprofloxacin in patients with non-cystic fibrosis bronchiectasis who are chronically colonized with *P. aeruginosa* and suffering from an acute exacerbation reduces bacterial load but has no clinical benefit compared with placebo. The authors postulated that the lack of clinical benefit might be due to the side effects of nebulized tobramycin. However, Drobnic *et al.* have shown that twice-daily administration of nebulized tobramycin over 6 months in patients with non-cystic fibrosis bronchiectasis chronically colonized with *P. aeruginosa* is effective in reducing bacterial density and hospital admissions for exacerbations. Scheinberg and Shore demonstrated that regular inhaled tobramycin treatment over 3 months in non-cystic fibrosis bronchiectasis had significant clinical benefits. There were, however, significant local adverse effects and patients should have a tobramycin challenge before therapy and be monitored for these complications during treatment. Further longitudinal studies are needed to determine whether there are long-term benefits in terms of symptoms, exacerbation frequency and health-related quality of life.

Pneumococcal vaccination is effective in preventing community-acquired pneumonia in patients with COPD who are less than 65 years old and in those with severe airflow obstruction with an FEV_1 <40% of predicted, as reported by Alfageme *et al.*

Steentoft *et al.* concluded that an increase in antibody level after pneumococcal vaccination could be expected in patients with COPD despite the use of systemic steroids. This study involved only a small number of patients; larger studies are needed to address the clinical efficacy of the vaccine. The systematic review by Poole *et al.* highlights the limited number of randomized controlled trials conducted in patients with COPD. It supports the use of this vaccination as part of a wider management plan to reduce exacerbation frequency. Although there are associated local side effects reported with vaccination, these are predominantly mild and transient. The study by Allegra *et al.* demonstrates that purulent sputum is associated with bacterial growth in acute exacerbations of COPD. The greater the purulence the greater the likelihood of isolating Gram-negative bacteria, *P. aeruginosa* and Enterobacteriaceae. These organisms are more likely to be present in those with FEV_1 <35% of predicted.

Wilson *et al.* identified significant prognostic factors of short- and long-term outcomes of antibiotic treatment in acute exacerbations of chronic bronchitis. Multivariate analysis indicated that clinical cure was positively influenced by treatment with moxifloxacin, the absence of cardiopulmonary disease, FEV_1 >50% of predicted, and fewer than four exacerbations in the preceding year. Multivariate analysis also indicated that the occurrence of a composite event was less likely if the patient was treated with moxifloxacin, aged <65, had FEV_1 >50% of predicted, had fewer than four exacerbations in the preceding year and had no need for acute bronchodilator use. Future studies should take these into account.

Further larger and longer-term studies are needed to address whether long-term antibiotics affect patients with COPD with recurrent exacerbations, as Banerjee *et al.* reported that 3 months of oral clarithromycin in stable moderate to severe COPD had no effect on health status, bacterial load or exacerbation frequency.

Reference

1. Wilson R, Allegra L, Huchon G, Izquierdo JL, Jones P, Schaberg T, Sagnier PP; MOSAIC Study Group. Short and long term outcomes of moxifloxacin compared to standard antibiotic treatment in acute exacerbations of chronic bronchitis. *Chest* 2004; **125**: 953–64.

Part III

Thoracic malignancy

7

Screening and staging of lung cancer

RON FERGUSSON

Introduction

Lung cancer remains the leading cause of death from malignant disease worldwide, the vast majority of patients (more than 90%) having a tumour related to tobacco use. Epidemiological studies of the condition show that the incidence of the disease increases dramatically when populations use tobacco for 30–40 years, and when smoking cessation is seen the incidence of the disease eventually starts to fall. This means that in many industrialized countries the disease is actually becoming less common, but there would appear to be a potential epidemic of lung cancer about to appear in underdeveloped countries, whose smoking habits have only increased in the last few decades.

Although the cause of lung cancer is known in the vast majority of patients, prolonged survival remains an elusive goal. Most treatments are ineffective because of advanced disease at presentation. This has led to much interest over the years in screening high-risk populations for lung cancer, the hope being that the detection of early-stage disease would mean that treatment should be more effective. Early studies using X-ray examinations at regular intervals failed to show any significant survival benefit in the screened population. In the last 5 years interesting results have been reported from groups using low-dose computed tomography (CT) scanning to pick up small nodules. Whilst this approach is attractive in that perhaps more surgical patients could be found, a major drawback has been encountered in that many individuals, especially in North America, have benign nodules present on their initial screening scan. As the early screening studies are now reporting their follow-up results at 2 and 3 years, better appreciation of the effectiveness of CT scanning as a screening tool is emerging. It is likely, however, that large population-based randomized trials of CT scanning as a screening tool for lung cancer will be required before it is known whether a survival benefit can be obtained with this technique.

As it is likely that current radiological techniques are too blunt a tool to find early lung cancer, newer methods for detecting malignant disease at an early stage are emerging. These include the use of 'electronic noses', which can sense volatile organic compounds in human breath. Also, the use of microarray technology allows the detection of biomarkers which may allow the early detection of cancer-related proteins in groups of high-risk patients. Data are appearing on the effectiveness of these techniques.

Once the diagnosis of lung cancer has been established the most important evaluation for the clinician is to accurately stage the patient's disease. This allows the correct planning of treatment modalities, an accurate indication of prognosis for the patient, and the rational design of clinical trials. Until fairly recently CT scanning has been the mainstay of lung cancer staging. This has allowed useful information to be obtained about the state of the primary tumour as well as the size of local lymph nodes and the presence or absence of distant metastases. Unfortunately, CT scanning is not the ideal tool in terms of sensitivity and specificity and, importantly, does not allow histological confirmation.

Two important advances in diagnosis and staging have emerged in the last decade in lung cancer. The first is the use of positron emission tomography (PET), which is an indirect measurement of metabolic activity within tumour tissues. Whilst a CT scan gives accurate information about structure, a PET scan adds a further dimension by enabling the metabolic activity of tissues to be assessed. This can allow the clinician to distinguish between enlarged reactive glands which are not metabolically active and normal-sized lymph glands which contain tumour. Clinicians are now using PET scanning to decide which patients are suitable for radical therapy.

Another important advance in the diagnostic armoury of lung cancer clinicians has been the development of endoscopic ultrasound techniques. This has allowed clinicians to directly visualize, using ultrasound, and biopsy using fine needles, tumour tissue outwith the lumen of both the oesophagus and the bronchial tree. These techniques have facilitated the sampling of mediastinal nodes and, when used with newer imaging techniques such as PET scanning, may provide the clinician with a more accurate diagnosis and staging. This will inevitably allow better planning of treatment for the lung cancer patient.

Epidemiology

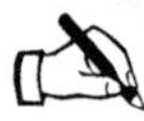

Effect of smoking reduction on lung cancer risk
Godtfredsen NS, Prescott E, Osler M. *JAMA* 2005; **294**: 1505–10

BACKGROUND. At least 90% of lung cancer cases are related to tobacco smoking. Reducing cigarette consumption rather than smoking cessation has not been shown to have a major impact on ischaemic heart disease and the incidence of chronic obstructive pulmonary disease (COPD). Smoking cessation strategies have a low level of success. It is not known whether reducing the number of cigarettes smoked will cut the risk of lung cancer. The object of this large observational population-based cohort study was to assess the effects of smoking reduction on lung cancer incidence.

INTERPRETATION. This was a huge study from Copenhagen which enrolled almost 20 000 people between 1964 and 1988. The study population was divided into six groups according to smoking habit, ranging from continuing heavy smokers (more than 15 cigarettes per day), reducers (50% reduction without quitting), light smokers (1–14 cigarettes per day), quitters, stable ex-smokers and never smokers. The outcome measure was the incidence of lung cancer in each group, assessed up to the end of 2003.

There were 864 lung cancers found in follow-up. The hazard ratio (HR) for lung cancer in reducers was 0.73 (95% confidence interval [CI] 0.054–0.98) compared with persistent heavy smokers. Hazard ratios were 0.44 for light smokers, 0.5 for quitters, 0.17 for stable ex-smokers and 0.09 (95% CI 0.06–0.13) for never smokers.

Comment

The results of the study would suggest that individuals who smoke 15 or more cigarettes per day could significantly reduce their risk of lung cancer if they could cut their cigarette consumption by 50%. This study has the strength of large size, a large proportion of smokers at baseline and almost complete follow-up. The weakness of the study lies in the fact that reduction in smoking could not be checked by biomarkers of tobacco exposure. Despite this, it would seem reasonable to conclude that reducing smoking from 20 to 10 cigarettes per day will cut the lung cancer risk by approximately 25%. Although smoking reduction has not been shown to reduce the risk of contracting COPD and ischaemic heart disease, the authors stress that cessation of smoking should be advocated as the ultimate method for reducing harm as this would also improve the outlook for patients with these conditions.

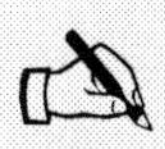

Risk of lung cancer among white and black relatives of individuals with early-onset lung cancer

Cote ML, Kardia SLR, Wenzlaff AS, *et al. JAMA* 2005; **293**: 3036–42

BACKGROUND. It has long been suspected that lung cancer aggregates in families and that lung cancer susceptibility has a genetic link. Whilst cigarette smoking has long been established as the main risk factor for the development of lung cancer in the population, few data exist to help relatives of patients with lung cancer quantify their risk. This study attempted to quantify the risk of lung cancer across a lifetime according to race, smoking status and family history of onset of the disease at an early age. The authors identified families through population-based lung cancer cases diagnosed before the age of 50 years. Population-based controls were also obtained with data collected from their family members. The study included 7576 parents and siblings of 692 early-onset lung cancer patients diagnosed between 1990 and 2003 in Detroit. There were 773 frequency-matched controls. A third of the population were of black race. The cumulative lifetime risk of lung cancer was assessed according to race and smoking habit. The incidences of other conditions, such as emphysema and allergy, were also determined.

INTERPRETATION. Not surprisingly, smokers with a family history of early-onset lung cancer had a higher risk of developing lung cancer themselves compared with smokers without a family history. Race also appeared to have a significant influence, with 25.1% of black case relatives developing the disease compared with 17.1% of white case relatives. The risk of a relative of a black patient compared with a white patient developing lung cancer was 2.07 (95% CI 1.29–3.32) after adjusting for age and sex, smoking history and other lung diseases (Fig. 7.1).

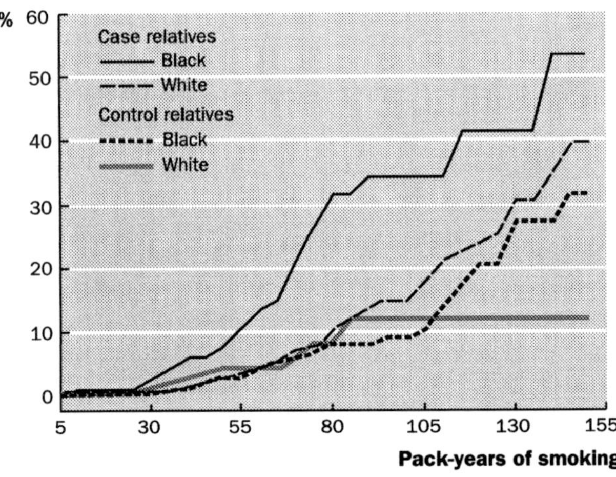

Fig. 7.1 Cumulative risk of lung cancer by pack-years and relation to early-onset case or control. Source: Cote *et al.* (2005).

Comment

This study showed a significant increase in lung cancer risk for individuals with a first-degree relative with the disease compared with those without a family history. This odds ratio of 1.71 was adjusted for race, age, sex and pack-years. The study provided further evidence that lung cancer aggregates in families and that aggregation is stronger in black families. The study has a number of limitations. The authors were unable to contact 37.2% of case relatives. Missing data had to be obtained by proxy, which clearly would have some inaccuracies. An accurate smoking history was not obtained in all relatives; black men, regardless of their relationship to a case or a control, were more likely to have missing information. Another major weakness was the fact that there may have been over-reporting of lung cancers in case relatives. The authors found it impossible to verify the correct diagnosis. In a small subset of patients ($n = 115$) for whom details were available, only 62.6% were confirmed as having lung cancer. Despite these limitations, the study provides significant data showing that there may be an important genetic link in the development of lung cancer and that this may be more important in the families of black individuals.

Screening for lung cancer

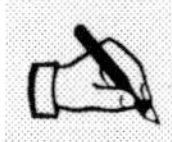 **Guidelines for management of small pulmonary nodules detected on CT scans: A statement from the Fleischner Society**

MacMahon H, Austin JHM, Gamsu G. *Radiology* 2005; **237**: 395–400

BACKGROUND. It is very common to detect lung nodules on CT of the chest. The vast majority of nodules turn out to have a benign cause but small tumours may appear as an incidental finding on a CT scan. In some parts of the USA almost 50% of smokers aged over 50 have pulmonary nodules. Existing guidelines for the management of these nodules are now outdated and affected patients require serial CT follow-up. This means substantial radiation exposure for the patient and increasing use of CT scanning time. Longitudinal studies of lung nodules performed over the last 5 years have allowed the formation of new guidelines for the follow-up and management of small pulmonary nodules detected on CT scans.

INTERPRETATION. The authors used data from large-scale, population-based screening studies for lung cancer using CT scanning in different locations around the world to construct guidelines for the management of lung nodules found on CT scans. The authors conclude that each year 10% of screening subjects develop a new nodule. The probability that a given nodule is malignant increases according to its size, such that a nodule smaller than 4 mm has a <1% chance of being a tumour whereas an 8 mm nodule has a 10–20% chance. Cigarette smokers were found to be at greater risk of lethal lung cancers and malignant nodules than non-smokers. Certain radiological features, such as ground-glass change, correlate with the likelihood of malignancy, the cell type and the growth rate. These features may predict a doubling time of the order of 2 years, which may have relevance if the patient is over 80 years of age. Using these data the authors have come up with a useful table of recommendations for the follow-up and management of small pulmonary nodules (Table 7.1).

Comment

The detection of small pulmonary nodules on CT scanning is a common occurrence for practising clinicians. CT scanning is being used in increasing numbers of patients with various medical conditions, often resulting in long waiting times for scans. Once they are detected, it is unclear how nodules need to be followed up. Many will prove to be benign and aggressive intervention at this stage is therefore inappropriate. In the past it was advised that nodules should be followed for up to 2 years. This resulted in multiple CT scans with high doses of radiation for the patient and increased cost for the healthcare providers. The Fleischner Society has come up with helpful recommendations for the management of small pulmonary nodules based on the interpretation of data from longitudinal studies of lung cancer screening. This will allow the detection at an early stage of suspicious

Table 7.1 Recommendations for follow-up and management of nodules smaller than 8 mm detected incidentally at non-screening CT

Nodule size (mm)*	Low-risk patient†	High-risk patient‡
≤4	No follow-up needed§	Follow-up CT at 12 mo; if unchanged, no further follow-up
>4–6	Follow-up CT at 12 mo; if unchanged, no further follow-up	Initial follow-up CT at 6–12 mo, then at 18–24 mo if no change
>6–8	Initial follow-up CT at 6–12 mo, then at 18–24 mo if no change	Initial follow-up CT at 3–6 mo, then at 9–12 and 24 mo if no change
>8	Follow-up CT at around 3, 9, and 24 mo, dynamic contrast-enhanced CT, PET, and/or biopsy	Same as for low-risk patient

Note: Newly detected indeterminate nodule in persons 35 years of age or older.
* Average of length and width.
† Minimal or absent history of smoking and of other known risk factors.
‡ History of smoking or of other known risk factors.
§ The risk of malignancy in this category (<1%) is substantially less than that in a baseline CT scan of an asymptomatic smoker.
Source: MacMahon *et al.* (2005).

nodules that will turn out to be tumours and enable patients who have nodules with benign features not to be over-investigated.

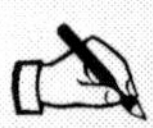

Final results of the Lung Screening Study, a randomised feasibility study of spiral CT versus chest X-ray screening for lung cancer

Gohagan JK, Marcus PM, Fagerstrom RM, *et al. Lung Cancer* 2005; **47**: 9–15

BACKGROUND. Low-dose helical CT screening is able to detect lung cancer at an early stage. Baseline screening always has a higher pick-up rate than subsequent annual testing. There are no data comparing low-dose spiral CT scanning with conventional chest X-ray used as a screening tool. The Lung Screening Study was a large randomized trial begun in 2000 which randomized smokers or ex-smokers between the ages of 55 and 74 to screening with either low-dose CT or chest X-ray. Diagnostic evaluation of images used a fairly standard screening protocol and the final results of the study were reported this year.

INTERPRETATION. More than 3200 subjects were randomized to the two arms of the study. Compliance with screening at year 1 was around 80% for each arm, having been between 93% (chest X-ray) and 96% (CT) at baseline. The positivity rates for the year 1 screen were 25.8% for CT screening and 8.7% for chest X-ray. The cancer yield for CT scanning was 1.9% of baseline falling to 0.57% at year 1. Corresponding rates for chest X-ray were 0.45% and 0.68%. Forty lung cancers in the CT arm and 20 in the chest X-ray arm were diagnosed over the study period. Distributions of stage and histopathological type were not significantly different between the two study arms.

Comment

This large study from the National Cancer Institute showed that it is feasible to randomize patients to two different screening modalities in lung cancer. Perhaps not surprisingly, more cancers were picked up in the CT arm. However, it is not known whether this will have a long-term impact on survival. The fact that many Stage III and IV cases were found by CT is a little surprising, suggesting the weakness of chest CT as a screening tool. This result would also cast doubt on whether a long-term screening programme will actually influence outcomes in terms of survival in this disease. It has, however, paved the way for the current ongoing randomized National Lung Screening Trial (NLST) in the USA, which should have the power to answer this important question.

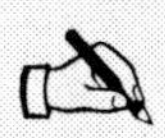

CT screening for lung cancer: five-year prospective experience

Swensen SJ, Jett JR, Hartman TE, *et al. Radiology* 2005; **235**: 259–65

BACKGROUND. It has been shown that screening with helical CT allows the detection of early-stage lung cancer which cannot be seen on chest radiography. The initial reports were greeted with great enthusiasm. Subsequent detection of early-stage lung cancers has been less impressive in interval scanning. The Mayo lung project has now enrolled 1520 individuals aged 50 years and older with a smoking history of >20 pack-years. Participants have undergone five annual (one initial and four subsequent) CT examinations. The 5-year results have now been published.

INTERPRETATION. In these 1520 individuals, 3356 uncalcified lung nodules were identified in 74% of the participants. Sixty-eight lung cancers were diagnosed in 66 participants (31 in the initial scan and 34 in subsequent interval scans). The mean diameter of cancer detected was 14 mm. The authors were unable to show a statistically significant shift in the proportion of Stage I tumour detection (the target was 50% shift). The authors conclude that although CT allows the detection of early-stage lung cancers and the benign nodule detection rate was high, results of subsequent scans suggest no stage shift.

Comment

This is a disappointing result. CT screening for lung cancer offers the possibility of reducing mortality by detecting early-stage tumours. The results of this study do not support this hypothesis and raise concerns that false-positive results and over-diagnosis could actually do more harm than good. The apparent high percentage of Stage I incidence tumours (61%) looks encouraging. However, the proportion of advanced stage cancers in the screened population was similar to that in previous studies using X-rays. This has important implications for ongoing randomized trials of CT scanning for the detection of early disease. Results of national lung screening trials in Europe and the USA are eagerly awaited, although they are unlikely to be reported for a number of years. They will answer the question whether CT screening for lung cancer meets the criteria for an effective screening test in terms of improving mortality.

Newer screening techniques

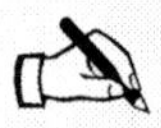

Detection of lung cancer by sensor array analyses of exhaled breath

Machado RF, Laskowski D, Deffenderfer O, *et al. Am J Respir Crit Care Med* 2005; **171**: 1286–91

BACKGROUND. **Electronic noses use chemical vapour sensors to detect volatile organic compounds. Human breath contains many hundreds of volatile organic compounds. Is it possible to use an electronic nose to identify and discriminate between lung diseases, both malignant and non-malignant?**

INTERPRETATION. This was a small study looking at the exhaled breath of 14 patients with lung cancer and 45 controls who had either had no respiratory problems or had chronic respiratory conditions such as α_1-antitrypsin deficiency or chronic beryllium disease. The authors used a support vector machine (SVM) analysis of each smell print of exhaled gas to create a cancer prediction model using a training set of exhaled breaths from individuals with cancer or other non-cancer lung disease. The discrimination power of the model was tested in an independent sample of 76 individuals. The electronic nose had a high specificity and moderately high sensitivity for detecting lung cancer (Table 7.2). The authors found that cigarette smoking did not influence the results of the study. The presence of a control group with lung disease suggests that the findings could not be explained by the presence of either airway inflammation or lung dysfunction.

Comment

This is a fascinating study suggesting that the exhaled breath characteristics of patients with bronchogenic carcinoma may be different from that of patients with other diseases. It also suggests that the use of an electronic nose could be a potentially simple, non-invasive and inexpensive screening tool for the disease. Little is known about the practicality of using this technique in patients with occult tumours as the lung cancer patients in the study had advanced disease. The fact that 18% of the validation patient cohort had tumours may also have affected the negative predicted value of the study compared with the normal population, which has a much lower incidence of lung cancer.

Table 7.2 Accuracy indices of the electronic nose for detection of lung cancer

Subgroup	Lung cancer present (n)	Lung cancer absent (n)	Sensitivity (95% CI)	Specificity (95% CI)	Positive predictive value (95% CI)	Negative predictive value (95% CI)
Positive exhaled breath test	10	5				
Negative exhaled breath test	4	57				
Total	14	62	71.4% (41.9–91.6) n = 10/14	91.9% (82.1–97.3) n = 57/62	66.6% (38.3–88.1) n = 10/15	93.4% (84–98.1) n = 57/61

CI, confidence interval
Source: Machado *et al.* (2005).

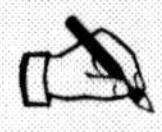

Using protein microarray as a diagnostic assay for non-small cell lung cancer

Zhong L, Hidalgo GE, Stromberg AJ. *Am J Respir Crit Care Med* 2005; **172**: 1308–14

B ACKGROUND. **The search for biomarkers for the early detection and diagnosis of non-small-cell lung cancer has not been particularly successful. The sensitivity and specificity of any marker identified has not been good enough to allow clinical use. Fluorescent microarray technology allows the grouping of thousands of proteins on a single glass slide, enabling simultaneous measurements of multiple non-small-cell lung cancer-associated antibodies to be combined in a single diagnostic assay. Does this new technique have any place in the prediction of a non-small-cell lung cancer diagnosis?**

I NTERPRETATION. DNA phage libraries of non-small-cell lung cancer were used to produce a microarray slide capable of detecting 212 immunogenic phage-expressed proteins. Samples from 20 patients with non-small-cell lung cancer and 21 normal subjects were randomly chosen and used for statistical determination of the predictive value of each putative marker. Seven unique phage-expressed proteins were found which were significantly different between the patient and normal groups. These selected markers were then independently tested for their predictive ability on 40 further samples (20 patients, 20 normal subjects). A logistic regression model was constructed to achieve 90% sensitivity and 95% specificity in the prediction of patient samples using the five most predictive phage proteins. This model achieved an overall diagnostic accuracy of just under 90% in all of the samples tested.

Comment

This is an interesting application of fluorescent protein microarray techniques. We wait to see whether this method of screening, identifying and measuring multiple circulating antibodies as markers of disease will have any clinical relevance. The technique requires validation and development.

Staging of lung cancer

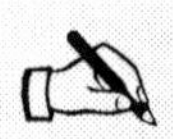

Comparison between clinical and pathological staging in 2,994 cases of lung cancer

López-Encuentra A, García-Luján R, Rivas J. *Ann Thorac Surg* 2005; **79**: 974–9

B A C K G R O U N D . Accurate clinical staging in lung cancer is necessary for planning treatment, giving an accurate prognosis to the patient and planning clinical trials. It is known from data already published that patients undergoing thoracotomy are often found to have a more advanced stage of disease at resection than that predicted by clinical evaluation. The accuracy of clinical staging can best be evaluated by comparison against the gold standard of pathological staging.

I N T E R P R E T A T I O N . This series of patients comprised 2994 lung cancer cases operated upon consecutively in various Spanish thoracic surgical units between 1993 and 1997. Ninety-three per cent were male and 80% underwent complete resection; 2377 patients had accurate clinical and pathological staging data. In only 47% of patients was there agreement between the clinical and the pathological stage. This was highest for Stage I tumours (75%). As expected, downstaging was more frequent than upstaging. The poorest correlation was seen in patients with Stage IIIa disease, in whom the clinical–pathological agreement was only 8%.

Comment

This is an impressive study but a disappointing result. The patients included in the trial constituted almost 50% of all lung cancer patients operated upon in Spain over a 4-year period in the mid-1990s. The poor correlation between clinical and pathological staging which had been reported many years previously remains. This is despite improvement in pre-operative CT scanning. This study did not include data from patients undergoing PET scanning prior to surgery. As this is now becoming a commonplace investigation before resection, it is likely that this study will represent a histological control for future studies that use pre-operative PET scanning.

Table 7.3 Comparison of clinical stages and pathological stages (c/p)

	pIA	pIB	pIIA	pIIB	pIIIA	pIIIB	pIV	Total
				Pathological stages				
cIA	198	136	25	29	68	15	0	471
cIB	51	672	10	235	228	172	0	1368
cIIA	–	–	–	–	–	–	–	–
cIIB	10	64	0	83	74	69	0	300
cIIIA	2	4	2	6	36	18	0	68
cIIIB	4	20	1	4	22	77	0	128
cIV	0	0	0	0	0	0	42	42
Total	265	896	38	357	428	351	42	2337
Agreement c/p	75%	75%	–	23%	8%	22%	–	
Under-estimation	–	15%	92%	74%	86%	–	–	
Over-estimation	–	10%	8%	3%	6%	–	–	

Source: López-Encuentra *et al.* (2005).

Staging using endoscopic techniques

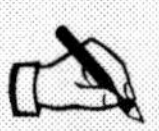

Endoscopic ultrasound in non-small cell lung cancer and negative mediastinum on computed tomography

Le Blanc JK, Devereaux BM, Imperiale F, *et al*. *Am J Respir Crit Care Med* 2005; **171**: 177–82

BACKGROUND. Endoscopic ultrasonography (EUS) has been shown to be useful to stage the mediastinum in patients with non-small-cell lung cancer and enlarged glands on CT scanning. Its role in patients in whom lymphadenopathy has not been detected on CT is less well defined. This study looked at the role of EUS in staging non-small-cell lung cancer in patients without lymphadenopathy on CT scanning.

INTERPRETATION. This study enrolled 76 patients with non-small-cell lung cancer who did not have enlarged mediastinal nodes on the CT and were thought to be operable candidates. Three patients had hilar (N1) nodes. PET scans were not performed. All patients underwent a standard EUS examination. Four patients were lost to follow-up or refused participation subsequently. Sixty-two (86%) of the 72 patients in the study underwent surgery. Nine patients were precluded from surgery on the basis of the EUS fine-needle aspiration. Eight patients had a benign left adrenal lesion confirmed by endoscopic ultrasonography and proceeded to surgery.

Of the 62 patients undergoing surgery, 23 (37%) had positive lymph nodes at operation, and 17 of these patients had N2 disease. EUS imaging identified five of these cases, resulting in a sensitivity of 29% for N2 disease. There was a statistically significant difference in the proportion of positive mediastinal lymph nodes detected by EUS between lower lobe and upper lobe lesions (10/10 lower lobe lesions found compared with 1/6 in the upper lobes).

Comment

This study showed the usefulness of EUS in preventing unnecessary surgery in a significant percentage (12%) of patients who were thought to be operable on CT alone. The low sensitivity of EUS in detecting N2 disease can be explained by the fact that EUS is unable to assess all mediastinal nodes. Anterior, hilar and paratracheal nodes are not easily seen by EUS because of air interference from air-filled airways. Obviously, the combining of endobronchial ultrasonography (EBUS) and EUS should overcome this weakness. It is likely that the better detection of mediastinal node involvement in lower lobe tumours is also explained by the anatomical difference in lymph drainage from the upper and lower lobes. Lymphatics from the upper lobes tend to drain to lymph nodes which cannot be detected by EUS whereas lower lobe tumours commonly drain to the subcarinal space, an area well seen by EUS. The numbers, however, in this study were perhaps too low to make a firm conclusion about whether only certain patients should have an EUS prior to resection (those with a normal mediastinum on CT but a lower lobe lesion). This study would suggest, however, that the addition of EUS may alter the management of 25% of patients with non-small-cell lung cancer without mediastinal lymphadenopathy on CT.

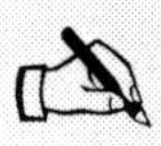

Transbronchial versus transoesophageal ultrasound guided aspiration of enlarged mediastinal lymph nodes

Herth FJF, Lunn W, Eberhardt R, *et al. Am J Respir Crit Care Med* 2005; **171**: 1164–7

BACKGROUND. Assessing mediastinal nodes is important for accurate staging in non-small-cell lung cancer. Mediastinoscopy has long been the mainstay of mediastinal lymph node sampling. Unfortunately, it requires general anaesthesia. The endoscopic needle aspiration of mediastinal lymph nodes is now possible either via the oesophagus or the airway wall. This allows the sampling of lymph nodes in parts of the mediastinum which cannot be reached by the mediastinoscope (hilar and posterior carinal nodes). The two ultrasound-guided techniques have been developed in parallel but never compared directly for their ability to reach specific lymph node stations.

INTERPRETATION. One hundred and fifty-six patients were enrolled into this study. All had enlarged mediastinal lymph nodes. Eight mediastinal lymph node stations (2R, 2L, 3, 4R, 4L, 7, 10R and 10L) were selected to allow direct comparison between the two techniques. Twenty patients were assigned to each of the lymph node station groups depending upon their initial contrast CT scan. Patients then underwent both EBUS and transoesophageal ultrasonography and enlarged nodes, once located, were aspirated. A successful aspiration was confirmed if lymphocytes were seen in the specimen. A successful puncture was obtained through the bronchial wall in 89% and the oesophagus in 78%. Combining the results of both approaches, a successful puncture of the included enlarged lymph node was achieved in 97% of subjects and a specific diagnosis was obtained in 94%.

Comment

This study confirmed that it is possible to sample all important lymph node stations in the mediastinum by combining the two endoscopic techniques. The trial showed a slight advantage of EBUS-guided transbronchial needle aspiration in right-sided mediastinal stations. The overall yield for the combined approach was at least as good as surgical mediastinoscopy. The authors recommend that if a clinician is going to learn EBUS they should also master the endo-oesophageal approach to allow complete sampling of the mediastinum.

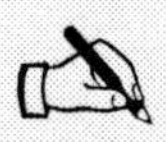

Endobronchial and endoscopic ultrasound-guided real time fine-needle aspiration for mediastinal staging

Rintoul RC, Skwarski KM, Murchison JT, *et al. Eur Respir J* 2005; **25**: 416–21

BACKGROUND. Accurate staging of the mediastinum in lung cancer is essential to allow the correct choice of treatment and to give an accurate prognosis. The gold standard test for assessing the mediastinum has historically been mediastinoscopy. This is obviously an invasive procedure and not all parts of the mediastinum can be reached. By applying ultrasound probes to bronchoscopes and endoscopes, it may be possible to sample most mediastinal nodes via the lumen of the bronchi or oesophagus. Data are now emerging concerning the accuracy of these techniques.

INTERPRETATION. Twenty patients with known or suspected lung cancer were enrolled in the study. All patients underwent EBUS and in seven patients sequential EUS was used. EUS was used to assess the posterior and inferior mediastinal nodes. All procedures were performed under sedation at the same time. Eighteen patients had lymph node sampling. Eleven had malignancy confirmed (non-small-cell in nine). Seven patients had a negative aspirate; aspirates from five patients were true negatives on follow-up and two whose aspirates were thought to be negative had mediastinal malignancy at thoracotomy. This gave an overall sensitivity, specificity and accuracy for EBUS/EUS of 85, 100 and 89% respectively.

Comment

There is now a fair amount of data in the literature concerning the accuracy of EBUS and EUS. This paper shows that the two procedures can be combined at the same sitting to provide good coverage of the mediastinum. This should hopefully reduce the number of patients proceeding to mediastinoscopy and will allow more accurate staging of nodal status at the initial diagnostic bronchoscopy. Obviously, these scopes are expensive and training to perform the tests is required. The fact that this can be done as an outpatient procedure with conscious sedation makes it an attractive way of assessing the mediastinum.

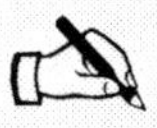

Ultrasound guided cytological aspiration of supraclavicular lymph nodes in patients with suspected lung cancer

Kumaran M, Benamore RE, Vaidhyanath R, *et al. Thorax* 2005; **60**: 229–33

BACKGROUND. Patients presenting with lung cancer require histological confirmation of their disease and accurate staging. This allows the correct treatment to be given, stage being the most important prognostic indicator. Detection of supraclavicular lymph node involvement puts the patient into the N3 category, meaning that their disease is largely incurable. Clinical examination is poor for the detection of supraclavicular lymph nodes and recently ultrasound has been used to detect and sample supraclavicular lymph nodes by fine needle cytology. This paper from a single centre enrolled 101 patients prospectively over a 1-year period to assess the usefulness of ultrasound-guided cytological aspiration of supraclavicular lymph nodes in patients who were suspected of having lung cancer.

INTERPRETATION. The study defined an enlarged node as having a short-axis diameter of more than 5 mm. Enlarged nodes were sampled using a capillary aspiration technique and cytospin preparations were prepared in the conventional way. Sixty-two patients were found to have enlarged nodes on ultrasonography (mean dimension 13.3 mm). All but one (68.4%) underwent fine needle aspiration. A positive malignant diagnosis was obtained in 44 patients (72% of those sampled). The overall malignancy yield was 46 of the 101 patients scanned (45.5%) and 46 of 61 patients sampled (75.4%). Four patients had an eventual diagnosis of lymphoma.

Comment

The authors describe a relatively non-invasive technique which can be used in virtually all patients with suspected lung cancer. The patients in this trial had CT evidence of mediastinal lymphadenopathy and would therefore be expected to have a higher than normal incidence of supraclavicular lymph node involvement. The overall yield of malignancy was high, but this does not represent the true incidence of N3 disease because of selection bias. The procedure appears relatively straightforward and easily learned. It allows patients to be staged accurately and a histological diagnosis to be obtained. It does not require expensive equipment and allows the rapid and accurate confirmation of N3 disease. Ten patients without known distant metastases were upstaged from N2 to N3 disease by the technique. This should have major implications for treatment options and prognosis for these patients.

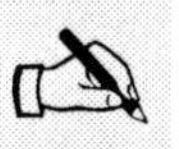

Accuracy of transbronchial needle aspiration for mediastinal staging of non-small cell lung cancer: a meta-analysis

Holty JEC, Kuschner WG, Gould MK. *Thorax* 2005; **60**: 949–55

BACKGROUND. The accuracy of transbronchial needle aspiration (TBNA) for staging the mediastinum in non-small-cell lung cancer has been reported to vary widely. The authors of this study performed a meta-analysis to estimate the accuracy of TBNA for mediastinal staging in non-small-cell lung cancer by searching commonly used medical databases for studies of TBNA accuracy. Standard meta-analytical methods were used to calculate sensitivity and specificity.

INTERPRETATION. Although 62 full-text reports of TBNA were evaluated, only 13 could be included in the meta-analysis because there were insufficient data to calculate sensitivity and specificity. The authors confirmed the extremely high specificity of TBNA (99%) but found a much lower sensitivity (around 39%) compared with previously reported series (76%). The authors concluded that the accuracy of TBNA depends critically upon the prevalence of mediastinal lymph node involvement and that in patients with a low prevalence of mediastinal disease (patients normally considered suitable for resection) the sensitivity of the technique is low. The authors reported that the safety of TBNA is extremely high, with a major complication rate of only 0.3%.

Comment

This is an important study looking at a technique which is not widely practised. It will be unfortunate if clinicians are discouraged from performing TBNA as a result of this meta-analysis. The sensitivity of the technique is high if mediastinal lymph node involvement is likely. The advantage of TBNA is that, when positive, it provides both histological confirmation and accurate mediastinal staging. It is relevant that 76% of the published papers on TBNA had to be excluded from this meta-analysis because the data were insufficient to calculate sensitivity and specificity. It is likely, therefore, that most clinicians are unaware of how useful this technique can be or how accurate the results are.

PET scanning in lung cancer

Cost effectiveness of routine mediastinoscopy in computed tomography – and positron emission tomography – screened patients with Stage I lung cancer

Meyers BF, Haddad F, Siegel BA. *J Thorac Cardiovasc Surg* 2006; **131**: 822–9

BACKGROUND. Accurate staging of the mediastinum in potentially resectable non-small-cell lung cancer patients is essential to prevent futile thoracotomy. Mediastinoscopy has always been the gold standard for assessment of the mediastinum. **Modern staging scanning using CT and PET together may detect the presence of N2 disease in the vast majority of patients, thereby rendering mediastinoscopy unnecessary. The key to such a change in surgical practice depends upon the level of false-negative assessments of the mediastinum using PET and CT scanning. Should mediastinoscopy now be routinely performed in patients with clinical Stage I lung cancer who have been assessed by CT and PET scans?**

INTERPRETATION. This is a retrospective view of 248 patients who were thought to have clinical Stage I tumours after PET and CT scanning. Seventy-two per cent had undergone mediastinoscopy before resection. Five of these 178 patients (3%) were found to have N2 disease at the procedure. An additional nine patients were found to have N2 disease in the final resected specimen, giving a total of 14 out of 248 (5.6%) with occult mediastinal lymph node metastases (i.e. false-negative CT/PET scans). The authors used a decision analysis tree with data reported in the literature on the prevalence of mediastinal lymph node metastases and the rate of unexpected benign disease to estimate the cost/benefit ratio of mediastinoscopy.

This analysis showed that mediastinoscopy in their group of patients added 0.008 years of life expectancy at a cost of $250 989 per life-year gained. They concluded that patients with clinical Stage I lung cancer assessed by CT and PET scanning benefit little from mediastinoscopy. The survival advantage conferred was very small but varied depending upon the prevalence of N2 metastases in the population at risk.

Comment

This is an interesting study which questions the dogma of performing routine mediastinoscopy in all patients undergoing resection for lung cancer. The data would suggest that the yield of mediastinoscopy is extremely low in patients who are considered to have Stage I tumours (T1NoMo or T2NoMo) on routine CT–PET scanning. One possible weakness in the conclusion of the study is that it is known that patients with T2 tumours have a much higher incidence of N2 disease compared with those with a T1 primary. This would suggest that the incidence of occult N2 disease in patients with T2 tumours is also higher, but it was not possible to determine this from the study as the data were not broken down for T stage.

Using the model postulated by the authors, the cost/benefit per life-year gained in this group of patients would be less than $100 000. The study also did not take into account the fact that N2 disease is commoner in patients with adenocarcinoma than in those with squamous carcinoma for the same size of primary tumour.

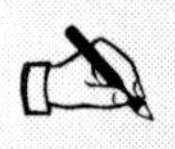

The size of mediastinal lymph nodes and its relation with metastatic involvement: a meta-analysis

de Langen AJ, Raijmakers P, Riphagen I, *et al. Eur J Cardiothorac Surg* 2006; **29**: 26–9

BACKGROUND. **Most reports have suggested that 18-fluorodeoxyglucose (FDG)-PET scanning is superior to standard CT scanning in staging the mediastinum in patients**

with non-small-cell lung cancer. This staging modality is becoming standard in the assessment of patients with the disease. More information is required about the negative predictive rate of PET scanning and its relationship to the initial size of mediastinal nodes on CT. Whilst positive predictive values may be poor with PET scanning (i.e. there are a number of false positives), if a low negative predictive value existed then patients with a negative PET scan might avoid further staging investigations, such as mediastinoscopy.

INTERPRETATION. This study was a meta-analysis including 14 trials looking at the relationship between mediastinal lymph node size, as measured by CT scanning, and the prevalence of metastatic involvement in patients with non-small-cell lung cancer. The authors then calculated the predicted positive and negative values of FDG-PET for identifying metastases in patients with enlarged lymph nodes of different size, based on the calculated post-test probabilities after CT scanning.

Patients with lymph nodes between 10 and 15 mm short-axis diameter on CT scanning and a negative FDG-PET result had a predicted post-test probability of malignancy of 5%. A positive FDG-PET result in this group of patients was likely to predict a post-test probability of 62%. In the group with larger lymph nodes (>16 mm) the post-test probability of malignancy was 21% when FDG-PET scanning was negative and 90% when it was positive. These results held for groups of patients with lymph nodes >20 mm in short-axis diameter.

Comment

This study provides data which have implications for the positioning of mediastinoscopy in patients with enlarged lymph glands on CT but negative PET scans. It would suggest that patients with nodes <15 mm on CT and a negative PET should proceed directly to thoracotomy as the expected yield at mediastinoscopy would be extremely low (5%). Patients whose nodes are larger than 16 mm on CT with a negative PET should undergo mediastinoscopy, although five patients will have to undergo this test to reveal one positive result.

Etiology of solitary extrapulmonary positron emission tomography and computed tomography findings in patients with lung cancer

Lardinois D, Weder W, Roudas M, *et al. J Clin Oncol* 2005; **23**: 6846–53

BACKGROUND. One of the strengths of scanning lung cancer patients with PET is that it is often possible to pick up extrapulmonary disease which is asymptomatic. The finding of such a lesion has a significant impact on management strategies. Whilst the accuracy of intrapulmonary PET scanning has been well documented, little is known about the accuracy of PET in detecting extrapulmonary disease.

INTERPRETATION. In this study reported from Switzerland and Russia, 350 patients with non-small-cell lung cancer underwent whole body PET-CT scanning. Extrapulmonary lesions were found in 110 patients. In 72 patients (21% of the total group) solitary lesions were present. These abnormalities were evaluated by histopathology, further imaging and clinical follow-up in order to try to obtain a final diagnosis. This was achieved in 69 of the 72 patients with solitary lesions. Just over half of these were found to be solitary metastases but in 32 (46%) of patients with solitary lesions abnormalities unrelated to the lung primary were found. Pathological confirmation of these 32 lesions showed a benign or inflammatory pathology in 26 (81%). Six patients (19%) had an unsuspected secondary malignancy or recurrence of a previously diagnosed carcinoma. Benign pathologies included colonic adenoma, Warthin's tumour and other, rarer abnormalities, including reflux oesophagitis, pancreatitis and arthritis.

Comment

This is an important study. The results would indicate that in patients with non-small-cell lung cancer, solitary extrapulmonary accumulations of FDG are almost as likely to be due to benign disease as to be definitive evidence of extrapulmonary spread. This would mean that patients should not be turned down for radical treatment on the basis of a solitary extrapulmonary lesion on PET until there is a definitive histological confirmation of malignancy at these distant sites. It is unfortunate that this process is likely to lead to much anxiety for both the clinician and the patient prior to undertaking lung cancer treatment.

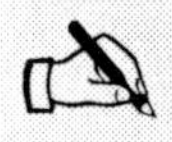

Is late diagnosis of lung cancer inevitable? Interview study of patients' recollections of symptoms before diagnosis

Corner J, Hopkinson J, Fitzsimmons D, *et al. Thorax* 2005; **60**: 314–19

BACKGROUND. Although there is much interest in reducing delays in the diagnosis of lung cancer, little is known about the pathways to diagnosis in terms of symptoms. Many clinicians are aware of the fact that patients often present with advanced disease and that late diagnosis is inevitable. Much work has been focused on general practitioner and hospital delays but little is known about the pattern of symptoms prior to presentation and diagnosis.

INTERPRETATION. This was a directed interview study performed in 22 patients diagnosed with lung cancer in two cancer centres in England. Patients were asked for symptoms leading up to the diagnosis of lung cancer and their accounts were verified from hospital and general practitioner records. Patients typically had symptoms for over a year before their diagnosis, irrespective of their disease stage at presentation. Chest and systemic symptoms were common and, with the exception of haemoptysis, were rarely interpreted as serious by patients at the time and were therefore not acted upon. Once the patient presented to their general practitioner or hospital, events were speedy and delays were rarely encountered. It seems, therefore, that patients' beliefs about their health may have played a part in the delay in diagnosis.

Comment

This is an interesting study in an area where there are few data. The authors found that patients did not readily attend general practitioner surgeries with symptoms until the disease became fairly advanced. The authors suggest that there may be a role for public education about the key symptoms of lung cancer and that this may lead to earlier presentation, faster diagnosis and perhaps better outcomes.

Conclusion

The papers covered in this chapter have addressed the important areas of the epidemiology, screening and staging of lung cancer. The close link between cigarette smoking and the development of the disease has been illustrated by the fact that smoking reduction reduces the subsequent risk of developing the disease. This is an important public health message. There is also evidence that there appears to be some genetic influence on the risk of developing lung cancer.

Lung cancer screening continues to provoke much interest and many of the early screening studies using low-dose helical CT scanning are now maturing. Definitive algorithms regarding the way that nodules picked up on routine screening should be managed have been formulated. A number of newer techniques aimed at picking up evidence of tumours before they are radiologically obvious provide an exciting insight into the future.

The importance of accurately staging lung cancer patients cannot be over-emphasized. Current clinical methods still tend to under-report disease in patients undergoing surgery. New endoscopic techniques employing ultrasound have improved the sensitivity and specificity of our current diagnostic tools. Their value is that they obtain histological confirmation of nodal disease within the mediastinum. Nodal involvement in this area is one of the most potent predictors of lung cancer survival.

Developments in PET scanning have also improved the accuracy of diagnosis and staging in lung cancer, although it is likely that its main role will be the detection of occult metastases. This may prevent patients from having futile but potentially toxic treatments, and although this will have no impact on the overall survival rate in lung cancer it will improve the selection of patients for radical treatments.

New advances in diagnosis and staging, however, are futile if patients continue to present with advanced disease. It appears that many patients tolerate symptoms for prolonged periods before seeking medical help. Although a public health campaign to improve earlier diagnosis may seem an obvious requirement, it is not known whether such an approach would actually result in improved survival.

8

Treatment of lung cancer

RON FERGUSSON

Introduction

Survival rates for patients with lung cancer have remained extremely low for decades. In the UK fewer than 10% of patients are alive 5 years after diagnosis, although other European countries and the USA report somewhat higher rates. The reasons for this are unclear but may be related to late presentation, higher comorbidity and lower treatment rates in the UK. Direct comparison between lung cancer services in the UK and Europe using standard methods are lacking. Ethnic differences in the uptake of treatment may also be important, although the reasons for such disparities remain unclear.

These poor survival rates could be improved if more effective treatment options were available to clinicians. Since most patients have advanced disease at presentation (Stage III or IV), newer systemic forms of treatment are urgently needed. Whilst chemotherapy has been shown to improve survival when it is added to modalities such as radiotherapy and surgery, most non-small-cell tumours are fairly chemoresistant. Drugs which have a targeted action against specific properties of malignant growth are now emerging. These treatments will hopefully have a better toxicity profile than standard anticancer chemotherapies. Drugs inhibiting the epidermal growth factor receptor (EGFR) are clinically available and would appear to have useful activity in lung cancer. They are given orally and have a good toxicity profile. One interesting fact that is emerging from their use is that there appear to be certain subgroups of patients who benefit most from their use.

Surgery remains the mainstay of lung cancer therapy. Unfortunately, many patients relapse following resection, presumably because micrometastases are present at the time of surgery. The use of systemic chemotherapy following surgery (adjuvant treatment) has long been thought to improve survival after resection. The evidence for such a benefit, however, has not been proven. In the last decade, large studies looking at the value of adjuvant chemotherapy following resection have been planned and are now being reported. Results are promising and this form of treatment has now become established. More information has been gained about the exact timing of chemotherapy with surgery and there is still interest in giving this prior to resection (neoadjuvant treatment), although the early trials looking at this effect were small and gave conflicting results.

Radiotherapy remains an important treatment in the management of lung cancer. Patients may be given high doses in an attempt to prolong survival or even to obtain a cure. However, the vast majority of patients who receive radiotherapy for this disease are treated with palliative intent. The planning of radiotherapy is extremely important as the irradiation of normal tissue results in increased toxicity with no antitumour effect. Interesting work is emerging in which newer imaging modalities, such as positron emission tomography (PET) scanning, can be used to give more effective planning of radiotherapy treatment.

Geographical and ethnic variation in lung cancer management

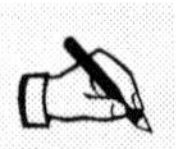

Lung cancer in Teesside (UK) and Varese (Italy): a comparison of management and survival

Imperatori A, Harrison RN, Leitch DN, *et al. Thorax* 2006; **61**: 232–9

BACKGROUND. It has been known for many years that the survival rates for lung cancer in the UK are significantly lower than in other European countries and the USA. Although there are several potential explanations for this, such as late presentation, comorbidity and lower resection rates, the precise causes for this apparent problem are unclear. No direct comparison of lung cancer management in the UK and another European centre has been made. This study compared lung cancer data prospectively for all new cases diagnosed in the year 2000 in the Teesside area of northern England and Varese in northern Italy. The areas were selected as they had similar incidences of lung cancer and well-established cancer registers.

INTERPRETATION. Two hundred and sixty-eight cases in Teesside were compared with 243 in Varese. The UK patients were older (*P* <0.05), had higher comorbidity and poorer performance status (*P* <0.001) and were more likely to have had higher smoking and occupational risks of cancer (*P* <0.001). The histological confirmation rate was lower in the UK, where there were fewer early-stage tumours. The resection rate was 7% in Teesside versus 25% in Varese. Patients were twice as likely to receive specific anticancer treatment in Italy than in the UK (50 vs 25%). Not surprisingly, the overall 3-year survival rate was 7% in Teesside and 14% in Varese (Fig. 8.1).

Comment

This is an ambitious study that highlights major differences in lung cancer management between the UK and Italy. Poorer survival is seen in English patients. On average, British patients are older, more symptomatic, have poorer performance status and are less likely to receive an operation than their Italian counterparts. The reason for these differences is not clear. The possibilities are that the English perhaps ignore symptoms for longer before seeking medical care and are perhaps less fit for surgery because of comorbidity. It may be that Italian physicians and surgeons are more aggressive in resecting tumours and treating their lung cancer patients, although the possibility that comorbidity has a major influence on these

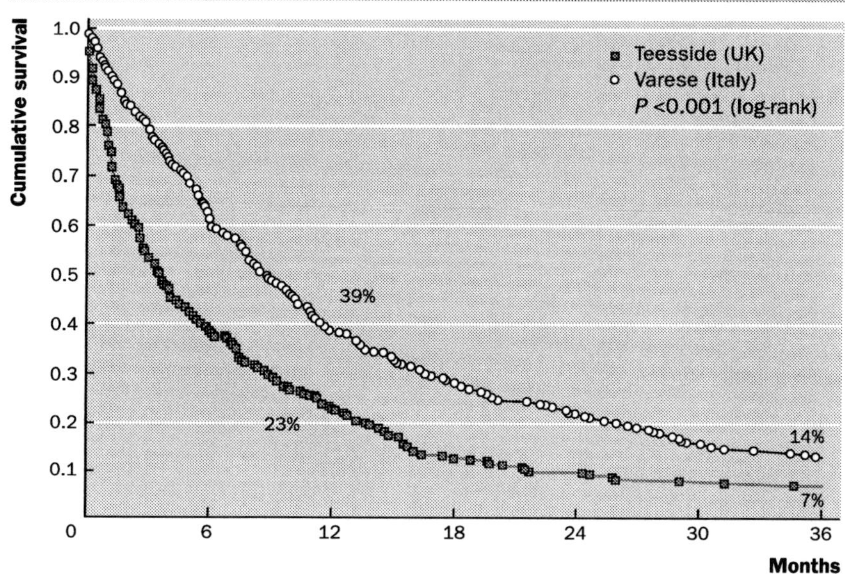

Fig. 8.1 Kaplan–Meier survival curves (from diagnosis) of all patients presenting with lung cancer in the year 2000 in Teesside, UK (*n* = 268) and in Varese, Italy (*n* = 243). Source: Imperatori *et al.* (2006).

factors remains. Further, more accurate data on comorbidity and physicians' attitudes are required.

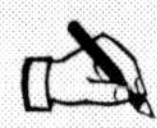

Ethnic disparities in the treatment of Stage I non-small cell lung cancer

Wisnivesky JP, McGinn T, Henschke C, *et al. Am J Respir Crit Care Med* 2005; **171**: 1158–63

BACKGROUND. **Variations in lung cancer treatment and survival as a result of racial and social factors have been reported in several studies. The reasons for this are not clear. Possible explanations include low surgical resection rates and more advanced disease at diagnosis. This study examined whether apparent disparities in survival between Hispanic and white patients with Stage I lung cancer were due to resection rates and stage distribution at the time of diagnosis.**

INTERPRETATION. More than 16 000 Hispanic and white patients with Stage I lung cancer diagnosed in the 10 years before the year 2000 were identified from the Surveillance, Epidemiology and End Results (SEER) programme registry. This is a national database in parts of the USA that collects data on all incident cancer cases. Standard statistical analysis was used to evaluate differences in survival and stage.

Hispanic patients had poor overall and lung cancer-specific survival compared with whites ($P = 0.04$ and 0.008, respectively). Five-year survival was 54% for Hispanics versus 62% for whites. Hispanic patients were more likely to be diagnosed with Stage Ib disease and less likely to undergo resection than white patients. After adjusting for surgery and stage there was no difference in survival between the two groups (Fig. 8.2).

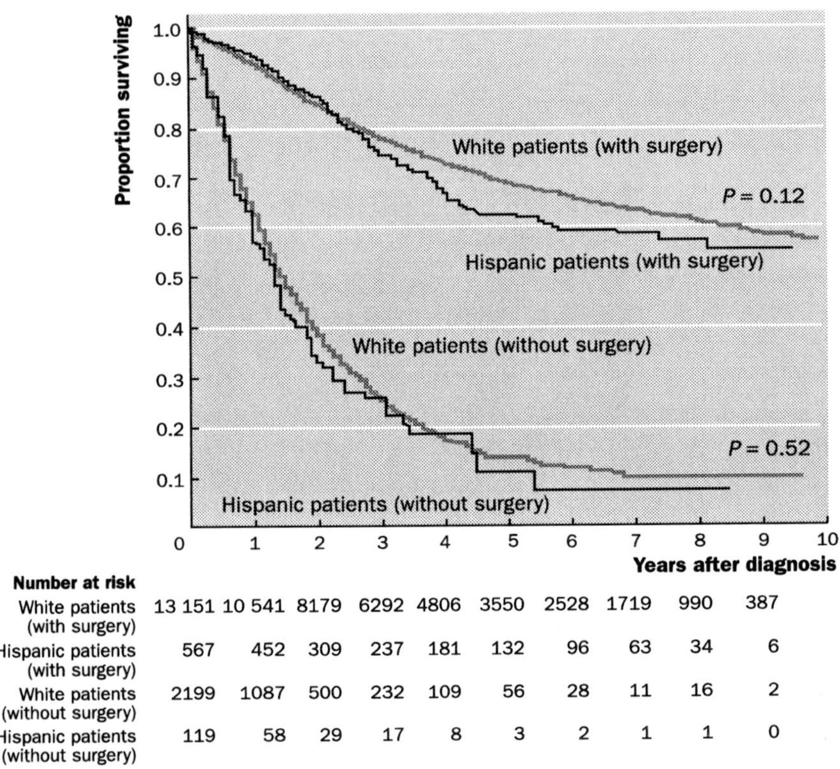

Number at risk										
White patients (with surgery)	13 151	10 541	8179	6292	4806	3550	2528	1719	990	387
Hispanic patients (with surgery)	567	452	309	237	181	132	96	63	34	6
White patients (without surgery)	2199	1087	500	232	109	56	28	11	16	2
Hispanic patients (without surgery)	119	58	29	17	8	3	2	1	1	0

Fig. 8.2 Lung cancer-specific Kaplan–Meier survival curves according to treatment and ethnicity. Lung cancer-specific survival was similar among Hispanic and white patients who underwent surgery (log-rank test, $P = 0.12$). Those who did not undergo surgery had similar survival (log-rank test, $P = 0.52$). Source: Wisnivesky *et al.* (2005).

Comment

This large study would suggest that Hispanic patients were less likely to receive surgery than white patients of a similar stage. The reasons for this were not clear. The SEER database which was used to collect the cases does not record comorbidity, which may have differed between the two groups. The effect of other patient-related factors on the decision to resect were not measured. These include cultural issues, insurance status and health beliefs. More in-depth prospective studies are needed to tease out which factors are present to explain these disparities in the treatment and diagnosis of potentially curable disease.

Blockade of epidermal growth factor receptor

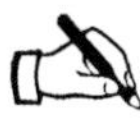

Erlotinib in previously treated non-small-cell lung cancer

Shepherd FA, Rodrigues Pereira J, Cinleanu T, *et al. N Engl J Med* 2005; **353**: 123–32

BACKGROUND. Chemotherapy has become an accepted treatment modality for Stage IIIb and IV non-small-cell lung cancer. The treatment is given with palliative intent and patients often relapse fairly quickly. In patients who have responded, however, there is a place for second- and even third-line treatments. The EGFR inhibitors have shown promising activity in this disease, although their exact place in the treatment algorithm has not been established. This trial was designed to investigate whether erlotinib could improve survival after relapse from standard first-line chemotherapy in non-small-cell lung cancer. The design of the study was an international Phase III randomized, double-blind, placebo-controlled trial. Patients were assigned in a 2:1 ratio to receive oral erlotinib (150 mg daily) or placebo. The primary end-point was overall survival. Secondary end-points included progression-free survival, response rate, toxic effects and quality of life.

INTERPRETATION. Seven hundred and thirty-one patients were randomized; 488 were allocated to active treatment with erlotinib. Half the patients had received two previous chemotherapy regimens. The response rate was 8.9% in the treatment group and <1% in the placebo. Overall survival was 6.7 months compared with 4.7 months in the placebo group (hazard ratio [HR] 0.70; P <0.001) in favour of erlotinib (Fig. 8.3). Rash was the commonest adverse event and was seen in 76% of treated patients. Treatment with erlotinib was associated with improvement in quality of life; there were increased times to progression of cough, dyspnoea and pain, which were of similar magnitude to the overall increase in survival.

Comment

This was a large randomized trial which had the strength of being placebo-controlled. The ethics of this design would seem reasonable in view of the extremely poor prognosis of patients with non-small-cell lung cancer who have relapsed from first- and second-line chemotherapy. A significant survival advantage was seen in the treatment group at the expense of fairly mild toxicity. Rash and diarrhoea were the main problems with erlotinib, as with other EGFR inhibitors. The response rate to this treatment was <10%, but despite this there were useful gains in terms of survival and symptom control. A further paper from the same group appeared in the same journal, looking at factors predicting clinical response.

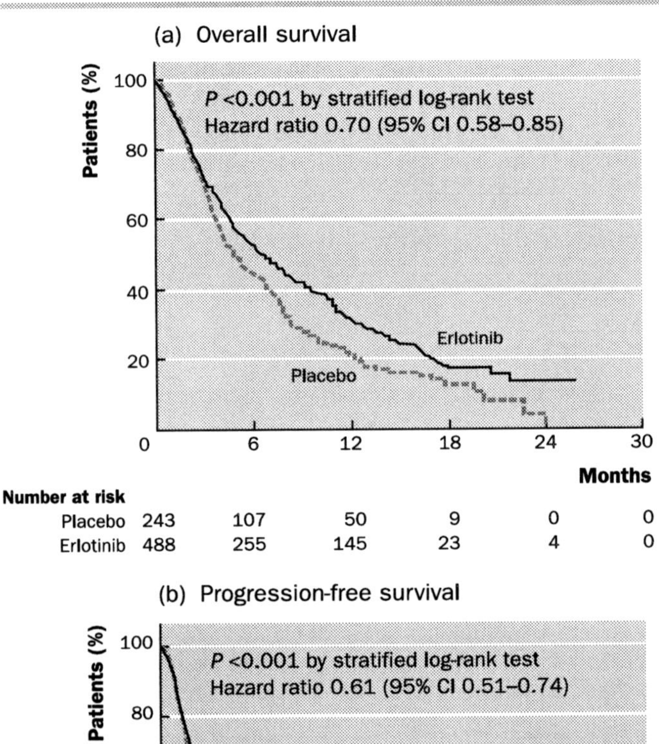

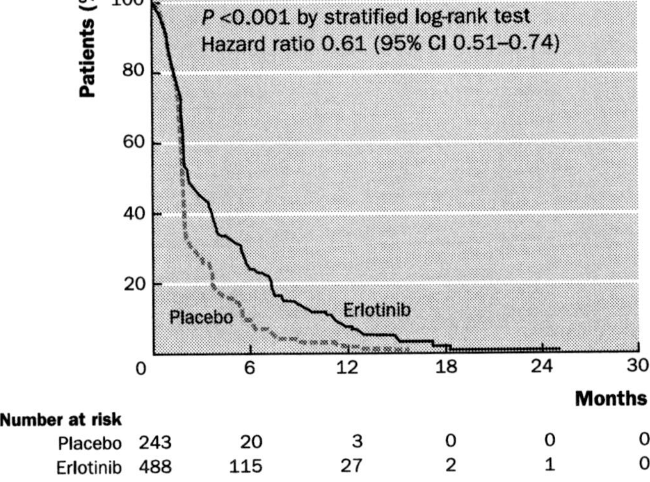

Fig. 8.3 Kaplan–Meier curves for overall survival (a) and progression-free survival (b) among all patients randomly assigned to erlotinib or placebo. Source: Shepherd *et al.* (2005).

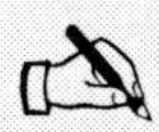

Erlotinib in lung cancer—molecular and clinical predictors of outcome

Tsao MS, Sakurada A, Cutz J-C, *et al*. *N Engl J Med* 2005; **353**: 133–44

BACKGROUND. The previous study showed that erlotinib, when compared with placebo, gave a survival benefit in patients with previously treated non-small-cell lung cancer. It is known that not all patients with non-small-cell lung cancer express EGFR and it is thought that EGFR gene amplification and mutation are important in predicting the response to EGFR inhibitors. This trial used biopsy specimens from patients in the clinical study to see whether there were important molecular predictors of response, and these were then correlated with other clinical markers in an attempt to identify patients who would benefit more from this form of treatment.

INTERPRETATION. Just under half the patients in the study (325 of 731) had their samples evaluated immunohistochemically for EGFR expression. One hundred and ninety-seven samples were analysed for EGFR mutation and in 221 the number of EGFR genes was assessed. Univariate analysis showed that survival was much longer in the group expressing EGFR (HR 0.68; $P = 0.02$) compared with placebo (Fig. 8.4). Amplification of EGFR was measured in only small numbers of patients but was the strongest predictor for survival (HR 0.44; 95% confidence interval [CI] 0.23–0.82) Multivariate analysis showed that adenocarcinoma, never having smoked and EGFR expression were associated with an objective response. However, survival after treatment was not influenced by the status of EGFR expression, the number of EGFR copies or the presence of EGFR mutation.

Comment

The results of this study are perhaps a little disappointing. The clinical trial showed good survival benefit with erlotinib and it would have been hoped that EGFR expression would have been an important predictor for survival. The presence of EGFR mutations is not required for survival benefit, although it may predict patients who may respond. The result of this trial, therefore, suggests that analysis of mutations is not necessary in standard clinical practice to decide which patients should receive this treatment. One disappointing factor is the small number of patients available for analysis from what was a very large randomized clinical trial. Another previously reported study suggested that rash may be an important predictor of the response.

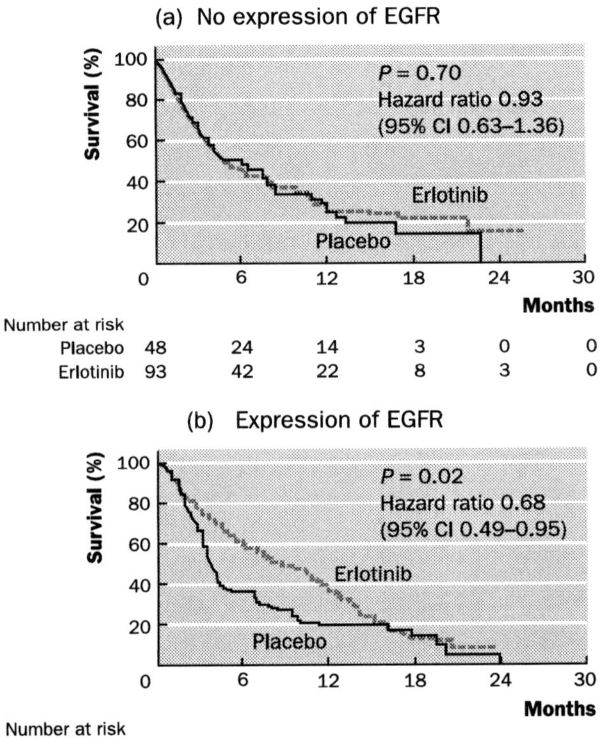

Fig. 8.4 Kaplan–Meier estimates of survival. Panel (a) shows the results for patients who did not have expression of EGFR on immunohistochemical analysis (<10% of tumour cells had membrane staining). Panel (b) shows the results for patients who had expression of EGFR on immunohistochemical analysis (≥10% of tumour cells had membrane staining). *P*-values were calculated with the log-rank test. Source: Tsao *et al.* (2005).

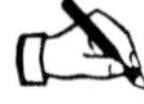

Determinant of tumor response and survival with erlotinib in patients with non-small-cell lung cancer

Pérez-Soler, R, Chachoua A, Hammond LA, *et al. J Clin Oncol* 2004; **22**: 3238–47

BACKGROUND. Data are now appearing concerning the clinical efficacy of EGFR receptor inhibitors in patients with non-small-cell lung cancer. One important result appears to be that only a small proportion of patients actually respond to treatment.

These responses, however, can be extremely impressive even in patients who have been pre-treated with standard chemotherapeutic regimens. A pattern appears to be emerging concerning the clinical characteristics of patients who respond well to this form of treatment. This study was one of the earlier reports of the activity of erlotinib in previously treated patients. Attempts were made to assess the treatment response according to a number of different parameters and thus to try to form a profile of the kind of non-small-cell lung cancer patient who may benefit from this new form of therapy. Fifty-seven patients received 150 mg of erlotinib. They had all been pre-treated with platinum-based chemotherapy. Tumour response, survival and symptom improvement using standard quality-of-life tools were used. Further analysis was performed to identify predictors of response and survival (Fig. 8.5).

INTERPRETATION. The response rate to treatment for the trial was 12.3%, median survival 8.4 months and the 1-year survival rate 40%. These figures are similar to those reported elsewhere. Treatment with the drug produced improvements in tumour-related symptoms. As with other studies, the most important toxic effect was a skin rash and diarrhoea (occurring in 75% and 56% of patients respectively). Good performance status and time since diagnosis were significant predictors of survival, although EGFR staining intensity, interestingly, was not. Survival was impressively correlated with the occurrence and severity of the skin rash.

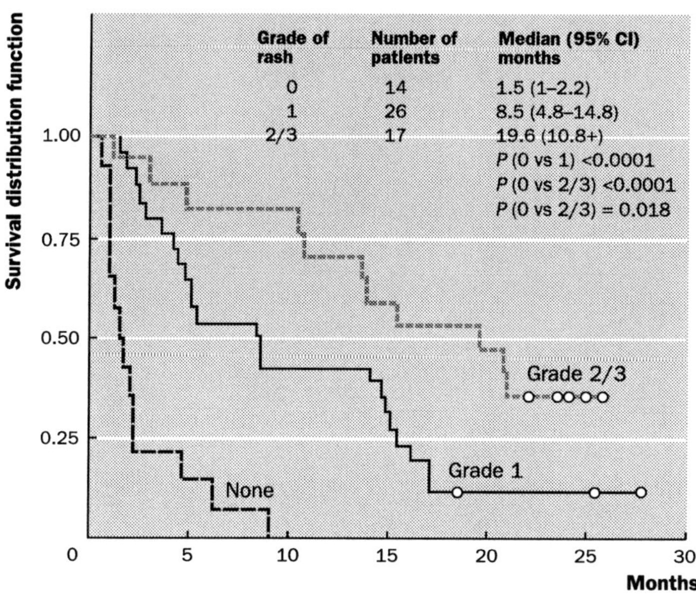

Fig. 8.5 Survival of patients by grade of rash. Bullets represent patients still alive at the time of analysis. Source: Pérez-Soler *et al.* (2004).

Comment

This was a fairly small study which pre-dated the important randomized clinical trial performed by Shepherd *et al.* described above. The authors were unable to show that previously suggested predictors of response and survival, such as smoking status, gender and Asian origin, were not important predictors of survival, although this was largely a result of the size of the study. One important result to emerge in the data was the usefulness of rash as a predictor of response and survival. Patients who did not develop skin rash fared extremely poorly, with little or no improvement with therapy. On the other hand, a small group of patients who had a grade 2/3 skin rash responded well to therapy. This effect was not seen in the two Phase II trials of gefitinib (Iressa) in larger groups of patients and may be a feature of erlotinib. Further studies are required to assess the precise relationship between rash and erlotinib response. This will require more analysis at the molecular level of skin and tumour tissue collected before and after therapy. The authors wondered, however, whether the presence of rash was a surrogate for the inability of a patient to mount an inflammatory response and may, therefore, be a surrogate of immunocompetence rather than receptor inhibition. One other effect of rash being required for the response is the problem this may pose in unblinding any future double-blind randomized trials. Patients would know that if they did not develop a rash it would be unlikely that they would respond to treatment.

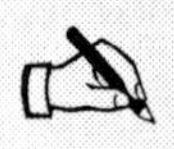

Gefitinib plus best supportive care in previously treated patients with refractory advanced non-small-cell lung cancer: results from a randomised, placebo-controlled, multicentre study (Iressa Survival Evaluation in Lung Cancer)

Thatcher N, Change A, Parikh P, et al. *Lancet* 2005; **366**: 1527–37

BACKGROUND. The EGFR inhibitor gefitinib has shown good activity in Phase II studies, with a response rate of approximately 12–18%, median survival 7–8 months and 1-year survival around 30% at a dose of 250 mg per day in previously treated patients. Randomized Phase III data are required to show whether the drug has activity as a second- and third-line treatment in this disease.

INTERPRETATION. This was a large, double-blind, placebo-controlled, parallel-group, multicentre, randomized Phase III survival study performed in 210 centres in 28 countries around the world. One thousand, six hundred and ninety-two patients who were refractory to or intolerant of standard non-small-cell lung cancer chemotherapy were randomly allocated to either gefitinib (250 mg per day) or placebo, all patients receiving best supportive care. The primary end-point was survival, with subgroup analysis for adenocarcinoma type.

One thousand, one hundred and twenty-nine patients were assigned the active treatment and 563 placebo. There was no difference in median survival rate between the two groups after a median follow-up of 7.2 months. The hazard ratio for death was

0.89 (95% CI 0.77–1.02; $P = 0.08$) for patients treated with gefitinib. There was prolongation of median survival in those with the adenocarcinoma cell type. A significant improvement in survival was seen in never-smokers (HR 0.67; 95% CI 0.49–0.92; $P = 0.012$) and patients of Asian origin (HR 0.66; 95% CI 0.48–0.91; $P = 0.01$).

Comment

This is a disappointing result, showing no survival advantage for gefitinib in previously treated patients. This result is at variance with the results of the paper published in the same year by Shepherd *et al.* (see above), in which, interestingly, similar levels of response to the treatment were seen. Once again, improved results were seen in a small subgroup of patients (never-smokers, adenocarcinoma subtype and Asian origin). There are a number of reasons why there are differences between these two trials. It is possible that the study populations differed in ethnic origin and smoking status, and there is some evidence that in the erlotinib study the patients had a better response to their previous chemotherapy.

The place of gefitinib in refractory non-small-cell lung cancer has been thrown into doubt by this trial. Other important studies which are currently under way may help to elucidate other points. The first is a comparison between gefitinib and docetaxel in the second- and third-line setting (Iressa™ NSCLC Trial Evaluating Response and Survival against Taxotere [INTEREST] study). The second is a Phase II trial comparing gefitinib with vinorelbine (Iressa™ versus vinorelbine [INVITE]), which involves prospective tissue collection and is likely to show more clearly the population of patients most likely to benefit from EGFR inhibitors.

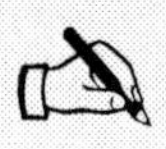

Survival impact of epidermal growth factor receptor overexpression in patients with non-small lung cancer: a meta-analysis

Nakamura H, Kawasaki N, Taguchi M, *et al. Thorax* 2006; **61**: 140–5

BACKGROUND. The EGFR is commonly activated in patients with non-small-cell lung cancer. This results in enhancement of cell proliferation and suppression of apoptosis. The EGFR has, therefore, become a target for drug treatment in lung cancer. Over-expression of EGFR is thought to be associated with poor survival. Details of the accurate evaluation of the clinical significance of EGFR over-expression are lacking, although this information will be important when considering future anti-EGFR therapy. This was a meta-analysis of published studies to quantitatively review the effect of EGFR over-expression on survival in patients with non-small-cell lung cancer.

INTERPRETATION. This study presents a meta-analysis of trials that were performed to review the relationship between EGFR over-expression and survival in patients with non-small lung cancer. Eighteen studies (2972 patients) were subjected to final analysis. Positivity for EGFR over-expression differed between histological types (39% in adenocarcinoma, 58% in squamous carcinoma, 38% in large-cell carcinoma and 32% in other cancers). The combined hazard ratio for survival was 1.14 (95% CI 0.97–1.34; $P = 0.103$). This suggests that EGFR over-expression has no significant impact on survival.

Comment

Most of the studies reported in this meta-analysis evaluated EGFR protein expression by immunohistochemistry and it is possible that different conclusions may result from differences in assay techniques. There was also no information in the study about whether EGFR expression based on gene copy number or EGFR gene mutation affects survival. This may be particularly relevant to the role of new EGFR receptor drugs, which appear to depend upon EGFR mutation for activity. It may be relevant that the status of EGFR protein expression was not predictive of survival benefit in response to erlotinib in a large randomized trial.

Adjuvant chemotherapy following surgery

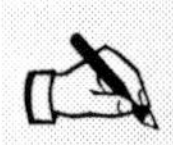

Vinorelbine plus cisplatin vs observation in resected non-small cell lung cancer

Winton T, Livingston R, Johnson D, *et al. N Engl J Med* 2005; **352**: 2589–97

BACKGROUND. Data are appearing concerning the place of adjuvant chemotherapy in patients with resectable non-small-cell lung cancer. The 1995 meta-analysis |1| has suggested that the addition of chemotherapy to surgery would improve survival in absolute terms by approximately 5% at 5 years. Data from prospective clinical studies are required to confirm this.

INTERPRETATION. This was a large study commenced in 1994 in Canada. Other large collaborative groups in the USA joined 4 years later. Over a 7-year period, 482 patients were randomly assigned to either observation or chemotherapy following apparent complete resection of their Stage Ib or Stage II non-small-cell tumours (Fig. 8.6). The chemotherapy used was vinorelbine plus cisplatin. Median follow-up was in excess of 5 years. The median number of cycles delivered to patients in the chemotherapy group was 3. Chemotherapy caused neutropenia in 88% of patients, with death from toxic effects in two patients (0.8%). Fatigue, nausea and anorexia were common in the chemotherapy group but severe toxicity was uncommon (<10%). Overall survival was significantly prolonged in the chemotherapy group (HR for death was 0.69; $P = 0.04$); the 5-year survival rate in the chemotherapy arm was 69% compared with 54% in the group receiving surgery alone ($P = 0.003$).

Comment

This is a large, prospective, randomized trial using reasonably modern chemotherapy. The results indicate that adjuvant treatment with this combination of chemotherapy (vinorelbine plus cisplatin) is associated with a significant improve-

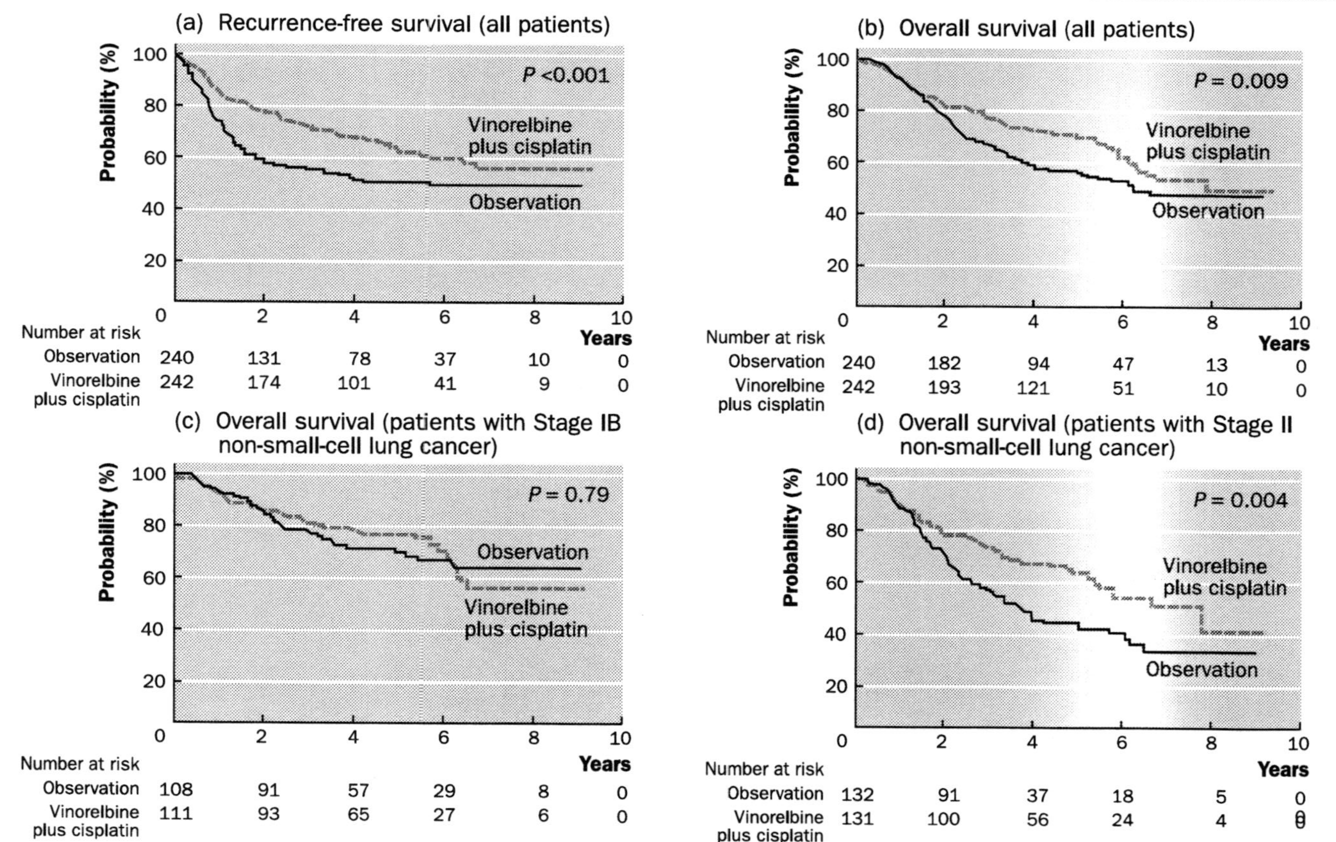

Fig. 8.6 Kaplan–Meier estimates of survival among patients who received adjuvant vinorelbine plus cisplatin and those who underwent observation alone. *P*-values are based on two-sided statistical analyses of differences between treatment groups after randomization. Source: Winton *et al.* (2005).

ment in survival after resection without significant toxicity. The authors found more benefit in patients with Stage II rather than Stage Ib disease. It is likely that the results of this study, and of others reported around the same time, will mean that post-operative chemotherapy will become the standard of care for patients with good performance status who undergo complete resection of early-stage non-small-cell disease.

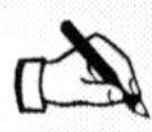

Meta-analysis of post-operative adjuvant chemotherapy with tegafur-uracil in non-small-cell lung cancer

Hamada C, Tamaka F, Ohta M, *et al. J Clin Oncol* 2005; **23**: 4999–5006

BACKGROUND. Results from clinical trials assessing the efficacy of adjuvant chemotherapy have appeared recently in the literature. In the Western world most of the studies have involved platinum-based chemotherapy following resection. In Japan, however, the standard adjuvant chemotherapy involves tegafur–uracil. This is an oral treatment which, in general, is well tolerated. Results of the studies using this treatment published so far have been inconclusive and a meta-analysis was therefore performed to give a better idea of the effectiveness of this treatment as an adjuvant therapy following complete resection of non-small-cell lung cancer. Standard meta-analytical methods were used.

INTERPRETATION. Of the nine trials of post-operative adjuvant tegafur–uracil chemotherapy, six compared surgery alone with surgery plus tegafur–uracil chemotherapy. These trials included more than 2000 patients, the vast majority having Stage I disease (65.3% had a T1 tumour and 33.6% had T2 disease, 95% had nodal status N0). The median duration of follow-up was 6.44 years. The 5- and 7-year survival rates were significantly higher in the adjuvant chemotherapy group (81.5 and 76.5% respectively) compared with the surgery alone group (77.2 and 69.5%; $P = 0.11$ and 0.001). The hazard ratio for death in the chemotherapy arm was 0.74 (95% CI 0.61–0.88; $P = 0.001$).

Comment

This meta-analysis confirms the activity of post-operative tegafur–uracil in patients with resectable non-small-cell lung cancer. It is interesting that two-thirds of the patients had Stage Ia disease. The activity of the treatment in this group is at variance with results from some platinum-based studies from European and American centres which have failed to show such benefit in these T1 patients. It is important to know whether a similar survival advantage would be conferred on surgical patients with a more advanced stage and whether non-Asian patients would benefit from this form of treatment.

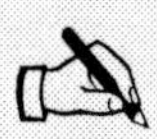

Adjuvant chemotherapy for completely resected non-small cell lung cancer. A systematic review

Alam N, Darling G, Evans WK, *et al. Crit Rev Oncol Hematol* 2006; **58**: 146–55

BACKGROUND. Individual trials looking at the effect of adjuvant chemotherapy in resected non-small-cell lung cancer have reported generally favourable results for this form of treatment. Some studies, however, have proved negative. The number of studies now available allows a meta-analysis approach to see whether this form of treatment is effective and safe.

INTERPRETATION. This systematic review was performed in the usual way with relevant randomized trials and meta-analysis identified through electronic and hand searches. Seven meta-analysis and 26 randomized trials comparing surgery with and without chemotherapy were included in the review. Predefined eligibility criteria were established. Studies involving non-platinum agents and immunotherapy were not considered.

The meta-analyses included in the review all showed a survival advantage for platinum or tegafur–uracil-based post-operative chemotherapy. Results, however, did not always achieve statistical significance. More recent trials have detected a large survival advantage with post-operative platinum-based chemotherapy. The authors of the review conclude that post-operative adjuvant platinum-based chemotherapy improves survival compared with surgery alone in completely resected non-small-cell lung cancer and that the survival benefits strongly outweigh the adverse effects of the treatment. The authors comment on the fact that survival improvement obtained with post-operative tegafur–uracil in early-stage disease had only been demonstrated in Japan and that this agent was not available in North America and Europe.

Comment

The results of this systematic review are perhaps not surprising. The authors confirm the current status of post-operative chemotherapy in completely resected disease. The survival advantage gained is approximately 5%, as predicted in the early meta-analysis, and suggests that post-operative chemotherapy should be standard practice in patients undergoing a complete resection of Stage Ib, II and IIIa non-small-cell lung cancer.

Other treatment advances

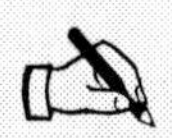

Morbidity and mortality in the surgery arm of EORTC 08941 trial

Van Schil P, Meerbeeck J Van, Kramer G, *et al. Eur Respir J* 2005; **26**: 192–7

BACKGROUND. Variable survival results of resection after induction chemotherapy or chemoradiotherapy have been reported. Some trials have shown high mortality rates, leading to loss of confidence in the principle of neoadjuvant treatment in some surgeons. Many of the early trials had small numbers of patients. EORTC 08941 is a multicentre, prospective, randomized, Phase III trial of surgical resection versus radiotherapy in patients with proven Stage IIIa (N2) non-small-cell lung cancer who respond to platinum-based induction chemotherapy. The results of the surgical arm were published in 2005.

INTERPRETATION. One hundred and sixty-seven patients were randomized to surgical resection and a similar number to radiotherapy. Patients had to have proven N2 disease prior to entry into the trial. All patients had three cycles of platinum-based induction-based chemotherapy, although no set regimen was specified. One hundred and twenty-seven patients (76%) proceeded to surgery alone, 22 having surgery following adjuvant radiotherapy. Radical resection with clear surgical margins was obtained in 74 patients (49.7%), with pathological downstaging of mediastinal nodal involvement to NO or N1 seen in 61 (40.9%). Thirty-day operative mortality in the surgical group was 4%, with predictable post-operative complications. Twelve patients (8.1%) underwent re-operation.

Comment

This trial, which had tight entry criteria, has shown that surgical resection after induction chemotherapy is feasible in patients with proven N2 disease. Some would question the high rate of incomplete resection and the increased rate of pneumonectomy (46.3%). This paper therefore re-opens the debate concerning neoadjuvant chemotherapy in patients with Stage IIIa disease. This is happening at a time when most clinical researchers are concentrating their efforts on the efficacy of post-operative adjuvant treatment in surgically managed patients.

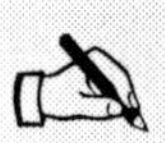

Increased therapeutic ratio by 18FDG-PET/CT planning in patients with clinical CT stage N2-N3M0 non-small-cell lung cancer: A modelling study

Van Der Wel A, Nijsten S, Hochstenbag M, *et al. Int J Radiat Oncol Biol Phys* 2005; **61**: 649–55

BACKGROUND. Accurate staging of the mediastinum with PET may allow computed tomography (CT) radiotherapy planning that would decrease the radiation dose to normal organs and perhaps reduce geographical misses. This might allow dose escalation, which would improve the chances of tumour control. Is this clinically feasible?

INTERPRETATION. This was a small clinical modelling study in which PET data were incorporated into CT radiotherapy planning for 21 consecutive patients with CT Stage III non-small-cell lung cancer. For each patient, radiation dose escalation for CT planning alone versus CT plus PET was calculated using constraints for lung, oesophageal and spinal cord toxicity. The impact of this dose escalation on local treatment control was estimated using dose–response parameters. The gross tumour volume of positive nodes decreased from 13.7 cm^3 on CT scan planning alone to 9.9 cm^3 on PET-CT. This allowed reduction of exposure of normal tissues such as the oesophagus, lung and spinal cord. For the same toxicity levels for these organs, the dose of radiotherapy given to the tumour could be increased from 56 ± 5.4 Gy with CT planning to 71 ± 13.7 Gy with PET scanning.

Comment

The authors conclude that the use of PET scanning reduced the radiation exposure of the oesophagus and lungs and allowed significant escalation of the radiation dose. They also felt there would be a reduced risk of geographical misses using PET-CT. They estimated the increase in tumour control probability, from 13 to 18% ($P = 0.009$), by using PET scanning in radiotherapy planning. The authors plan a larger prospective clinical study.

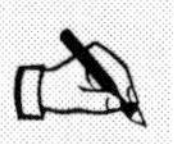

Selective mediastinal node irradiation based on FDG-PET scan data in patients with non-small-cell lung cancer: a prospective clinical study

De Ruysscher D, Wanders S, van Haren E, *et al*. *Int J Radiat Oncol Biol Phys* 2005; **62**: 988–94

BACKGROUND. Radiotherapy is an effective treatment in the management of non-small-cell lung cancer. Unfortunately, most patients will eventually fail locally, with tumour recurrence being observed in the field of radiotherapy. Dose escalation or intensification may improve the prognosis and reduce the incidence of local failure. This benefit is obviously achieved at the cost of increased toxicity. The diagnostic accuracy of mediastinal staging with fluorodeoxyglucose (FDG)-PET scanning is higher than that with CT scanning. It would seem reasonable, therefore, to irradiate only FDG-positive mediastinal areas, which should result in more successful treatment but should limit toxicity by reducing field size as a result of PET scanning. This study was a prospective clinical trial to investigate whether selective radiation of FDG-PET-positive mediastinal areas would be safe in terms of local failure and whether escalation of the radiation dose in a short overall treatment time would be feasible.

INTERPRETATION. Forty-four patients with histologically proven non-small-cell lung cancer (Stage I–IIIb) were included in the study. Sixty-five per cent of patients were also given chemotherapy. The radiotherapy regimen was either 61.2 Gy in 34 fractions over 23 days or 64.8 Gy in 36 fractions over 24 days, administered to the primary tumour and positive mediastinal areas on the pre-treatment FDG-PET scan. Isolated nodal failure was defined as recurrence in the regional nodes outside the clinical target volume in the absence of in-field failure. After a median follow-up of 16 months, eleven patients (25%) developed a local recurrence, only one patient developing an isolated nodal failure.

Comment

This is an important study. PET scanning has raised hopes of more accurate mediastinal staging. It is important that this increased knowledge is used for better targeting of therapies. This trial shows that reliance on PET positivity allows patients to receive more specifically localized doses of radiotherapy which will obviously minimize toxicity to normal tissues. The worry about false negatives, however, is important. This would mean that areas which may normally have been included in a field would be missed if the PET scan was falsely negative. This study suggests that reliance on PET positivity would not result in under-treatment. The numbers in the trial were small and larger studies are required to ensure that this is a reasonable approach. Histological confirmation of mediastinal involvement is important but until recently a fairly invasive procedure. It is to be hoped that endobronchial and endoscopic ultrasound techniques when applied in tandem with PET scanning may allow even more precise mapping of mediastinal disease and better-targeted radiotherapy.

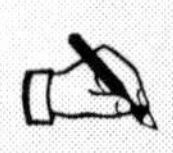

Vinorelbine plus cisplatin versus docetaxel plus gemcitabine in advanced non-small lung cancer: a Phase III randomized trial

Georgoulias V, Ardavanis A, Tsiafaki X, *et al. J Clin Oncol* 2005; **23**: 2937–45

BACKGROUND. Combination chemotherapy has become the mainstay of management of most patients with advanced non-small-cell lung cancer. Gold standard regimens include platinum treatments. Many of these regimens have considerable toxicity for patients who are being treated with palliative intent. Novel regimens with combinations of newer drugs are appearing which may offer a better therapeutic index for these patients. Prolonged survival and improving tumour-related symptoms and quality of life are the usual main objectives of palliative chemotherapy in this disease. Non-platinum regimens may have less toxicity but it is not known whether they confer similar survival benefit. Prospective multicentre randomized trials comparing different platinum and non-platinum regimens are required.

INTERPRETATION. Four hundred and thirteen patients with chemotherapy-naive advanced non-small-cell lung cancer were randomly assigned to receive either gemcitabine plus docetaxel or vinorelbine plus cisplatin (with prophylactic granulocyte colony-stimulating factor). Median survival was similar in the two groups (9 vs 9.7 months). The 1-year survival rates were 34.3 and 40.8% respectively. Toxicity was more common in the platinum-containing regimen; significant anaemia was seen in 55% in this group vs 34% of those in the group receiving gemcitabine plus docetaxel and neutropenia was seen in 37% (platinum-containing) vs 16% (gemcitabine plus docetaxel), with double the number of febrile episodes (11 vs 6%) compared with the gemcitabine plus docetaxel group. Nausea and vomiting, not surprisingly, was also more common in the platinum regimen (15 vs 1%). Quality of life using a standard symptom scale questionnaire improved in patients receiving the docetaxel plus gemcitabine regimen but not in the vinoralbine plus cisplatin arm. The authors concluded that the non-platinum chemotherapy regimen had efficacy comparable to that of the platinum-containing regime in terms of survival, but a better toxicity profile.

Comment

The data from this study would favour the use of docetaxel and gemcitabine as first-line treatment in advanced-stage non-small-cell lung cancer patients. This would appear to be certainly true in patients unlikely to tolerate cisplatin or in those with significant comorbidity or poor performance status. A significant rider on this conclusion is the cost of the docetaxel/gemcitabine regimen compared with the much cheaper, though perhaps more toxic, cisplatin/vinorelbine combination.

Conclusions

Advances continue to be made in the management of patients with lung cancer. The emergence of specific targeted therapies which should produce enhanced anticancer activity with less toxicity is to be welcomed. Although numerous targets are being developed, most of the clinical activity involves the EGFR inhibitors. The clinical results to date have perhaps been disappointing but drugs such as erlotinib do appear to have a place, especially if the patients are non-smokers, of female gender, have the adenocarcinoma subtype and are of Asian ethnicity. As new treatments emerge it may be possible to tailor them for specific subgroups with easily measured demographic and tumour characteristics.

The evidence for administering chemotherapy following surgery cannot be doubted. It is likely that this form of treatment will become standard in certain groups of patients undergoing apparent complete resection. The toxicity of the chemotherapy regimens seems reasonable and the improvement of around 5% in survival is to be welcomed.

Newer treatments for lung cancer are emerging constantly. It is hoped that these advances will improve the outcome of patients with lung cancer irrespective of geographical and ethnic variations. Indeed, it may be necessary in the future to tailor certain treatments to patients of a specific ethnicity and with certain tumour characteristics.

References

1. Non-small Cell Lung Cancer Collaborative Group. Chemotherapy in non-small-cell lung cancer, a meta-analysis using updated data on individual patients from 52 randomized clinical trials. *BMJ* 1995; **311**: 899–909.

Part IV

Obstructive sleep apnoea/hypopnoea syndrome

9

Genetic aspects of the sleep apnoea/hypopnoea syndrome

RENATA RIHA

Introduction

Obstructive sleep apnoea/hypopnoea syndrome (OSAHS) is a common condition affecting approximately 2–4% of the middle-aged population and is defined on the basis of symptoms of daytime sleepiness and objective measures of disordered breathing during sleep [1]. Characteristic of OSAHS is obstruction of the upper airway during sleep, resulting in repetitive breathing pauses accompanied by oxygen desaturation and arousal from sleep. This results in diurnal sleepiness leading to cognitive impairment.

OSAHS occurs throughout the entire lifespan, from infancy to old age. The frequency of disordered breathing during sleep increases with age and is poorly associated with an increased incidence of daytime sleepiness or other symptoms of OSAHS [2–4].

A number of studies have shown that OSAHS runs in families [5–10]. Mechanisms contributing to the aetiology of OSAHS include genetically and environmentally induced changes in craniofacial dimensions, differential deposition of adipose tissue, abnormalities in upper airway control and differential susceptibility to sleepiness. All potential intermediate phenotypes have come under scrutiny at a genetic level [10].

The following papers have been chosen to highlight the progress, albeit limited, made in examining the intermediate phenotypes and mechanisms of OSAHS on a molecular basis over the last 2 years.

Craniofacial morphology

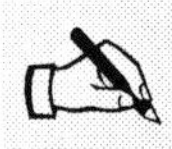

Family aggregation of upper airway soft tissue structures in normal subjects and patients with sleep apnea

Schwab RJ, Pasirstein M, Kaplan L, *et al*. *Am J Resp Crit Care Med* 2006; **173**: 453–63

BACKGROUND. The craniofacial complex is probably one of the most important heritable determinants of OSAHS. A number of morphological features have been described, including changes in cranial base dimensions, displacement of the hyoid bone inferiorly, macroglossia, adenotonsillar hypertrophy, bulkier soft tissue in the upper airway resulting in narrowing, and increases in lower facial height |11–13|. Retroposed maxillae and short mandibles have been consistently shown to predispose to OSAHS |7, 14–16|. Such differences in jaw size can be inherited or acquired—for example, following nasal occlusion in childhood |17–19|.

INTERPRETATION. The structure of the soft tissues of the upper airway has a strong heritable component in both normal subjects and subjects without sleep apnoea, even after adjustment for the confounding variables of age, sex, ethnicity, craniofacial structure and visceral fat.

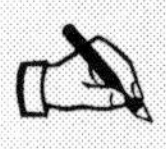

A cephalometric comparison of patients with the sleep apnea/hypopnea syndrome and their siblings

Riha RL, Brander P, Vennelle M, Douglas NJ. *Sleep* 2005; **28**: 315–20

BACKGROUND. This study was carried out to define differences in the skeletal components of facial structure predisposing to OSAHS by a comparison of the craniofacial complex between people with OSAHS and their siblings without OSAHS. One hundred and four patients with OSAHS living in Scotland and 107 of their siblings participated. Sleep studies, clinical review and cephalometry were performed in all subjects. All measurements were scored blind to index/control status.

INTERPRETATION. There were few differences between males with OSAHS and non-apnoeics. Significantly, the hyoid bone was lower in relation to the mandibular plane in those with OSAHS (*P* = 0.01). Previous cephalometric studies support this observation |12–15|. In 22 pairs of brothers discordant for OSAHS, those with the diagnosis had a trend to a shorter mandibular corpus and mandibular ramus and a lower-swung hyoid in relation to the mandibular plane. Those without OSAHS, however, were largely snorers, thus limiting the likelihood of finding cephalometric differences. Although siblings share the same characteristics that predispose to snoring and sleep-disordered breathing in relation to the rest of the population, additional morphological characteristics may be necessary to cause OSAHS.

Comment

These two studies suggest that there is a heritable component to craniofacial structure that predisposes to OSAHS in both the soft tissues and the bony structures.

The use of volumetric magnetic resonance imaging (MRI) was shown to be extremely effective in phenotyping the upper airway, transcending the limitations of previous two-dimensional techniques in the characterization of upper airway anatomy. This is an important advance in evaluating anatomical risk factors for OSAHS.

By contrast, the use of cephalometry in the second study represents the application of a two-dimensional technique in examining a three-dimensional structure. Despite this limitation, the method is sufficiently powerful to allow the recognition of trends and changes in the craniofacial skeleton in a way that makes it comparable to other studies in similar populations. Furthermore, its relative simplicity, ease of access, low radiation exposure and low cost as well as its routine use in the practice of prosthodontics and orthodontics makes cephalometry a more practical tool in the investigation of the craniofacial complex than more sophisticated techniques.

Head shape and size are determined genetically but compensatory mechanisms that prevent extreme development are also at work. A partial failure in these compensatory mechanisms may be responsible for the observation of certain anatomical features that are noted more frequently in the OSAHS population, most notably lower facial height and overbite as well as brachycephaly [7, 20–21]. Mandibular size and position seem to play the greatest role in determining facial alignment and predisposition to sleep-related breathing disorders. A lower position of the hyoid bone in both males and females is also associated with greater propensity to OSAHS.

Environmental mechanisms affecting growth include habits such as thumb-sucking and abnormal tongue posturing; nasopharyngeal disease and disturbed respiratory function, which may produce mouth-breathing; oral/gingival tumours; dental caries with loss of teeth; loss of permanent teeth; malnutrition; and endocrinopathy.

Such factors are difficult to control for in large studies that are cross-sectional in design, and may be significant confounders. Genes responsible for determining overall craniofacial structure and development in humans are still the subject of intense investigation. Likewise, genes controlling postnatal bone and soft tissue growth, obesity and final adult height and stature may play significant roles in the development of the skull and face.

Obesity

Obesity is the most commonly identified risk factor for OSAHS [22, 23]. Obesity is thought to contribute to the development/expression of OSAHS as a result of reduction in nasopharyngeal calibre secondary to fat deposition or of hypoventilation due to a decrease in chest wall compliance. Twin studies have shown that up to 70% of the variance in obesity within a population may be attributable to genetic factors. Adoption studies, by contrast, have generated the lowest heritability estimates (of the order of 30%). Family studies showing a level of heritability intermediate between the latter and twin studies [24]. The heritability of body mass index in large samples has been estimated to lie between 25 and 40% [25]. Susceptibility to becoming obese therefore seems to be determined significantly by genetic factors, but a favourable 'obesogenic' environment is necessary for phenotypic expression [24].

The regulation of appetite and energy expenditure constitutes an extremely complex system, with a large number of redundant pathways biased towards weight gain. Obesity develops when energy intake exceeds energy expenditure over time. Accumulated information regarding obesity susceptibility genes is so extensive that it is currently published in updated form on an annual basis as The Human Obesity Gene Map and is now available as a website (http://obesitygene.pbrc.edu). The most current update [26] incorporates published results on single-gene mutation obesity cases, Mendelian disorders exhibiting obesity as a feature, quantitative trait loci from human genome-wide scans and animal crossbreeding experiments as well as association and linkage studies with candidate genes and other markers. In total, more than 300 genes, markers and chromosomal regions have been associated or linked with human obesity phenotypes.

No studies are currently available looking specifically at the genetic basis of obesity in the context of sleep-disordered breathing.

Sleepiness and inflammation

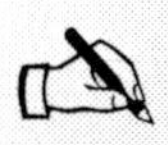

Predictors of elevated nuclear factor-kappaB-dependent genes in obstructive sleep apnea syndrome

Ryan S, Taylor CT, McNicholas WT. *Am J Respir Crit Care Med* 2006; **174**: 824–30

BACKGROUND. Epidemiological studies have shown that sleepiness does not necessarily correlate with the severity of sleep-disordered breathing. There also appears to be differential susceptibility to somnolence between individuals [27]. Sleep is regulated by neuronal and humoral mechanisms that are interdependent [28]. Cytokines have an integral role in the generation and promotion of sleep [29]. The mediation of a large number of neurohumoral factors by interleukin (IL)-1 and tumour necrosis factor-α (TNF-α) appears to be central to the sleep activation pathway and their roles in OSAHS have been the subject of much work [30, 31]. Other cytokines thought to induce sleep include IL-10, IL-6, interferon, IL-2, IL-4, granulocyte-macrophage colony-stimulating factor and fibroblast growth factor [31]. Current knowledge indicates that IL-6 is more important in the genesis of somnolence than was previously thought [29, 32]. OSAHS is also considered a state of low-grade inflammation, which may predispose to the development of hypertension and metabolic dysregulation. Pro-inflammatory cytokines may play a large part in this.

INTERPRETATION. This paper demonstrates the effects of intermittent hypoxia in cell culture on the development of pathways predisposing to increased production of pro-inflammatory cytokines. Circulating levels of TNF-α were higher in OSAHS patients than in normal controls at baseline and normalized with the use of continuous positive airway pressure (CPAP) after 6 weeks. Circulating neutrophil levels were also elevated in patients with OSAHS compared with controls, suggesting that a low-grade inflammatory state is present.

Comment

Tumour necrosis factor-α and IL-6 are elevated in OSAHS independently of obesity, and the circadian rhythm of TNF-α secretion is disrupted |33, 34|. Other mediators of inflammation are also elevated, including intercellular adhesion molecule-1 and C-reactive protein |35|. TNF-α, C-reactive protein and IL-6 appear to produce their harmful effects by inducing endothelial dysfunction. TNF-α damages endothelial cells, causes apoptosis of these cells and triggers procoagulant activity and fibrin deposition. TNF-α also enhances the production of reactive oxygen species, including inducible nitric oxide, and decreases myocardial contractility in a dose-dependent fashion |36|.

Sleep disruption in OSAHS may be one factor driving increased susceptibility to cardiovascular diseases in this condition. A genetic propensity to increased pro-inflammatory cytokine production may exacerbate these effects. The driving forces leading to elevations of pro-inflammatory cytokines in OSAHS may be related to increased activity of both branches of the autonomic nervous system, intermittent hypoxia, localized inflammation in the oropharynx leading to increased cytokine induction, and increased visceral adiposity |35|. Ryan *et al.* elegantly demonstrated in a cell culture model the selective activation of nuclear factor κB (NFκB)-dependent inflammatory pathways through intermittent hypoxia and reoxygenation |37|. They went on to show in a clinical study that reversing OSAHS by the use of CPAP resulted in a drop in the levels of circulating NFκB-dependent cytokines, specifically TNF-α and IL-8 |38|. Other circulating inflammatory cytokines, including IL-1, IL-12, IL-6, IL-8, IL-10 and interferon γ, showed no consistent association with OSAHS.

Apolipoprotein E: a role in OSAHS?

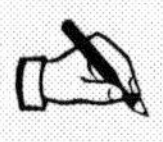

Apolipoprotein E and obstructive sleep apnea: evaluating whether a candidate gene explains a linkage peak

Larkin EK, Patel SR, Redline S, Mignot E, Elston RC, Hallmayer J. *Genet Epidemiol* 2006; **30**: 101–10

BACKGROUND. Apolipoprotein E (*APOE* = gene; ApoE = protein) occurs in all lipoproteins and its major role is thought to be the conversion of low-density lipoproteins to intermediate-density lipoproteins |40|. The three major isoforms of human ApoE (ApoE2; ApoE3 and ApoE4) are encoded by three alleles (ε2, ε3 and ε4).

The *APOE3* allele is the most frequent in human populations |41|. *APOE4* may be a 'thrifty' allele and exposure of the allele to the environmental conditions of a Western diet and longer lifespan may have rendered it a susceptibility allele for atherosclerosis and Alzheimer disease |41|.

INTERPRETATION. A variety of techniques was employed to examine the role of ApoE in OSAHS: genotyping, association studies and linkage analysis in a cohort previously recruited as part of the Cleveland Family Study, a longitudinal study of sleep apnoea in families (2426 individuals from 346 families). Two hundred and one Caucasian families were examined. No significant association was found between the ApoE E4 allele and subjects with OSAHS. An association-based analysis on 1211 individuals showed a higher prevalence of sleep apnoea in those with the *ApoE2* allele! The *APOE* locus on the genome is unlikely to be causal in the development of sleep-disordered breathing.

Comment

Four other studies have examined the *APOE4* genotype in the context of sleep-disordered breathing. The earliest study showed no significant difference in allelic variants between 291 patients with obstructive sleep apnoea and 728 random controls |42|. A study in 718 Japanese-American men in Hawaii (aged 79–97 years) investigating the possible linkage of apnoea/hypopnoea index (AHI) with *APOE4* likewise showed no significant association |43|. Kadotani *et al.* |44| stratified patients as *APOE4*-positive or -negative ($n = 222$ vs 569). There were significantly higher AHIs in the E4-positive group (see also comment in *JAMA* 2001; **286**: 1447–8). The most recent study showed one *APOE4* allele present in 25% of subjects undergoing sleep studies in a community-based sample ($n = 1775$; 40–100 years old) |45|. Of this population, 1.3% were E4/E4 homozygotes, which is approximately the normal and expected distribution of this genotype. The strongest statistical effect of *APOE4* was found in subjects aged less than 65 years who had sleep-disordered breathing (OR 3.08; 95% CI 1.43–6.64) and the effect was stronger in association with hypertension or cardiovascular disease. However, only 19% of the study population as a whole had an AHI greater than 15 events/hour and symptoms were not elicited, so the true prevalence of OSAHS was in all likelihood much lower.

ApoE is inconsistently associated with the presence of atherosclerosis, Alzheimer's disease and potentially neuropathy, and the association with sleep apnoea is even more problematic. No controls without OSAHS have been examined in the positive studies. Furthermore, OSAHS is associated with a number of comorbidities that have independently been shown to associate with increased frequency of the E4 allele, such as atherosclerosis, and coronary artery disease, irrespective of the presence of sleep-disordered breathing. There also appears to be no biologically plausible mechanism currently under consideration that would link ApoE with the development of OSAHS.

The upper airway in OSAHS

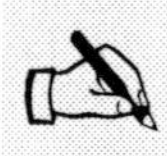

Contribution of 5-HT2 receptor subtypes to sleep-wakefulness and respiratory control, and functional adaptations in knock-out mice lacking 5-HT2A receptors

Popa D, Lena C, Fabre V, *et al J Neurosci* 2005; **25**: 11231–8

BACKGROUND. Sleep-related reductions in pharyngeal muscle activity are considered integral to the pathogenesis of OSAHS. A decrement in pharyngeal muscle activity leads to snoring and upper airway obstruction, which in turn leads to arousal from sleep. These arousals activate the pharyngeal muscles, thereby restoring airway patency and more effective breathing. The genioglossus muscle, innervated by the hypoglossal nerve, is considered to be the major upper airway dilator. The loss of activity of the genioglossus, especially during rapid eye-movement (REM) sleep, is thought to contribute to the onset of airway narrowing and occlusion, but some controversy exists |46|. Non-REM sleep and especially REM sleep are associated with the withdrawal of tonic excitation of the hypoglossal motor neurones via reduced firing of predominantly serotonergic medullar raphe neurons, and to a lesser extent of noradrenergic locus coeruleus neurones |47|. Molecular dissection techniques have shown the 5-HT2A receptor (5-hydroxytryptamine [serotonin] receptor 2A) to be the predominant receptor subtype in hypoglossal motor neurones |48, 49|. Pharmacological trials of 5-HT receptor agonists and antagonists support this receptor subtype as well as 5-HT2C (found in much smaller quantities) as the predominant post-synaptic facilitator of hypoglossal motor neurones, thereby being instrumental in the regulation of upper airway tone |50|. 5-HT2A receptor stimulation also excited the respiratory motor system at the level of the pre-Botzinger complex (still not identified in humans, but identified in rodent models) |51|.

INTERPRETATION. This is a rodent model for assessing sleep–wakefulness and breathing characteristics in relation to the 5-HT2 receptors. The balance between the 5-HT2A and 5-HT2B receptors in regulating the amount of non-REM and REM sleep was ascertained in greater detail than has previously been published. In terms of respiration, it was expected that 5-HT2A blockade would increase the occurrence of apnoeas, but this did not occur in the normal mice. The 5-HT2 receptors mediate the Hering–Breuer reflex, which can produce a transient bradypnoea via the afferent vagal system. Activation of the nucleus tractus solitarius results in baroreceptor-like reflexes that result in a reduction in respiratory frequency. It is therefore postulated that blockade of 5-HT2A receptors could reduce the contribution of the serotonergic system to the generation of apnoea.

Comment

Despite being a rodent model, this study has important implications for further research into pharmacological mediators of apnoea in sleep. The search for a 'magic pill' to replace CPAP for the treatment of OSAHS has been long and generally fruitless.

Attempts have been made to alleviate obstructive apnoeas by using selective serotonin reuptake inhibitors (SSRIs) |52, 53|. The results have been mixed, with incomplete responses to the SSRIs despite the demonstration of increased genioglossal activity, as measured by EMG in the awake state. To some extent this may be accounted for by the incompleteness of our current knowledge of the exact mechanisms regulating pharyngeal motor control during sleep and the roles of other upper airway muscle stabilizers and dilators in humans.

It might be of potential therapeutic and scientific value to explore whether gene polymorphisms in the 5-HT2A receptor may play a role in the modulation of serotonin metabolism, potentially affecting upper airway responsiveness. However, the issue is complicated by imprinting, which affects the expression of this gene, and the fact that such a study would require over 3000 subjects to be adequately powered. More promising may be examination of the serotonin transporter (5-HTT) molecule, which is the initial site of action of SSRIs. A number of polymorphisms have been identified, but the two most important ones are located in the promoter region and the second intron of the gene (variable number tandem repeat; VNTR) |54|. One of the best studies to date has examined the SSRI dose–response relationship to 5-HTT kinetics and demonstrated significant associations of the long promoter allele with placebo and drug response in comparison with the short allele |55|. A recent study in a small Turkish population showed no association of the serotonin transporter gene polymorphism with OSAHS, but the study was underpowered |56|.

Control of ventilation

Genetic influences may play a role in determining the wide variability in the magnitude of response to hypoxia and hypercapnia in the adult human. Studies in adult monozygotic twins have shown concordance in responses to hypoxia, but not consistently to hypercapnia |57, 58|. A high degree of heritability of the peripheral chemoreceptor response to hypoxia and hyperoxia in monozygotic twins during infancy compared with dizygotic twins exposed to similar environmental conditions has also been shown |59|.

Family studies examining ventilatory responses have suggested that healthy family members share a reduction in ventilatory response to hypoxia with the index case |60, 61|. Examination of the ventilatory drive in OSAHS patients and their healthy relatives as well as healthy unrelated controls has been undertaken by a number of investigators, with conflicting results. Based on this information, it is difficult to conclude that there is one single abnormality in ventilation in sleep-disordered breathing, making the search for a candidate gene currently untenable. Knowledge with regard to the neural control of breathing in vertebrates is still in its relative infancy |62|. Models of gene deletion and their effects on ventilatory responses in transgenic mice have been investigated at length |63| but the genes examined potentially play their most important role during early embryonic development and for a brief and transient period only |64|. Gene expression in the cardiorespiratory sites of the brainstem during development and in later life may be modified by responses to hypoxia in the context of environmental constraints. The hypoxia-inducible factors (HIF), such as HIF-1a, are upregulated in the mammalian brainstem in response to a hypoxic stress, compatible with normal respiratory physiology [65]. HIF-1 is recognized now as the master regulator of oxygen homeostasis during hypoxia. By regulating the expression of hundreds of genes, it controls innumerable physiological processes [66]. Limited evidence has suggested a role for HIF-1 in carotid body activation under conditions of chronic intermittent hypoxia (as in OSAHS), but these studies have been performed only in rodents to date and the identity of genes regulated downstream that contribute to these changes remains obscure [67]. The role of neurotrophins, such as brain-derived neurotrophic factor, during development of the brainstem has also been found to be integral to the establishment of functional respiratory control [62].

The outstanding issue remains whether respiratory control is implicated in the pathogenesis of OSAHS. Although there are abnormalities of respiratory control in OSAHS [68–70], these reverse with continuous positive airway pressure [71, 72]. Thus, the changes may be secondary rather than causal.

Conclusion

OSAHS is likely to be a polygenic disease. The degree of environmental influence on its development is currently unknown but is almost certainly considerable, including effects on obesity and craniofacial structure.

The major factor affecting progress in genetic studies remains a sturdy definition of OSAHS phenotype. At present, we are limited to studying the phenotype at a single point in time—when it calls clinical attention to itself.

Longitudinal studies – firstly identifying those who have OSAHS in childhood and following them through, and secondly continuing to follow those with sleep-disordered breathing identified in adult life – could be useful in clarifying this issue. There may be large differences in the underlying genotype, for instance, between those progressing into old age with asymptomatic sleep-disordered breathing, compared with those who develop symptoms and require treatment. We may discover that we are dealing with a range of diseases that manifest as a single phenotype at a particular point in time in the individual's life. Further study is needed to determine the best variables to be used to define the phenotype, including age and gender-related criteria.

At present, it is probably premature to use genome-wide scans in OSAHS owing to phenotype complexity. Choosing candidate genes for OSAHS in case–control studies is also difficult because a large number of disparate co-aetiologies need to be considered. Future work attempting to unravel the genetic basis of OSAHS may be better served by using a combination of investigative methods.

References

1. Young T, Palta M, Dempsey J, Skatrud J, Weber S, Badr S. The occurrence of sleep-disordered breathing among middle-aged adults. *N Engl J Med* 1993: **328**: 1230–5.

2. Ancoli-Israel S, Kripke DF, Mason W, Kaplan OJ. Sleep apnea and periodic movements in an aging sample. *J Gerontol* 1985; **40**: 419–25.

3. Duran J, Esnaola S, Rubio R, Iztueta A. Obstructive sleep apnea-hypopnea and related clinical features in a population-based sample of subjects aged 30 to 70 yr. *Am J Respir Crit Care Med* 2001; **163**: 685–9.

4. Bixler EO, Vgontzas AN, Ten Have T, Tyson K, Kales A. Effects of age on sleep apnea in men: I. Prevalence and severity. *Am J Respir Crit Care Med* 1998; **157**: 144–8.

5. Manon-Espaillat R, Gothe B, Adams N, Newman C, Ruff R. Familial 'sleep apnea plus' syndrome: report of a family. *Neurology* 1988; **38**: 190–3.

6. Douglas NJ, Luke M, Mathur R. Is the sleep apnoea/hypopnoea syndrome inherited? *Thorax* 1993; **48**: 719–21.

7. Mathur R, Douglas NJ. Family studies in patients with the sleep apnea-hypopnea syndrome. *Ann Intern Med* 1995; **122**: 174–8.

8. Ferini-Strambi L, Calori G, Oldani A, Della MG, Zucconi M, Castronovo V, Gallus G, Smirne S. Snoring in twins. *Respir Med* 1995; **89**: 337–40.

9. Holberg CJ, Natrajan S, Cline MG, Quan SF. Familial aggregation and segregation analysis of snoring and symptoms of obstructive sleep apnea. *Sleep Breath* 2000; **4**: 21–30.

10. Redline S, Tishler PV. The genetics of sleep apnea. *Sleep Med Rev* 2000; **4**: 583–602.

11. Schwab RJ, Gupta KB, Gefter WB, Metzger LJ, Hoffman EA, Pack AI. Upper airway and soft tissue anatomy in normal subjects and patients with sleep-disordered breathing. Significance of the lateral pharyngeal walls. *Am J Respir Crit Care Med* 1995; **152**: 1673–89.

12. Tangugsorn V, Skatvedt O, Krogstad O, Lyberg T. Obstructive sleep apnoea: a cephalometric study. Part I. Cervico-craniofacial skeletal morphology. *Eur J Orthod* 1995; **17**: 45–56.

13. Tangugsorn V, Krogstad O, Espeland L, Lyberg T. Obstructive sleep apnea (OSA): a cephalometric analysis of severe and non-severe OSA patients. Part I: Multiple comparisons of cephalometric variables. *Int J Adult Orthodon Orthognath Surg* 2000; **15**: 139–52.

14. Miles PG, Vig PS, Weyant RJ, Forrest TD, Rockette HE Jr. Craniofacial structure and obstructive sleep apnea syndrome—a qualitative analysis and meta-analysis of the literature. *Am J Orthod Dentofacial Orthop* 1996; **109**: 163–72.

15. Riha RL, Brander P, Vennelle M, Douglas NJ. A cephalometric comparison of patients with the sleep apnea/hypopnea syndrome and their siblings. *Sleep* 2005; **28**: 315–20.

16. Lowe AA, Ono T, Ferguson KA, Pae EK, Ryan CF, Fleetham JA. Cephalometric comparisons of craniofacial and upper airway structure by skeletal subtype and gender in

patients with obstructive sleep apnea. *Am J Orthod Dentofacial Orthop* 1996; **110**: 653–64.

17. Trask GM, Shapiro GG, Shapiro PA. The effects of perennial allergic rhinitis on dental and skeletal development: a comparison of sibling pairs. *Am J Orthod Dentofacial Orthop* 1987; **92**: 286–93.

18. Linder-Aronson S. Adenoids. Their effect on mode of breathing and nasal airflow and their relationship to characteristics of the facial skeleton and the dentition. A biometric, rhino-manometric and cephalometro-radiographic study on children with and without adenoids. *Acta Otolaryngol Suppl* 1970; **265**: 1–132.

19. Harvold EP. Neuromuscular and morphological adaptations in experimentally induced oral respiration. *Cranio-facial Growth Series No.9*. Ann Arbor, Michigan: Center for Human Growth and Development, University of Michigan, 1979; pp.149–64.

20. Pae EK, Ferguson KA. Cephalometric characteristics of nonobese patients with severe OSA. *Angle Orthod* 1999; **69**: 408–12.

21. Cakirer B, Hans MG, Graham G, Aylor J, Tishler PV, Redline S. The relationship between craniofacial morphology and obstructive sleep apnea in whites and in African-Americans. *Am J Respir Crit Care Med* 2001; **163**: 947–50.

22. Kushida CA, Efron B, Guilleminault C. A predictive morphometric model for the obstructive sleep apnea syndrome. *Ann Intern Med* 1997; **127**: 581–7.

23. Hoffstein V, Szalai JP. Predictive value of clinical features in diagnosing obstructive sleep apnea. *Sleep* 1993; **16**: 118–22.

24. Ravussin E, Bouchard C. Human genomics and obesity: finding appropriate drug targets. *Eur J Pharmacol* 2000; **410**: 131–45.

25. Bouchard C. Obesity in adulthood—the importance of childhood and parental obesity. *N Engl J Med* 1997; **337**: 926–7.

26. Perusse L, Rankinen T, Zuberi A, Chagnon YC, Weisnagel SJ, Argyropoulos G, Walts B, Snyder EE, Bouchard C. The human obesity gene map: the 2004 update. *Obes Res* 2005; **13**: 381–490.

27. Cluydts R, De Valck E, Verstraeten E, Theys P. Daytime sleepiness and its evaluation. *Sleep Med Rev* 2002; **6**: 83–96.

28. Krueger JM, Obal F Jr, Fang J. Humoral regulation of physiological sleep: cytokines and GHRH. *J Sleep Res* 1999; **8** (Suppl 1): 53–9.

29. Opp MR, Toth LA. Neural-immune interactions in the regulation of sleep. *Front Biosci* 2003; **8**: d768–779.

30. Entzian P, Linnemann K, Schlaak M, Zabel P. Obstructive sleep apnea syndrome and circadian rhythms of hormones and cytokines. *Am J Respir Crit Care Med* 1996; **153**: 1080–6.

31. Vgontzas AN, Papanicolaou DA, Bixler EO, Kales A, Tyson K, Chrousos GP. Elevation of plasma cytokines in disorders of excessive daytime sleepiness: role of sleep disturbance and obesity. *J Clin Endocrinol Metab* 1997; **82**: 1313–16.

32. Redwine L, Hauger RL, Gillin JC, Irwin M. Effects of sleep and sleep deprivation on interleukin-6, growth hormone, cortisol, and melatonin levels in humans. *J Clin Endocrinol Metab* 2000; **85**: 3597–603.

33. Vgontzas AN, Papanicolaou DA, Bixler EO, Hopper K, Lotsikas A, Lin HM, Kales A, Chrousos GP. Sleep apnea and daytime sleepiness and fatigue: relation to visceral

obesity, insulin resistance, and hypercytokinemia. *J Clin Endocrinol Metab* 2000; **85:** 1151–8.

34. Entzian P, Linnemann K, Schlaak M, *et al.* Obstructive sleep apnea syndrome and circadian rhythms of hormones and cytokines. *Am J Respir Crit Care Med* 1996; **153:** 1080–6.

35. Mills PJ, Dimsdale JE. Sleep apnea: a model for studying cytokines, sleep, and sleep disruption. *Brain Behav Immun* 2004; **18:** 298–303.

36. Das UN. Is obesity an inflammatory condition? *Nutrition* 2001; **17:** 953–66.

37. Ryan S, Taylor CT, McNicholas WT. Selective activation of inflammatory pathways by intermittent hypoxia in obstructive sleep apnea syndrome. *Circulation* 2005; **112:** 2660–7.

38. Ryan S, Taylor CT, McNicholas WT. Predictors of elevated nuclear factor-{kappa}B-dependent genes in obstructive sleep apnea syndrome. *Am J Respir Crit Care Med* 2006; **174:** 824–30.

39. Riha RL, Brander P, Vennelle M, McArdle N, Kerr SM, Anderson NH, Douglas NJ. Tumour necrosis factor-alpha (-308) gene polymorphism in obstructive sleep apnoea-hypopnoea syndrome. *Eur Respir J* 2005; **26:** 673–8.

40. Davignon J, Gregg RE, Sing CF. Apolipoprotein E polymorphism and atherosclerosis. *Arteriosclerosis* 1988; **8:** 1–21.

41. Corbo RM, Scacchi R. Apolipoprotein E (APOE) allele distribution in the world. Is APOE*4 a 'thrifty' allele? *Ann Hum Genet* 1999; **63:** 301–10.

42. Saarelainen S, Lehtimaki T, Kallonen E, Laasonen K, Poussa T, Nieminen MM. No relation between apolipoprotein E alleles and obstructive sleep apnea. *Clin Genet* 1998; **53:** 147–8.

43. Foley DJ, Masaki K, White L, Larkin EK, Monjan A, Redline S. Sleep-disordered breathing and cognitive impairment in elderly Japanese-American men. *Sleep* 2003; **26(5):** 596–9.

44. Kadotani H, Kadotani T, Young T, Peppard PE, Finn L, Colrain IM, Murphy GM Jr, Mignot E. Association between apolipoprotein E epsilon4 and sleep-disordered breathing in adults. *JAMA* 2001; **285:** 2888–90.

45. Gottlieb DJ, DeStefano AL, Foley DJ, Mignot E, Redline S, Givelber RJ, Young T. APOE epsilon4 is associated with obstructive sleep apnea/hypopnea: the Sleep Heart Health Study. *Neurology* 2004; **63:** 664–8.

46. Remmers JE, deGroot WJ, Sauerland EK, Anch AM. Pathogenesis of upper airway occlusion during sleep. *J Appl Physiol* 1978; **44:** 931–8.

47. Parkis MA, Bayliss DA, Berger AJ. Actions of norepinephrine on rat hypoglossal motoneurons. *J Neurophysiol* 1995; **74:** 1911–19.

48. Fonseca MI, Ni YG, Dunning DD, Miledi R. Distribution of serotonin 2A, 2C and 3 receptor mRNA in spinal cord and medulla oblongata. *Brain Res Mol Brain Res* 2001; **89:** 11–19.

49. Zhan G, Shaheen F, Mackiewicz M, Fenik P, Veasey SC. Single cell laser dissection with molecular beacon polymerase chain reaction identifies 2A as the predominant serotonin receptor subtype in hypoglossal motoneurons. *Neuroscience* 2002; **113:** 145–54.

50. Fenik P, Veasey SC. Pharmacological characterization of serotonergic receptor activity in the hypoglossal nucleus. *Am J Respir Crit Care Med* 2003; **167:** 563–9.

51. Pena F, Ramirez JM. Endogenous activation of serotonin-2A receptors is required for respiratory rhythm generation in vitro. *J Neurosci* 2002; **22**: 11055–64.

52. Hanzel DA, Proia NG, Hudgel DW. Response of obstructive sleep apnea to fluoxetine and protriptyline. *Chest* 1991; **100**: 416–21.

53. Kraiczi H, Hedner J, Dahlof P, Ejnell H, Carlson J. Effect of serotonin uptake inhibition on breathing during sleep and daytime symptoms in obstructive sleep apnea. *Sleep* 1999; **22**: 61–7.

54. Serretti A, Lilli R, Smeraldi E. Pharmacogenetics in affective disorders. *Eur J Pharmacol* 2002; **438**: 117–28.

55. Rausch JL, Johnson ME, Fei YJ, Li JQ, Shendarkar N, Hobby HM, Ganapathy V, Leibach FH. Initial conditions of serotonin transporter kinetics and genotype: influence on SSRI treatment trial outcome. *Biol Psychiatry* 2002; **51**: 723–32.

56. Ylmaz M, Bayazit YA, Ciftci TU, Erdal ME, Urhan M, Kokturk O, Kemaloglu YK, Inal E. Association of serotonin transporter gene polymorphism with obstructive sleep apnea syndrome. *Laryngoscope* 2005; **115**: 832–6.

57. Kobayashi S, Nishimura M, Yamamoto M, Akiyama Y, Kishi F, Kawakami Y. Dyspnea sensation and chemical control of breathing in adult twins. *Am Rev Respir Dis* 1993; **147**: 1192–8.

58. Arkinstall WW, Nirmel K, Klissouras V, Milic-Emili J. Genetic differences in the ventilatory response to inhaled CO2. *J Appl Physiol* 1974; **36**: 6–11.

59. Thomas DA, Swaminathan S, Beardsmore CS, McArdle EK, MacFadyen UM, Goodenough PC, Carpenter R, Simpson H. Comparison of peripheral chemoreceptor responses in monozygotic and dizygotic twin infants. *Am Rev Respir Dis* 1993; **148**: 1605–9.

60. Kawakami Y, Yamamoto H, Yoshikawa T, Shida A. Chemical and behavioral control of breathing in adult twins. *Am Rev Respir Dis* 1984; **129**: 703–7.

61. Mountain R, Zwillich C, Weil J. Hypoventilation in obstructive lung disease. The role of familial factors. *N Engl J Med* 1978; **298**: 521–5.

62. Fortin G, del Toro ED, Abadie V, Guimaraes L, Foutz AS, Denavit-Saubie M, Rouyer F, Champagnat J. Genetic and developmental models for the neural control of breathing in vertebrates. *Respir Physiol* 2000; **122**: 247–57.

63. Gaultier C, Guilleminault C. Genetics, control of breathing, and sleep-disordered breathing: a review. 2001; **2**: 281–95.

64. Lumsden A, Krumlauf R. Patterning the vertebrate neuraxis. *Science* 1996; **274**: 1109–15.

65. Pascual O, Denavit-Saubie M, Dumas S, Kietzmann T, Ghilini G, Mallet J, Pequignot JM. Selective cardiorespiratory and catecholaminergic areas express the hypoxia-inducible factor-1alpha (HIF-1alpha) under in vivo hypoxia in rat brainstem. *Eur J Neurosci* 2001; **14**: 1981–91.

66. Manalo DJ, Rowan A, Lavoie T, Natarajan L, Kelly BD, Ye SQ, Garcia JG, Semenza GL. Transcriptional regulation of vascular endothelial cell responses to hypoxia by HIF-1. *Blood* 2005; **105**: 659–69.

67. Peng YJ, Yuan G, Ramakrishnan D, Sharma SD, Bosch-Marce M, Kumar GK, Semenza GL, Prabhakar NR. Heterozygous HIF-1alpha deficiency impairs carotid

body-mediated systemic responses and reactive oxygen species generation in mice exposed to intermittent hypoxia. *J Physiol* 2006; **577**: 705–16.

68. Ayappa I, Berger KI, Norman RG, Oppenheimer BW, Rapoport DM, Goldring RM. Hypercapnia and ventilatory periodicity in obstructive sleep apnea syndrome. *Am J Respir Crit Care Med* 2002; **166**: 1112–15.

69. Garcia-Rio F, Pino JM, Ramirez T, Alvaro D, Alonso A, Villasante C, Villamor J. Inspiratory neural drive response to hypoxia adequately estimates peripheral chemosensitivity in OSAHS patients. *Eur Respir J* 2002; **20**: 724–32.

70. Asyali MH, Berry RB, Khoo MC. Assessment of closed-loop ventilatory stability in obstructive sleep apnea. *IEEE Trans Biomed Eng* 2002; **49**: 206–16.

71. Moura SM, Bittencourt LR, Bagnato MC, Lucas SR, Tufik S, Nery LE. Acute effect of nasal continuous positive air pressure on the ventilatory control of patients with obstructive sleep apnea. *Respiration* 2001; **68**: 243–9.

72. Verbraecken J, Willemen M, De Cock W, Wittesaele W, Govaert K, Van de HP, De Backer W. Influence of longterm CPAP therapy on CO(2) drive in patients with obstructive sleep apnea. *Respir Physiol* 2000; **123**: 121–30.

10

Sleep-disordered breathing; congestive cardiac failure and cardiac pacemakers

ANNE JONES, RENATA RIHA

Introduction

There has been much research into the interaction between sleep-disordered breathing and cardiovascular disease. In this chapter we will examine two particular aspects in which there has been recent interest: the treatment of sleep-disordered breathing in association with congestive cardiac failure (CCF) and the possible role of cardiac pacemakers in the treatment of sleep-disordered breathing.

Congestive cardiac failure

Obstructive sleep apnoea/hypopnoea syndrome (OSAHS) is common in the general population, affecting 2–4% of the middle-aged population [1–3]. Congestive cardiac failure is also common, and may share similar risk factors. The prevalence of OSAHS in stable congestive cardiac failure has been reported at around 11% [4,5], and in these circumstances is less likely to present with excessive daytime sleepiness [6]. Whilst OSAHS and congestive cardiac failure undoubtedly share some risk factors, there is some evidence that OSAHS acts as an independent risk factor for systolic [7,8] and diastolic [8,9] impairment. It has been suggested that OSAHS leads to the progression of congestive cardiac failure. Possible mechanisms for this include swings in intrathoracic pressure during respiratory effort, leading to increased venous return and left ventricular afterload, increased activation of the sympathetic nervous system secondary to arousals and hypoxia, and endothelial dysfunction. However, it has not been shown that the prognosis of congestive cardiac failure is poorer in patients with OSAHS [10], nor that the progression of congestive cardiac failure in these patients is conclusively attenuated by continuous positive airway pressure (CPAP) therapy. Two studies with limited numbers of patients [11,12] have demonstrated small improvements in left ventricular ejection fraction (LVEF) (5% ± 4.4 [SD] and 8.8% ± 5.5 in the two studies respectively) in patients with OSAHS and congestive cardiac failure treated with CPAP compared with those continuing on medical therapy alone.

Whilst it is known that OSAHS is associated with hypertension [13] and all-cause cardiovascular mortality [14], more work is required to clarify the relationship between OSAHS and congestive cardiac failure, and any potential benefits associated with CPAP treatment.

Central sleep apnoea or Cheyne–Stokes respiration (CSA-CSR) is commoner than OSAHS in congestive cardiac failure, with prevalence rates of 29–40% [4,5,15]. Central sleep apnoea is characterized by apnoea associated with absence of respiratory effort and may coexist with OSAHS [16]. Central sleep apnoea in congestive cardiac failure is thought to be associated with resting hyperventilation caused by pulmonary vagal irritant receptors, leading to chronic hypocapnia [5]. This, along with alterations in chemosensitivity to carbon dioxide [17], can lead to levels of carbon dioxide falling below the apnoeic threshold. Risk factors for central sleep apnoea in congestive cardiac failure include male gender, age greater than 60 years, atrial fibrillation and hypocapnia [15].

Congestive cardiac failure associated with central sleep apnoea confers a worse prognosis than congestive cardiac failure alone [18,19]. With the exception of the swings in intrathoracic pressure, the postulated mechanisms are similar to those proposed in OSAHS [20].

There have been three relatively small randomized controlled trials examining the benefits of positive pressure ventilation in treating central sleep apnoea in patients with congestive cardiac failure [21–23]. These have shown varying results with only one showing a statistically significant increase (7.7% ± 8.7 [SD]) in LVEF [21]. In the only trial to look at death or heart transplantation as an outcome measure, 49% of patients in the control group either died or underwent heart transplantation compared with 29% in the CPAP-treated group. However, this did not reach statistical significance, presumably because of the limited size of the study ($n = 66$) [22].

The recently published multicentre CANPAP (Canadian Continuous Positive Airway Pressure for Patients with Central Sleep Apnea and Heart Failure) trial is the largest study to date to examine the effect of CPAP on central sleep apnoea in patients with congestive cardiac failure and will be reviewed in depth below.

Most research concentrates on CPAP therapy as the treatment of central sleep apnoea, but more recently a new form of positive airway pressure, termed adaptive servoventilation, has become available [24] and this will be discussed below. Other treatments, including nocturnal oxygen therapy and cardiac pacing, have also been investigated. Nocturnal oxygen has been shown in small studies to reduce central sleep apnoea [25], improve nocturnal oxygen desaturation [26] and reduce sympathetic activity [27]. However, this has not translated into improvements in clinical outcomes [27].

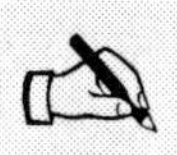

Nocturnal continuous positive airway pressure improves ventilatory efficiency during exercise in patients with chronic heart failure

Arzt M, Schulz M, Wensel R, *et al. Chest* 2005; **127**: 794–802

BACKGROUND. This study looked at the role of CPAP in improving ventilatory efficiency and cardiac function in patients with congestive cardiac failure and central sleep apnoea. Congestive cardiac failure is associated with impaired cardiorespiratory reflex control, manifesting as central sleep apnoea |4,5,15| and impaired ventilatory response to exercise |28,29|. Ventilatory efficiency can be measured at cardiopulmonary exercise testing as the V_E/V_{CO_2} slope, which is the slope of the regression line relating minute ventilation (V_E) to carbon dioxide production (V_{CO_2}) |28|. In patients with congestive cardiac failure and central sleep apnoea this slope is augmented |30|. Increased V_E/V_{CO_2} slope is associated with a worse prognosis in congestive cardiac failure |28,31,32|. The aim of this study was to test the hypothesis that, in contrast to nocturnal oxygen, CPAP therapy can improve cardiac function and ventilatory efficiency during exercise in chronic heart failure patients with central sleep apnoea.

INTERPRETATION. This was a prospective, non-randomized, controlled trial. Patients with stable New York Heart Association (NYHA) class II and III cardiac failure with an LVEF of <45% were eligible for inclusion if they had polysomnographic evidence of central sleep apnoea. Outcome measures included V_E/V_{CO_2} slope, LVEF, V_{O_2} and NYHA functional class. Twenty-six patients were recruited. The first ten patients received nocturnal oxygen therapy and the remaining 16 received CPAP therapy. Polysomnography, cardiopulmonary exercise testing and echocardiography were conducted at baseline and at 12 weeks. Adequate compliance with CPAP was taken to be ≥3 h per night; two patients were withdrawn as they did not achieve this. Both CPAP and oxygen therapy led to reductions in the apnoea/hypopnoea index (AHI) and nocturnal oxygen desaturation. Only CPAP was shown to reduce the V_E/V_{CO_2} slope significantly (from 31.2 ± 6.0 [SD] to 26.2 ± 3.7; $P = 0.005$) (Fig. 10.1).

A relevant reduction in V_E/V_{CO_2} slope was defined as >2.6 for this study. This is said to be based on an earlier study finding a difference of 3.2 between controls and patients with NYHA class I cardiac failure |33|. Based on this, 50% of those in the CPAP-treated group were considered to be responders. These patients had a significantly lower ventilatory efficiency at baseline and a trend towards lower LVEF than non-responders (Fig. 10.2). A small but statistically significant improvement in LVEF in the CPAP-treated group was also reported (from 31.7% ± 9.7 [SD] to 35.7% ± 10.1). Neither CPAP nor oxygen improved NYHA class or peak V_{O_2}.

Comment

This study demonstrates an improvement in ventilatory efficiency and LVEF in CPAP-treated patients with central sleep apnoea and congestive cardiac failure. However, only 50% of those within the CPAP-treated group had clinically relevant improvement in ventilatory efficiency. Those who responded in this trial were said

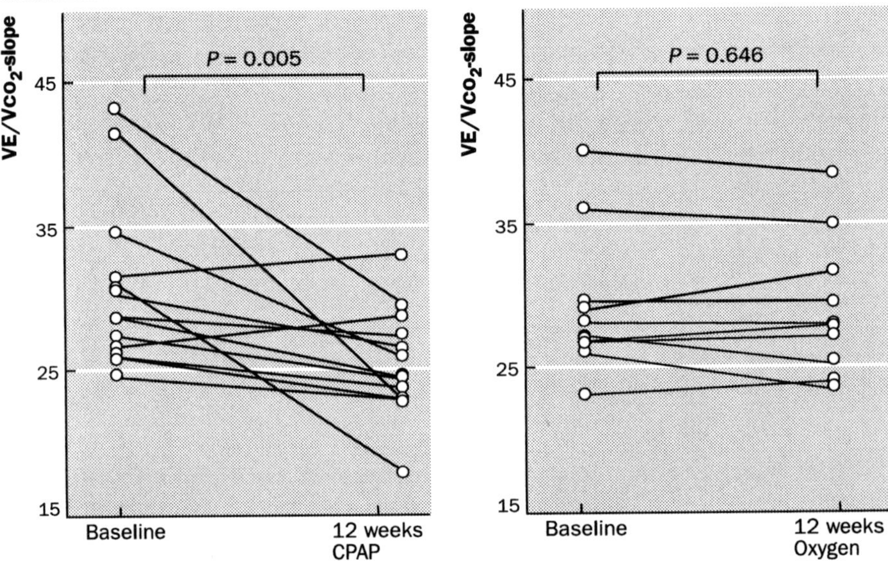

Fig. 10.1 Individual values of ventilatory efficiency (V_E/V_{CO_2} slope) of patients with chronic heart failure and central sleep apnoea before (baseline) and after 12 weeks of CPAP ($n = 14$) and oxygen therapy ($n = 10$). Source: Arzt *et al.* (2005).

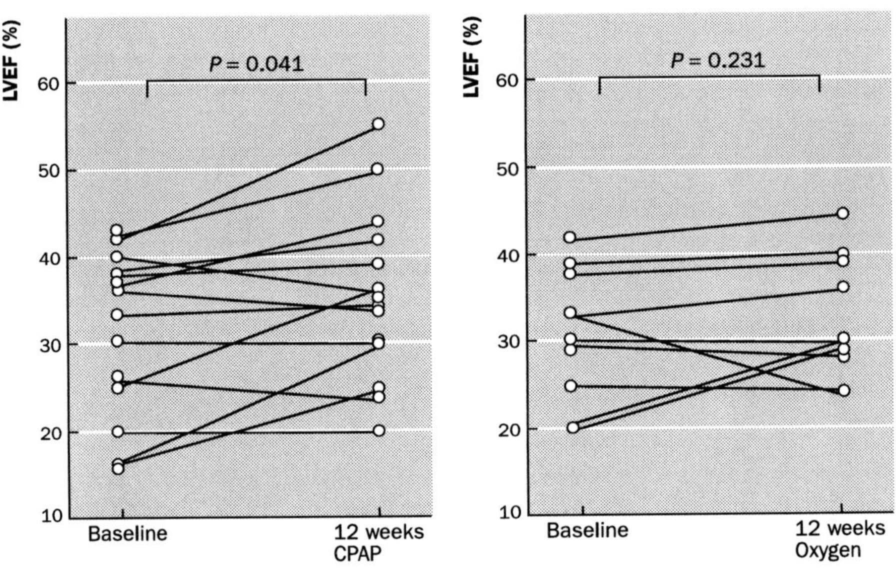

Fig. 10.2 Individual values of LVEF in patients with chronic heart failure and central sleep apnoea before (baseline) and after 12 weeks of CPAP ($n = 14$) and oxygen therapy ($n = 10$). Source: Arzt *et al.* (2005).

to have the greatest impairment in ventilatory efficiency at baseline, compared with non-responders (data not presented). However, this is based on data from a small number of patients within a non-randomized trial. Despite improvement in V_E/V_{CO_2} slope, no improvement in exercise capacity, as measured by peak V_{O_2}, was seen. As will be discussed below, such improvements in physiology have yet to be translated into survival benefit.

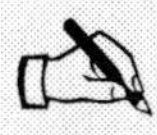

Continuous positive airway pressure for central sleep apnea and heart failure (CANPAP trial)

Bradley TD, Logan AG, Kimoff RJ, *et al. N Engl J Med* 2005; **353**: 2025–33

BACKGROUND. Prior to this study, there have been only a small number of randomized controlled trials looking at the impact of positive airway pressure treatment on central sleep apnoea in patients with congestive cardiac failure |21–23,34|. Sin *et al.* |22| looked at patients with congestive cardiac failure, both with and without central sleep apnoea, and randomized them to receive CPAP or standard medical therapy alone. Overall, a non-significant increase in LVEF (2.5% ± 0.1 [SD]) was noted in those treated with CPAP. Subgroup analysis (*n* = 14), however, suggested that there was a more significant increase in LVEF in those with central sleep apnoea who received CPAP treatment. A non-significant decrease in death/heart transplant rate was also described. Pepperell *et al.* |23| did not demonstrate a significant increase in LVEF in patients with central sleep apnoea who were treated with adaptive servoventilation. Significant improvements in serum brain natriuretic peptide (BNP) in the CPAP-treated group were noted. Naughton *et al.* |21| reported a statistically significant improvement in LVEF of 7.7% ± 8.7 (SD) in those treated with CPAP compared to no significant change in the control group. The work of Arzt *et al.* |34| is discussed in detail above. These were all small studies (*n* = 66, 30, 29 and 26 respectively) The aim of this study was to conduct a multicentre trial to test the hypothesis that long-term treatment of central sleep apnoea with CPAP in patients with heart failure on optimal medical therapy reduces the combined rates of death and heart transplantation.

INTERPRETATION. This was a prospective, randomized, controlled, multicentre trial. Patients with stable NYHA class II–IV heart failure and an LVEF of <40% were eligible for inclusion if they had polysomnographic evidence of central sleep apnoea. The primary outcome measure was the combined rate of death and heart transplantation. Secondary outcome measures included hospitalization rates, LVEF change, submaximal exercise capacity, quality of life, and levels of atrial natriuretic peptide and norepinephrine. Patients were randomized to continue optimal medical therapy alone or to receive CPAP plus optimal medical therapy. In total, 258 patients were recruited (96% male) between 1998 and 2004, with a mean follow-up period of 2 years. Recruitment was halted early because interim analyses suggested early divergence of the two groups in favour of the control arm, changes in the primary event rate and a poorer than expected rate of recruitment. In the CPAP-treated group, average CPAP usage was 4.3 h/night for the first 3 months and 3.6 h/night at 1 year, with an average pressure between 8 and 9 cm H_2O. A 50% decrease was seen in AHI in the CPAP-treated group, with improvement in nocturnal oxygen saturation.

In the CPAP-treated group there were 27 deaths and five heart transplants, compared with 28 deaths and four transplants in the control arm. (Fig. 10.3). A small increase in LVEF (2.2% ± 5.4 [SD]) was noted in the CPAP-treated group. There was no difference in hospitalization rate, quality of life or atrial natriuretic peptide level between the two groups. An initial improvement in the 6-min walk was noted, but this was not sustained. A small but statistically significant reduction in plasma norepinephrine was noted.

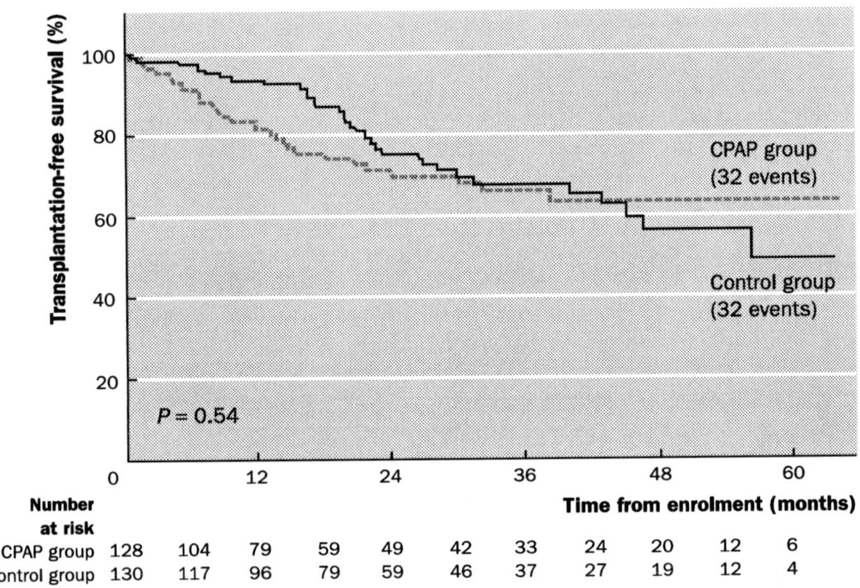

Number at risk										
CPAP group	128	104	79	59	49	42	33	24	20	12	6
Control group	130	117	96	79	59	46	37	27	19	12	4

Fig. 10.3 Heart transplantation-free survival. There was no difference in transplantation-free survival rates between the control group and the CPAP group (hazard ratio [HR] for transplantation-free survival 1.16; $P = 0.54$). However, there was an early divergence in the event rates that favoured the control group (HR for transplantation-free survival 1.5; $P = 0.02$); after 18 months the difference favoured the CPAP group (HR for transplantation-free survival 0.66; $P = 0.06$). Source: Bradley *et al.* (2005).

Comment

This trial, the largest to date, did not show any survival benefit associated with the use of CPAP in treating central sleep apnoea in patients with congestive cardiac failure. One problem was the sharp fall in the primary event rate during the course of the trial (falling from 20 per 100 person-years to just 4), related to improvements in pharmacological therapies, particularly the widespread introduction of β-blockers. As a result of this, had the trial continued it would still have been significantly underpowered to detect any change in the primary event rate. CPAP did reduce the AHI and improve nocturnal oxygen saturations, but the reduction in AHI was only 50%.

The authors discuss the early divergence in primary outcome rates favouring the control arm and consider the possibility that CPAP had an early adverse effect in some patients by reducing cardiac output in patients with low filling pressures.

This trial does not support the routine use of CPAP as treatment of central sleep apnoea in patients with congestive cardiac failure.

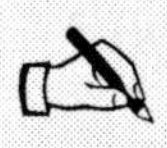

Compliance with and effectiveness of adaptive servoventilation versus continuous positive airway pressure in the treatment of Cheyne-Stokes respiration in heart failure over a six month period

Philippe C, Stoïca-Herman M, Drouot X, *et al. Heart* 2006; **92**: 337–42

BACKGROUND. Of the papers discussed above I21–23,34,35I, all but one I23I used CPAP as the method of delivering positive airway pressure. In two, a compliance of greater than 3 h was considered acceptable I22,34I, and a third reported an average compliance of 4.3 h/night initially, dropping to 3.6 h by the end of the trial I35I. In the two trials to report the change in AHI following CPAP treatment, a reduction of between 50 and 66% was described I34,35I. In these trials CPAP reduced, but did not abolish, central sleep apnoea. This has been put forward as a possible contributing factor to the lack of benefit seen I35I. There has been interest in a newer form of positive airway pressure: adaptive servoventilation. This provides positive inspiratory and expiratory pressures and is servocontrolled (with a backup respiratory rate) on detection of central sleep apnoea, providing higher pressures till respiration recommences I24I. In a small crossover study (*n* = 14), adaptive servoventilation was shown to significantly reduce AHI compared with CPAP or bi-level ventilation I24I. However despite this, Pepperell *et al.* I23I found no significant improvement in LVEF when comparing adaptive servoventilation with subtherapeutic adaptive servoventilation. Significant improvements in serum BNP and daytime wakefulness were seen, however. This trial sought to compare adaptive servoventilation with CPAP in the treatment of central sleep apnoea in congestive cardiac failure.

INTERPRETATION. This was a prospective, randomized, multicentre trial. Patients with stable NHYA class II–IV heart failure (receiving optimal medical therapy) with an LVEF of ≤45% were eligible for inclusion if they had polysomnographic evidence of central sleep apnoea. Outcome measures included AHI, daytime sleepiness, LVEF and quality of life. After CPAP titration, patients were randomized to either CPAP or adaptive servoventilation for 6 months. Twenty-five patients were initially recruited, eight of whom later dropped out, leaving nine in the adaptive servoventilation group and eight in the CPAP group. Whilst both treatments significantly reduced the AHI, the effect was most marked with adaptive servoventilation, and this persisted at 6 months (Fig. 10.4). Compliance with adaptive servoventilation at 6 months was significantly higher than with CPAP. A significant improvement in LVEF was seen with adaptive servoventilation compared with CPAP; however, data were not available for all patients so this is based on small numbers. Improvements in quality of life were seen with both treatments, but a significant difference between the two, favouring adaptive servoventilation, was seen at 6 months. No changes in daytime sleepiness were evident in either group.

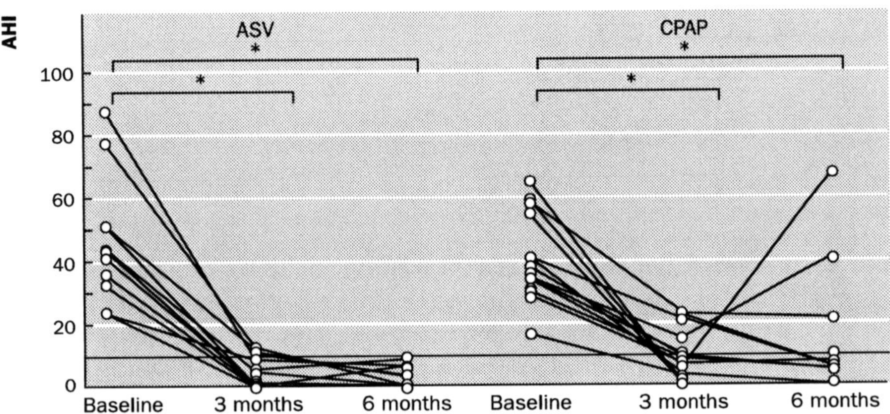

Fig. 10.4 Effect of nocturnal ventilation on the apnoea/hypopnoea index (AHI [/h]). Individual AHIs are shown at baseline and after 3 and 6 months of treatment with either adaptive servoventilation (ASV) (left) or continuous positive airway pressure (CPAP) (right). Source: Philippe *et al.* (2006).

Comment

Although small, this study confirms the previously noted observation |24| that adaptive servoventilation is superior to CPAP in reducing AHI in patients with congestive heart failure and central sleep apnoea. Longer-term compliance also seems to be improved when using adaptive servoventilation. Despite small studies suggesting some survival benefit |22|, small improvements in LVEF |21,22| and a reduction in serum BNP |23|, this has not translated into survival benefit in the largest trial to date |35|. Larger studies of adaptive servoventilation are required to determine whether the greater reduction in AHI and improved compliance lead to better patient outcomes.

Cardiac pacemakers and sleep-disordered breathing

Changes in cardiac rhythm are common in sleep apnoea, bradycardias often occurring during the apnoeic period followed by tachycardia as the apnoea resolves. Bradyarrythmias have been reported in up to 20% of patients with severe sleep apnoea |36|. Based on clinical observations, Garrigue *et al.* undertook a randomized crossover trial to investigate the efficiency of atrial overdrive pacing in the treatment of sleep apnoea syndrome |37|. They recruited 15 patients with previously implanted dual chamber pacemakers for bradyarrythmias, symptoms of sleep-disordered breathing and evidence of either obstructive ($n = 7$) or central ($n = 8$) sleep apnoea. They were then randomized to one night with their pacemakers set at 40 b.p.m. (to record as much spontaneous rhythm as possible) followed by a night with the pacemaker set 15 b.p.m. above their mean nocturnal heart rate, or vice versa. A significant reduction in AHI was demonstrated, the AHI falling from 28 ± 22 (SD) on the non-paced nights to 11 ± 14 on the paced nights. The AHI fell in all patients, 13 of the 15 patients experiencing a reduction in AHI greater than 50% |37|, which is similar to that seen with CPAP treatment in the CANPAP trial |35|.

A reduction in arousals and an increase in oxygen saturations were also seen. The reduction in central apnoeas is perhaps not surprising as atrial overdrive pacing improves cardiac output, which may reduce pulmonary congestion, and these may in turn reduce the hyperventilation and hypocapnia associated with central sleep apnoea |38|. Garrigue *et al.* postulated that high vagal tone could contribute to obstructive apnoeas through changes in upper airway musculature and that in bradycardic patients this high vagal tone may be counteracted by maintaining sympathetic activity using atrial overdrive pacing |38|.

Although the mechanism was largely speculative, the finding that, in this population, atrial overdrive pacing improved OSAHS was novel and merited further investigation. This is of particular importance because CPAP, though an effective treatment for OSAHS, is not universally tolerated by patients and compliance varies |39|. There have been many studies examining this further, two of which will be discussed in more detail below.

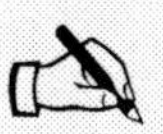

Overdrive atrial pacing does not improve obstructive sleep apnoea syndrome

Pépin JL, Defaye P, Garrigue S, Poezevara Y, Lévy P. *Eur Respir J* 2005; **25**: 343–7

BACKGROUND. Following the unexpected reduction in obstructive apnoeas with atrial overdrive pacing, it was proposed that this may have been secondary to a reduction in central apnoeas. The authors of this paper postulated that periods of central apnoea, associated with a reduction in cardiac output, could lead to obstructive episodes in those with susceptible upper airways. Garrigue *et al.* included seven patients with predominantly obstructive apnoeas |38|, but all patients also had evidence of central sleep apnoea. In this study, the authors tested the hypothesis that in patients with obstructive sleep apnoea, bradyarrythmia and normal left ventricular function, atrial overdrive pacing would not be effective in reducing AHI.

INTERPRETATION. This was a randomized crossover trial. Seventeen patients requiring permanent pacemakers for symptomatic bradyarrythmias were recruited from a pacemaker clinic. None were known to have sleep-disordered breathing prior to recruitment. One month after pacemaker insertion they underwent polysomnography and were then randomized to receive either 1 month of nocturnal overdrive pacing as previously, followed by 1 month with the pacemaker switched off or vice versa. Polysomnography was repeated at the end of each limb. Two patients dropped out, leaving 15 in the analysis. The prevalence of OSAHS in this population was high, 87% having an AHI of >15. No improvement was seen in AHI or sleep architecture associated with atrial overdrive pacing in this study.

Comment

This study does not support atrial overdrive pacing as an effective treatment for OSAHS. Although similar in terms of age, sex and body mass index to those studied by Garrigue *et al.* |**37**|, the two study populations were quite different. The patients in this study all had OSAHS rather than a mix of central sleep apnoea and OSAHS, their LVEF (± SD) was significantly higher (64 ± 11 vs 54 ± 11%) and their inclusion was not dependent on the presence of symptoms of sleep-disordered breathing. The results lend support to the theory that improvements in OSAHS with atrial overdrive pacing may be secondary to improvements in central sleep apnoea. The lack of improvement in AHI with atrial overdrive pacing has been confirmed in further studies. Both Luthje *et al.* |**40**| and Simantirakis *et al.* |**41**| found no benefit of atrial overdrive pacing, and Sharafkhaneh *et al.* |**42**| reported only a small, non-significant reduction in AHI.

Also of interest in this study was the high prevalence of patients with OSAHS, none of whom had previously sought investigation. Given this high prevalence, it has been suggested that the minute ventilation sensors within pacemakers could be used to detect OSAHS in this population |**43,44**|.

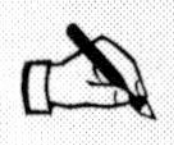

Atrial overdrive pacing compared to CPAP in patients with obstructive sleep apnoea syndrome

Unterberg C, Luthje L, Szych J, Vollmann D, Hasenfuss G, Andreas S. *Eur Heart J* 2005; **26**: 2568–75

BACKGROUND. In the trials discussed above, all patients had an indication for pacemaker insertion and had not previously sought medical attention for symptoms of sleep-disordered breathing. This trial concentrated on patients with known symptomatic OSAHS in whom there was no conventional indication for pacemaker insertion, and hence was more representative of the OSAHS population as a whole. Comparison was made with conventional CPAP therapy.

INTERPRETATION. This was a randomized crossover study. Patients who had initially reported daytime sleepiness and were subsequently diagnosed with OSAHS and commenced on CPAP therapy were eligible for inclusion. After baseline polysomnography, patients were randomized to either a night of standard CPAP therapy followed by a night of atrial overdrive pacing (with a temporary pacing wire) set at 15 b.p.m. above their previously determined mean nocturnal heart rate or vice versa. Twelve patients were recruited but the trial was stopped after ten because of the detection of significant differences in the primary outcome. The AHI was significantly higher during the pacing night than the CPAP night (39.1 vs 2.2; *P* = 0.002) (Fig. 10.5). Oxygen saturations were significantly higher and arousals significantly lower on the CPAP night.

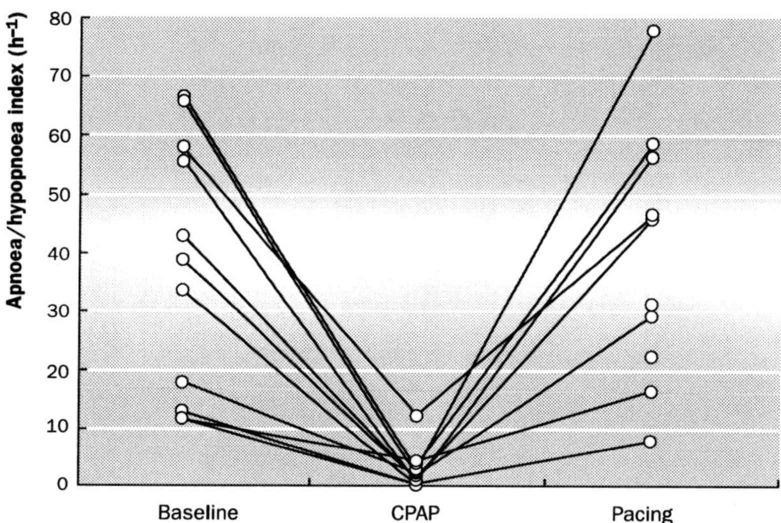

Fig. 10.5 Effect of CPAP and pacing on the apnoea/hypopnoea index (AHI). The *circles* represent the AHI of all individual patients. Source: Unterberg *et al.* (2005).

Comment

This study confirms the lack of effect of atrial overdrive pacing on AHI in a typical OSAHS population. Similarly, in a randomized crossover trial of patients with known OSAHS who had refused or were unable to tolerate CPAP, no improvement in AHI was seen with atrial overdrive pacing [45]. These studies, along with others [40–42] demonstrate no role for atrial overdrive pacing in the treatment of OSAHS.

References

1. Bearpark H, Elliott L, Grunstein R, Cullen S, Schneider H, Althaus W, Sullivan C. Snoring and sleep apnea. A population study in Australian men. *Am J Respir Crit Care Med* 1995; **151**: 1459–65.

2. Young T, Palta M, Dempsey J, Skatrud J, Weber S, Badr S. The occurrence of sleep-disordered breathing among middle-aged adults. *N Engl J Med* 1993; **328**: 1230–5.

3. Stradling JR, Barbour C, Glennon J, Langford BA, Crosby JH. Prevalence of sleepiness and its relation to autonomic arousals and increased inspiratory effort in a community based population of men and women. *J Sleep Res* 2000; **9**: 381–8.

4. Javaheri S, Parker TJ, Liming JD, Corbett WS, Nishiyama H, Wexler L, Roselle GA. Sleep apnea in 81 ambulatory male patients with stable heart failure: Types and their prevalences, consequences, and presentations. *Circulation* 1998; **97**: 2154–9.

5. Solin P, Bergin P, Richardson M, Kaye DM, Walters EH, Naughton MT. Influence of pulmonary capillary wedge pressure on central apnea in heart failure. *Circulation* 1999; **99**: 1574–9.

6. Arzt M, Young T, Finn L, Skatrud JB, Ryan CM, Newton GE, Mak S, Parker JD, Floras JS, Bradley TD. Sleepiness and sleep in patients with both systolic heart failure and obstructive sleep apnoea. *Arch Intern Med* 2006; **166**: 1716–22.

7. Hedner J, Ejnell H, Caidahl K. Left ventricular hypertrophy independent of hypertension in patients with obstructive sleep apnoea. *J Hypertens* 1990; **8**: 941–6.

8. Alchanatis M, Tourkohoriti G, Kosmas EN, Panoutsopoulos G, Kakouros S, Papadima K, Gaga M, Jordanoglou JB. Evidence for left ventricular dysfunction in patients with obstructive sleep apnoea syndrome. *Eur Respir J* 2002; **20**: 1239–45.

9. Arias MA, García-Río F, Alonso-Fernández A, Mediano O, Martínez I, Villamor J. Obstructive sleep apnea syndrome affects left ventricular diastolic function: Effects of nasal continuous positive airway pressure in men. *Circulation* 2005; **112**: 375–83.

10. Roebuck T, Solin P, Kaye DM, Bergin P, Bailey M, Naughton MT. Increased long-term mortality in heart failure due to sleep apnoea is not yet proven. *Eur Respir J* 2004; **23**: 735–40.

11. Mansfield DR, Gollogly NC, Kaye DM, Richardson M, Bergin P, Naughton MT. Controlled trial of continuous positive airway pressure in obstructive sleep apnea and heart failure. *Am J Respir Crit Care* 2004; **169**: 361–6.

12. Kaneko Y, Floras JS, Usui K, Plante J, Tkacova R, Kubo T, Ando S, Bradley TD. Cardiovascular effects of continuous positive airway pressure in patients with heart failure and obstructive sleep apnea. *N Engl J Med* 2003; **348**: 1233–41.

13. Stradling JR, Pepperell JCT, Davies RJO. Sleep apnoea and hypertension: proof at last? *Thorax* 2001; **56** (Suppl 11): ii45–ii9.

14. Marin JM, Carrizo SJ, Vicente E, Agusti AG. Long-term cardiovascular outcomes in men with obstructive sleep apnoea-hypopnoea with or without treatment with continuous positive airway pressure: an observational study. *Lancet* 2005; **365**: 1046–53.

15. Sin DD, Fitzgerald F, Parker JD, Newton G, Floras JS, Bradley TD. Risk factors for central and obstructive sleep apnea in 450 men and women with congestive heart failure. *Am J Respir Crit Care Med* 1999; **160**: 1101–6.

16. Tkacova R, Niroumand M, Lorenzi-Filho G, Bradley TD. Overnight shift from obstructive to central apneas in patients with heart failure: Role of PCO2 and circulatory delay. *Circulation* 2001; **103**: 238–43.

17. Javaheri S. A mechanism of central sleep apnea in patients with heart failure. *N Engl J Med* 1999; **341**: 949–54.

18. Lanfranchi PA, Braghiroli A Bosimini E, Mazzuero G, Colombo R, Donner CF, Giannuzzi P. Prognostic value of nocturnal Cheyne-Stokes respiration in chronic heart failure. *Circulation* 1999; **99**: 1435–40.

19. Hanly PJ, Zuberi-Khokhar NS. Increased mortality associated with Cheyne-Stokes respiration in patients with congestive heart failure. *Am J Respir Crit Care Med* 1996; **153**: 272–6.

20. Cormican LJ, Williams A. Sleep disordered breathing and its treatment in congestive heart failure. *Heart* 2005; **91**: 1265–70.

21. Naughton MT, Liu PP, Benard DC, Goldstein RS, Bradley TD. Treatment of congestive heart failure and Cheyne-Stokes respiration during sleep by continuous positive airway pressure. *Am J Respir Crit Care* 1995; **151**: 92–7.

22. Sin DD, Logan AG, Fitzgerald FS, Liu PP, Bradley TD. Effects of continuous positive airway pressure on cardiovascular outcomes in heart failure patients with and without Cheyne-Stokes respiration. *Circulation* 2000; **102**: 61–6.

23. Pepperell JCT, Maskell NA, Jones DR, Langford-Wiley BA, Crosthwaite N, Stradling JR, Davies RJO. A randomised controlled trial of adaptive ventilation for Cheyne-Stokes breathing in heart failure. *Am J Respir Crit Care* 2003; **168**: 1109–14.

24. Teschler H, Dohring J, Wang Y-M, Berthon-Jones M. Adaptive pressure support servo-ventilation. A novel treatment for Cheyne-Stokes respiration in heart failure. *Am J Respir Crit Care* 2001; **164**: 614–19.

25. Franklin KA, Eriksson P, Sahlin C, Lundgren R. Reversal of central sleep apnea with oxygen. *Chest* 1997; **111**: 163–9.

26. Krachman SL, D'Alonzo GE, Berger, TJ, Eisen HJ. Comparison of oxygen therapy with nasal continuous positive airway pressure on Cheyne-Stokes respiration during sleep in congestive heart failure. *Chest* 1999; **116**: 1550–7.

27. Staniforth AD, Kinnear WJM, Starling R, Hetmanski DJ, Cowley AJ. Effect of oxygen on sleep quality, cognitive function and sympathetic activity in patients with chronic heart failure and Cheyne-Stokes respiration. *Eur Heart J* 1998; **19**: 922–8.

28. Ponikowski P, Francis DP, Piepoli MF, Davies LC, Chua TP, Davos CH, Florea V, Banasiak W, Poole-Wilson PA, Coats AJS, Anker SD. Enhanced ventilatory response to exercise in patients with chronic heart failure and preserved exercise tolerance. *Circulation* 2001; **103**: 967–72.

29. Metra M, Dei Cas L, Panina G, Visioli O. Exercise hyperventilation in chronic congestive heart failure and its relation to functional capacity and haemodynamics. *Am J Cardiol* 1992; **70**: 622–8.

30. Arzt M, Harth M, Luchner A, Muders F, Holmer SR, Blumberg FC, Riegger GAJ, Pfeifer M. Enhanced ventilatory response to exercise in patients with chronic heart failure and central sleep apnea. *Circulation* 2003; **107**: 1998–2003.

31. Chua TP, Ponikowski P, Harrington D, Anker SD, Webb-Peploe K, Clark AL, Poole-Wilson PA, Coats AJS. Clinical correlates and prognostic significance of the ventilatory response to exercise in chronic heart failure. *J Am Coll Cardiol* 1997; **29**: 1585–90.

32. Arena R, Myers J, Aslam SS, Varughese EB, Peberdy MA. Peak VO2 and VE/VCO2 slope in patients with heart failure: a prognostic comparison. *Am Heart J* 2004; **147**: 354–60.

33. Kleber FX, Vietzke G, Wernecke KD, Bauer U, Opitz C, Wensel R, Sperfeld A, Glaser S. Impairment of ventilatory efficiency in heart failure: Prognostic impact. *Circulation* 2001; **101**: 2803–9.

34. Arzt M, Schulz M, Wensel R, Montalvan S, Blumberg FC, Riegger GAJ, Pfeifer M. Nocturnal continuous positive airway pressure improves ventilatory efficiency during exercise in patients with chronic heart failure. *Chest* 2005; **127**: 794–802.

35. Bradley TD, Logan AG, Kimoff RJ, Series F, Morrison D, Ferguson K, Belenkie I, Pfeifer M, Fleetham J, Hanly P, Smilovitch M, Tomlinson G, Floras JS. Continuous positive airway pressure for central sleep apnea and heart failure. *N Engl J Med* 2005; **353** (19): 2025–33.

36. Becker HF, Koehler U, Stammnitz A, Peter JH. Heart block in patients with sleep apnoea. *Thorax* 1998; **53** (Suppl 3): S29–S32.

37. Garrigue S, Bordier P, Jais P, Shah DC, Hocini M, Raherison C, Tunon De Lara M, Haissaguerre M, Clementy J. Benefit of atrial pacing in sleep apnoea syndrome. *N Engl J Med* 2002; **346**: 404–12.

38. Garrigue S, Bordier P, Barold SS, Clementy J. Sleep apnoea: A new indication for cardiac pacing. *Pacing Clin Electrophysiol* 2004; **27**: 204–11.

39. McArdle N, Devereux G, Heidarnejad H, Engleman HM, Mackay TW, Douglas NJ. Longterm use of CPAP therapy for sleep apnoea/hypopnoea syndrome. *Am J Respir Crit Care Med* 1999; **159**: 1108–14.

40. Luthje L, Unterberg-Buchwald C, Dajani D, Vollmann D, Hasenfuss G, Andreas S. Atrial overdrive pacing in patients with sleep apnea with implanted pacemaker. *Am J Respir Crit Care Med* 2005; **172**: 118–22.

41. Simantirakis EN, Schiza SE, Chrysostomakis SI, Chlouverakis GI, Klapsinos NC, Siafakas NM, Vardas PE. Atrial overdrive pacing for the obstructive sleep apnea-hypopnea syndrome. *N Engl J Med* 2005; **353**: 2568–77.

42. Sharafkhaneh A, Sharafkhaneh H, Bredikus A, Guilleminault C, Bozkurt B, Hirshkowitz M. Effect of atrial overdrive pacing on obstructive sleep apnea in patients with systolic heart failure. *Sleep Med* 2007; **8**: 31–6.

43. Scharf C, Cho YK, Bloch KE, Brunckhorst C, Duru F, Balaban K, Foldvary N, Liu L, Burgess RC, Candinas R, Wilkoff BL. Diagnosis of sleep-related breathing disorders by visual analysis of transthoracic impedance signals in pacemakers. *Circulation* 2004; **110**: 2562–7.

44. Defave P, Pepin J-L, Poezevara Y, Mabo P, Murgatroyd F, Levy P, Garrigue S. Automatic recognition of abnormal respiratory events during sleep by a pacemaker transthoracic impedance sensor. *J Cardiovasc Electrophysiol* 2004; **15**: 1034–40.

45. Krahn AD, Yee R, Erickson MK, Markowitz, Gula LJ, Klein GJ, Skanes AC, George CF, Ferguson KA. Physiologic pacing in patients with obstructive sleep apnea: a prospective, randomized crossover trial. *J Am Coll Cardiol* 2006; **47**: 379–83.

11

The metabolic syndrome, disorders of glucose control and the obstructive sleep apnoea/ hypopnoea syndrome

RENATA RIHA

Introduction

The link between metabolic syndrome, disorders of glucose metabolism and apnoea/hypopnoea syndrome (OSAHS) is currently the subject of intensive research. The contextual basis for these forays into non-respiratory fields of medicine lies in the observation that obesity is the commonest predisposing factor for OSAHS [1]. OSAHS has been shown in many epidemiological studies to result in several long-term sequelae, such as hypertension, cardiovascular disease, and increased morbidity and mortality [2,3]. There is mounting evidence that intermittent hypoxia has adverse effects on the biological regulation of the vascular endothelium and results in increased oxidative stress [4–6].

Since obesity is integral to the definition of metabolic syndrome as well as being a risk factor for disorders of glucose metabolism, it remains to be ascertained whether the observed associations with sleep-disordered breathing are causal or simply correlated as a result of having a shared confounder.

The metabolic syndrome

Definitions of the metabolic syndrome vary, but generally the following criteria should be met in order to make this diagnosis: fasting hyperglycaemia, high blood pressure, central obesity (visceral adiposity), a decreased concentration of high-density lipoprotein cholesterol and elevated triglycerides. The entire area, however, is complicated by the existence of four accepted definitions, which makes it difficult to reproduce studies (Table 11.1). The definition from the International Diabetes Federation (IDF) in May 2005 was intended to replace the 1999 World Health Organization (WHO) definition.

The true prevalence of metabolic syndrome varies according to the definition used. Other factors contributing potentially to its development, such as ageing, smoking, alcohol consumption, diet and physical inactivity, are difficult to factor into the equation. However, it is well accepted that obesity is the driving force for the development of metabolic syndrome [7] and that metabolic syndrome *per se* is the major risk factor for the development of diabetes mellitus [8] and cardiovascular disease [9]. A number of paradoxes remain. Not all obese people have metabolic syndrome, although a reduction in obesity leads to resolution of the metabolic syndrome [10] and insulin resistance can occur independently of obesity [11]. Intra-abdominal fat is associated with the vast majority of risk factors [12].

Table 11.1 Definitions of the metabolic syndrome

WHO criteria (1999)

Presence of diabetes mellitus, impaired glucose tolerance, impaired fasting glucose or insulin resistance, *and* two of the following:
blood pressure $\geq$140/90 mmHg
dyslipidaemia: triglycerides $\geq$1.695 mmol/l *and/or* HDL-C $\leq$0.9 mmol/l (male), $\leq$1.0 mmol/l (female)
central obesity: waist:hip ratio >0.90 (male), >0.85 (female), *and/or* body mass index >30 kg/m^2
microalbuminuria: urinary albumin excretion ratio $\geq$20 mg/min *or* albumin:creatinine ratio $\geq$30mg/g

European Group for the Study of Insulin Resistance (1999)

Insulin resistance defined as the top 25% of the fasting insulin values among non-diabetic individuals *and* two or more of the following:
central obesity: waist circumference $\geq$94 cm (male), $\geq$80 cm (female)
dyslipidaemia: triglycerides $\geq$2.0 mmol/l *and/or* HDL-C <1.0 mg/dl *or* treated for dyslipidaemia
hypertension: blood pressure $\geq$140/90 mmHg or antihypertensive medication
fasting plasma glucose $\geq$6.1 mmol/l

National Cholesterol Education Program—Adult Treatment Panel III (2001, 2005)

At least three of the following:
central obesity: waist circumference $\geq$102 cm (male), $\geq$88 cm (female)
dyslipidaemia: triglycerides $\geq$1.695 mmol/l
dyslipidaemia: HDL-C <40 mg/dl (male), <50 mg/dl (female)
blood pressure $\geq$130/85 mmHg
fasting plasma glucose $\geq$6.1 mmol/l

International Diabetes Federation (2005)

Central obesity
Waist circumference: ethnicity-specific[a]
plus any two of the following:
Raised triglycerides
>150 mg/dl (1.7 mmol/l)
Specific treatment for this abnormality
Reduced HDL-C
<40 mg/dl (1.03 mmol/l) in men
<50 mg/dl (1.29 mmol/l) in women

International Diabetes Federation (2005) (*cont.*)

Specific treatment for this abnormality
Raised blood pressure
Systolic ≥130 mmHg
Diastolic ≥85 mmHg
Treatment of previously diagnosed hypertension
Raised fasting plasma glucose[b]
Fasting plasma glucose ≥100 mg/dl (5.6 mmol/l)
Previously diagnosed type II diabetes
If above 5.6 mmol/l or 100 mg/dl, oral glucose tolerance test is strongly recommended, but is not necessary to define presence of syndrome

HDL-C, high-density lipoprotein cholesterol.
[a]If body mass index is over 30 kg/m^2, central obesity can be assumed and waist circumference does not need to be measured.
[b]In clinical practice impaired glucose tolerance is acceptable, but all reports of prevalence of metabolic syndrome should use only fasting plasma glucose and presence of previously diagnosed diabetes to define hyperglycaemia. Prevalences also incorporating 2-h glucose results can be added as supplementary findings.

Is apnoea/hypopnoea syndrome a manifestation of the metabolic syndrome?

Some have argued this to be the case, based largely on the presence of hypercytokinaemia, hyperleptinaemia, insulin resistance, hypertension and visceral obesity in disproportionate measure in the population with OSAHS [13]. When obesity has been controlled for, OSAHS has still been shown to be highly significantly associated with hypercytokinaemia, higher leptin levels, insulin resistance and hypertension [13,14].

Should hypertension be a diagnostic criterion of metabolic syndrome in OSAHS?

Sleep-disordered breathing alone has been shown to be an independent factor in the development of hypertension. The pathophysiology of hypertension in this situation may be more complex, involving mechanisms related to repetitive episodes of airway occlusion, periodic hypoxaemia and hypercapnia, changes in intrathoracic pressure and increases in sympathetic tone. Inflammation as a consequence of elevated levels of circulating pro-inflammatory cytokines may also play a contributory role. Tumour necrosis factor -α (TNF-α) and interleukin 6 (IL-6) are elevated in OSAHS independently of obesity and the circadian rhythm of secretion is disrupted [13,15]. Additionally, other mediators of inflammation are also elevated, including intercellular adhesion molecule 1 and C-reactive protein (CRP) [16].

Disorders of glucose metabolism

The area of disordered glucose metabolism is complex. In this chapter the focus will be on type II diabetes mellitus and pre-diabetic states. The most recent revision of the diagnostic criteria for diabetes mellitus from the American Diabetes Association, in 2003, maintained the following criteria: elevated fasting plasma glucose, random elevated glucose concentration with symptoms, or an abnormal oral glucose tolerance test (OGTT). Elevated fasting glucose is considered to be a glucose concentration of 5.6–6.9 mmol/l (100–125 mg/dl); impaired glucose tolerance as a 2-h post-challenge glucose level of 7.8–11.1 mmol/l (140–199 mg/dl); and type II diabetes is diagnosed as a fasting glucose level in excess of 6.9 mmol/l (125 mg/dl) or if the 2-h glucose after a 75 g oral glucose load is a minimum of 11.0 mmol/l (200 mg/dl) [18].

The risk of developing diabetes mellitus in states of impaired glucose tolerance is very high. At present it is estimated that type II diabetes affects about 5.9% of adults in the USA and this figure is predicted to rise by 50% in the next 3 years [19,20]. Methods of measuring insulin resistance and glucose tolerance rely heavily on the technique and the population setting in which they are employed. Insulin resistance is currently considered a major risk factor for the development of type II diabetes, hypertension, dyslipidaemia and atherosclerosis. For over 20 years, methods have been devised to measure the status of insulin resistance. The 'gold standard' against which all indices have been tested is the hyperinsulinaemic–euglycaemic clamp (HEC), which suffers from methodological problems [21]. The most commonly used of all derived indices is the homeostasis model assessment of insulin resistance (HOMA-IR), largely owing to its simplicity. This model was initially derived in 1985 and since then has been found to have correlations with estimates obtained by the HEC ranging from 0.88 to 0.59 [22,23]. The HOMA-IR is computed using the following equation:

$$\text{IR HOMA} = \text{insulin level fasting} \times \text{glucose level fasting}/22.5$$

The most common application is for large epidemiological studies where only fasting glucose and insulin levels are available, so its utility in small-scale studies is less validated. Neither the HOMA-IR nor any other derived index of insulin sensitivity is an appropriate measure in a frankly diabetic population. Furthermore, the application of the HOMA-IR in clinical practice is limited because of the lack of reference values. Use of these indices should ideally be restricted to predicting the risk of developing type II diabetes in a healthy population under study compared with individuals with impaired glucose metabolism, and to assessing the degree of insulin sensitivity in non-diabetic populations with risk factors for the development of diabetes [21]. No index has been found to be useful in small-scale studies, in individual patients or in studies looking at specific treatment effects and outcomes in detail.

Is obstructive sleep apnoea/hypopnoea syndrome a state of insulin resistance?

The association of OSAHS with disordered glucose metabolism is even more problematic than its association with metabolic syndrome.

The presence of sleep-disordered breathing in patients with type I diabetes mellitus was noted several decades ago [24]. Recently, interest has been diverted to sleep-disordered breathing in the context of type II diabetes mellitus. Several epidemiological studies have also suggested an independent association of OSAHS with impaired glucose tolerance and insulin resistance [25, 26].

In established type II diabetes, significant relationships have been found among sleep-disordered breathing, fasting insulin, glucose and haemoglobin A_{1c} (glycosylated haemoglobin, HbA_{1c}) levels, independently of obesity as determined by the waist–hip ratio [27].

A review of studies examining the effect of continuous positive airway pressure (CPAP) treatment in sleep apnoea patients on insulin resistance has shown largely negative results (Table 11.2). However, the total number of patients treated is small and, apart from one study, no matched controls were included. Of the studies looking specifically at sleep-disordered breathing in the context of type II diabetes, the results appear to favour treatment with CPAP (Table 11.3). Once again, the number of patients treated is minute, bearing in mind that type II diabetes and OSAHS occur with nearly equal frequency in the adult population of industrialized countries.

Table 11.2 The effects of CPAP on glucose metabolism in OSAHS

n	Control group	Parameter studied	Duration	Results	Reference
31	31 with OSAHS	OGTT Insulin measurements	6 months	No change except with weight loss	[28]
6	None	Invasive glucose, insulin and C-peptide sampling during sleep	One night	No change during sleep	[29]
10	Matched controls	Fasting insulin	3 months	No change in levels	[30]
40	None	HEC	3 months	Improved insulin sensitivity at 2 days and 3 months	[31]
9	None	Fasting glucose and insulin	6 months	No change	[32]
7	None	HEC	3 months	No change	[33]
8	None	Glucose insulin samples in sleep	1 night	No change	[34]
16	None	OGTT in 10 patients HEC in 6 patients	2 months	No change	[35]
5	None	Fasting glucose and insulin Glucose insulin samples during sleep	2 months	Increase in fasting and nocturnal glucose No change in fasting or nocturnal insulin levels	[36]

HEC, hyperinsulinaemic–euglycaemic clamp; OGTT, oral glucose tolerance test.

Table 11.3 The effects of CPAP on glucose metabolism in type II diabetics with sleep-disordered breathing

n	Control group	Parameter studied	Duration	Results	Reference
10	None	HEC Fasting glucose and insulin	4 months	Improvement in insulin responsiveness No change in fasting glucose or insulin	|27|
9	None	HEC	3 months	Improved insulin sensitivity	|37|
38	None	HbA$_{1c}$	Variable	Reduction in HbA$_{1c}$	|38|

HEC, hyperinsulinaemic–euglycaemic clamp; HbA1c, glycosylated haemoglobin.

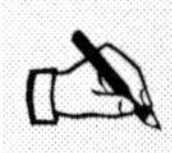

Obstructive sleep apnoea is independently associated with the metabolic syndrome but not insulin resistance state

Gruber A, Horwood F, Sithole J, Ali NJ, Idris I. *Cardiovasc Diabetol* 2006; **5**: 22–8

BACKGROUND. **Obstructive apnoea/hypopnoea syndrome has many features in common with metabolic syndrome and is associated with increased cardiovascular morbidity and mortality. The authors addressed the component parts of metabolic syndrome, including insulin resistance, albuminuria and cardiovascular risk factors, in patients with and without sleep-disordered breathing.**

INTERPRETATION. In this study, patients with OSAHS had a greater body mass index, waist circumference, systolic blood pressure, fasting glucose, fasting triglyceride, fasting insulin, HOMA and Epworth sleepiness score (ESS) compared with patients without OSAHS. Surprisingly, adjustment of confounding factors in logistic regression analysis showed no statistically significant association of OSAHS with insulin resistance alone (as defined by the HOMA score), although there was an association with metabolic syndrome as defined by the IDF guidelines.

Comment

This prospective study from Nottingham, UK, recruited 38 subjects with OSAHS (diagnosed using the VISI-3 sleep diagnosis system [Stowood Scientific Instruments Ltd, Oxford, UK]) and 41 patients without OSAHS. Daytime sleepiness was assessed using the ESS. Insulin resistance was defined using the HOMA-IR index and metabolic syndrome using the IDF guidelines. Unsurprisingly, patients in this small cohort had a greater body mass index, waist circumference, systolic blood pressure, fasting glucose, fasting triglyceride, fasting insulin, HOMA and ESS compared with non-OSAHS patients. The prevalence of metabolic syndrome was thus significantly higher in OSAHS compared with non-OSAHS patients (73 vs

37%; $P <0.001$). The prevalence of microalbuminuria ranged from 6.7% in the non-OSAHS group to 10.8% in the OSAHS group. When the findings were adjusted for significant confounders, such as age, body mass index and smoking history, only fasting glucose and triglycerides and ESS were independently associated with a diagnosis of OSAHS. The risk of metabolic syndrome was increased nearly 6-fold (odds ratio [OR] 5.88; 95% confidence interval [CI] 1.96–17.63; $P = 0.002$). There was no independent association for OSAHS and insulin resistance (OR 0.54; 95% CI 0.54–1.64; $P = 0.3$). Adjustment was also made for waist circumference as it is strongly correlated with body mass index ($r = 0.86$). The association between OSAHS and metabolic syndrome persisted despite this adjustment ($P = 0.002$).

The study had several shortcomings, including a small cohort, no prospective matching of the controls, and potential intrasubject confounding related to treatment of cardiovascular disease in the context of metabolic syndrome.

Although the value of teasing out the component parts of metabolic syndrome and analysing them separately is questionable, the finding that there is little correlation between insulin resistance and metabolic syndrome may explain why so many studies examining the effects of CPAP treatment on insulin sensitivity in OSAHS subjects have shown little effect (the number of subjects is small and the severity of OSAHS may vary). Despite a strong correlation with the gold standard insulin-clamp technique ($r = 0.82$) |39|, HOMA-IR may be an insufficiently sensitive method of documenting the insulin resistance state. Studies from more general population cohorts support this view |40|.

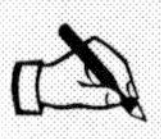

Type 2 diabetes, glycaemic control, and continuous positive airway pressure in obstructive sleep apnoea

Babu AR, Herdegen J, Fogelfeld L, Shott S, Mazzone T. *Arch Intern Med* 2005; **165**: 447–52

BACKGROUND. Treatment of sleep-disordered breathing in patients with type II diabetes mellitus has been shown to improve glucose control and insulin resistance. The effects of CPAP treatment on glycaemic control in a group of obese patients with type II diabetes were assessed in the context of CPAP adherence and more practical clinical measures, such as HbA$_{1c}$, as well as an invasive measure using a 24-h glucose monitoring system.

INTERPRETATION. Obese patients with type II diabetes mellitus and sleep-disordered breathing who were adherent with CPAP treatment had significant reductions in post-prandial glucose measurements and in HbA$_{1c}$. These changes were not seen in those using CPAP for less than 4 h a night or less.

Comment

This prospective study of the effects of CPAP on glucose homeostasis in obese type II diabetics with sleep-disordered breathing used both simple measures of assessing glucose control and a more invasive 72-h monitoring system to measure interstitial glucose levels. Using the invasive measurements, there was a significant mean reduction for the group as a whole in post-prandial glucose values compared with baseline. In 17 patients with an HbA_{1c} of >7% (consistent with moderate control), there was a significant reduction in their HbA_{1c} levels after a mean usage time of CPAP of 83 ± 50 days. Those who used CPAP for more than 4 h a day had an incrementally greater decrease compared with those who were not so adherent with treatment.

Overall, the patient group was very obese, with an average body mass index of 42.7 ± 8.7. The duration of diabetes was 8.3 ± 6.8 years and the baseline HbA_{1c} level was $8.3 \pm 2.2\%$. Seventeen patients were taking oral hypoglycaemics, four were on insulin and four were taking a combination of the two. Patients were sleepy (ESS 14 ± 6) and the apnoea/hypopnoea index (AHI) was 56 ± 37, therefore moderate to severe.

The biggest strength of the study was the use of an invasive monitor which recorded blood glucose every 5 min for 72 h. Thus, post-prandial glucose changes were clearly demonstrated. This approach is potentially more sensitive than fasting glucose levels and may be preferable for small group sizes. The limitations of the study include the small sample size, which may make subgroup analysis more hazardous unless the effect demonstrated is large. There was also no placebo group and no blinding to outcomes of the study, so it must be interpreted with some caution. Nevertheless, the authors point out that in this field of research, which is very flawed at present, most studies have not controlled for adherence with CPAP and thus positive treatment effects may be masked.

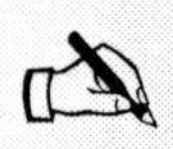

Obstructive sleep apnoea syndromes, plasma adiponectin levels, and insulin resistance

Makino S, Handa H, Suzukawa K, *et al*. *Clin Endocrinol* 2006; **64**: 12–19

BACKGROUND. Adiponectin is an adipocytokine discovered in 1996 and produced abundantly in adipocytes. There is an inverse correlation between plasma adiponectin levels and obesity. Low plasma adiponectin levels are thought to be a risk factor for cardiovascular, metabolic and cerebrovascular disorders due to reduced antagonism to the insulin resistance-producing effect of TNF-α.

INTERPRETATION. Adiponectin is one of several adipocytokines investigated in the context of OSAHS largely on the basis of its novelty. Sleep-disordered breathing in this study was found to be correlated with insulin resistance independently of obesity. Plasma adiponectin levels were found to be more closely correlated with obesity than sleep-disordered breathing. Plasma adiponectin levels were also independent determinants of insulin resistance, as measured using HOMA-IR. The role of adipocytokines in the generation of insulin resistance requires further study outwith the field of sleep-disordered breathing.

Comment

In a bid for novelty, much recent work in the area of OSAHS has focused on assaying plasma levels of various inflammatory markers, some of whose roles and pathways are as yet unclear. How sleep-disordered breathing affects plasma levels of these markers and vice versa is even more obscure. Additionally, it is probably unhelpful to study them in isolation. The aims of this Japanese study were to evaluate insulin resistance, as measured using HOMA-IR, in patients with various degrees of OSAHS (defined as mild, moderate or severe using the criteria of the American Sleep Disorders Association) and also measure plasma adiponectin levels to explore any association between these three variables.

Consecutive patients were recruited to the study from a sleep disorders laboratory; blood was taken whilst the patients were supine and the patients fasted the morning after overnight polysomnography. Only patients diagnosed with diabetes mellitus were excluded from the study. Intra-abdominal visceral fat area and subcutaneous fat area were measured by computed tomography (CT). Factors associated with metabolic syndrome were significantly more common in severe sleep-disordered breathing and, not surprisingly, the HOMA-IR of the patients with severe OSAHS was higher than that of the patients with mild ($P<0.05$) or moderate ($P<0.01$) OSAHS. In this study, the HOMA-IR was weakly but positively correlated with HbA_{1c}, diastolic blood pressure and triglycerides. Plasma adiponectin level did not differ among the three groups of patients and was not correlated with any other variables examined except for visceral fat area on CT scanning. Further modelling using stepwise multiple regression analysis was employed and the results suggested that the AHI as well as the plasma adiponectin level was strongly correlated with HOMA-IR. This study had several limitations, including the lack of a control group, single measurements of insulin and adiponectin levels, and a large number of uncontrolled variables in the group studied, including medication for cardiovascular disease. At best it suggests an association of insulin resistance with the severity of sleep apnoea. Reader, beware of statistical magic!

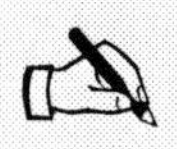

Prevalence of obstructive sleep apnoea in men with type 2 diabetes

West SD, Nicoll DJ, Stradling JR. *Thorax* 2006; **61**: 945–50

BACKGROUND. The prevalence of impaired glucose tolerance and type II diabetes mellitus is known to be high in patients with OSAHS. The prevalence of sleep-disordered breathing in patients with type II diabetes is currently unknown.

INTERPRETATION. The prevalence of obstructive sleep apnoea in a population of men with type II diabetes was significantly higher (17%) than in a general male population (6%) from the same region of England. Body mass index and diabetes were also shown to be significant predictors of the presence of obstructive sleep apnoea. The severity of obstructive sleep apnoea was also weakly correlated with the HbA_{1c} level and remained significant after correction for obesity.

Comment

This thoughtfully executed study examined the prevalence of OSAHS in male patients with type II diabetes in comparison with the prevalence in a general male population from the same area. It is surprising that other large cohorts of patients had not been interrogated previously, such as the NHANES (National Health and Nutrition Examination Survey) cohort in the USA.

Screening questionnaires were sent to 1676 men with type II diabetes from local hospital and selected general practice databases, with a 56% response rate. Of the responders, 4% were already known to have OSAHS. The remainder of the group were split into those with a high risk of OSAHS and those with a low risk of OSAHS (a slightly modified version of the Berlin questionnaire was used [41]). High-risk patients constituted 56% of the cohort. Screening oximetry was performed in 124 high-risk men and 116 low-risk men. In total, 44 patients had OSAHS on a portable sleep study system (18%); 17 of the men commenced CPAP. Interestingly, the HbA_{1c} level showed no significant correlation between the high-risk and low-risk groups. Patients from the hospital database did, however, have a positive but weak correlation of their HbA_{1c} levels with dips of more than 4% in arterial oxygen saturation on overnight oximetry when body mass index was controlled for ($r = 0.2$; $P = 0.03$). Table 11.4 demonstrates the characteristics of patients from the study diagnosed with OSAHS from the high- and low-risk groups.

The importance of this study lies in alerting clinicians who are managing patients with type II diabetes to the possibility of OSAHS in this population and to directing specific enquiries about snoring, witnessed apnoeas, nocturnal choking arousals and excessive daytime sleepiness appropriately to the patient (and

Table 11.4 Characteristics of known OSA, 'high' and 'low' risk questionnaire respondents

	Known OSA ($n = 39$)	'High' risk ($n = 528$)	'Low' risk ($n = 362$)	p-value between groups
Age	61.1 (10.5, 30–75)[1]	60.5 (9.7, 30–76)[1]	62.3 (9.5, 31–76)[1]	0.03
BMI	34.9 (5.8, 24–50)[1]	30.8 (5.6, 17.4–53.2)[2]	27.5 (3.9, 18.1–42.6)[3]	<0.001
Neck size	45.5 (3.6, 35.6–53.3)[1]	43.4 (3.0, 35.6–55.9)[2]	41.7 (2.8, 33.0–50.8)[3]	<0.001
HbA1c%	8.1 (1.9, 5.8–14.7)	8.3 (1.5, 5.1–13.5)	8.3 (1.7, 5.2–14.2)	0.9

Results are shown as mean (SD, 0–100% range). Groups with different superscript numbers are significantly different from each other.
Source: West *et al.* (2006).

partner). Apart from obesity and possible autonomic neuropathy, the mechanism of sleep-disordered breathing in this group requires further elucidation, especially regarding fat distribution. Epidemiological work also needs to be carried out in the female population.

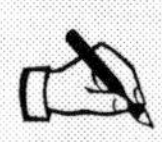

Treatment with continuous positive airway pressure may affect blood glucose levels in nondiabetic patients with obstructive sleep apnea syndrome

Czupryniak L, Loba J, Pawlowski M, Nowak D, Bialasiewicz P. *Sleep* 2005; **28**: 601–3

BACKGROUND. In several cohort and epidemiological studies, OSAHS has been associated with increased insulin resistance. Data on the early or late effects of CPAP treatment on glucose metabolism in OSAHS have yielded largely conflicting results.

INTERPRETATION. In a group of nine non-diabetic but obese subjects with OSAHS, one night of CPAP treatment resulted in raised fasting insulin, overnight glucose levels and HOMA-IR, despite correction of sleep-disordered breathing. This may be the result of a surge in growth hormone (due to re-establishment of normal sleep architecture) leading to growth-hormone-induced lipolysis. However, this is merely speculation.

Comment

This is a small study using a continuous glucose monitoring system (CGMS) to document glucose levels in non-diabetic patients with moderate to severe sleep apnoea on two separate nights; initially in the diagnostic study, then in a CPAP titration study. In the oral glucose tolerance test, two patients were found to have impaired OGTT. There were no statistically significant changes in the results for fasting insulin resistance and HOMA-IR after the CPAP night compared with baseline, but there was a tendency for values to be higher. Mean glucose values using CGMS were significantly higher on the CPAP night.

Strangely, no statistically significant correlations were noted for 60- and 120-min plasma glucose levels in the OGTT or CGMS readings. No food diaries were kept.

The authors speculated that CPAP, in correcting previously disordered sleep architecture on the first treatment night, might contribute to increased secretion of growth hormone. Cooper *et al.* |29| have shown that CPAP treatment causes significant increases in growth hormone levels, which in turn can result in elevations in plasma free fatty acids and 3-hydroxybutyrate, products of growth-hormone-stimulated lipolysis. Growth hormone is secreted during slow-wave sleep. Because this study did not use polysomnography, these comments remain conjectural at best.

Overall, the value of the study lies in highlighting the difficulties in measuring parameters of glucose intolerance accurately, but it adds further to the confusion regarding the true effects of CPAP on glucose metabolism in non-diabetic patients with OSAHS.

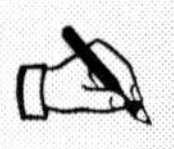

CPAP treatment of a population-based sample – what are the benefits and the treatment compliance?

Lindberg E, Berne C, Elmasry A, Hedner J, Janson C. *Sleep Med* 2006; **7**: 553–60

BACKGROUND. One cohort study has shown that CPAP can improve insulin sensitivity in severe obstructive sleep apnoea |37|. There is limited evidence that this is the case in subjects who have fewer symptoms or who have just mild–moderate OSAHS. Furthermore, studies looking at subjects who deny sleepiness with sleep-disordered breathing show that compliance with CPAP usage is limited |48|.

INTERPRETATION. Three weeks of CPAP treatment, even in subjects with an AHI >10, irrespective of symptoms resulted in reductions in serum insulin and insulin resistance and an increase in insulin-like growth factor 1 (IGF-1). Further improvements occurred in quality of life. However, adherence with CPAP at 6 months was present in only 29% of the group who initially started it, and these subjects had been subjectively sleepier at baseline. Despite physiological benefits, long-term CPAP adherence is largely determined by the perception of sleepiness.

Comment

This was a well-conducted, albeit small, study addressing several questions regarding the use of CPAP in less symptomatic subjects. Thirty-eight men with an AHI >10 were treated with CPAP irrespective of symptoms. Controls had an AHI <10 and were matched for age and hypertension. Evaluation of metabolic parameters was carried out at 3 weeks and 6 months. Interestingly, the reason for the significant reductions in serum insulin and insulin resistance in the CPAP group compared with controls may reside in the fact that glucose, HOMA-IR and serum insulin rose in the control group over the 3-week period. What the authors did find was that the men who were considerably more sleepy at the start of the study (ESS >8) were more likely to have a greater increase in their serum IGF-1 concentration compared with men with an ESS <8. The change in IGF-1 was maintained in those who continued to be compliant with CPAP at 6 months. Once again, this study confirms that adherence to CPAP was significantly more likely to be maintained if there was a baseline level of sleepiness.

The major limitation of the study is the low power for detecting a difference in metabolic parameters, but the differences reported suggest that the effect is sufficiently large to be valid. Since CPAP may have beneficial effects even in asymptomatic subjects, further developments of equivalently efficacious treatments need to continue.

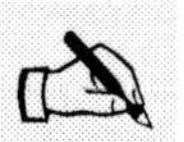

Cardiovascular and metabolic effects of CPAP in obese males with OSA

Coughlin SR, Mawdsley L, Mugarza JA, Wilding JPH, Calverley PMA. *Eur Respir J* 2007; **29**: 720–7

BACKGROUND. Although much work still needs to be done to establish cause and effect, metabolic syndrome occurs commonly in the context of OSAHS. Treatment of OSAHS with CPAP has been shown to reduce daytime sleepiness and improve health status in randomized, placebo-controlled trials l42,43l. The literature on the effects of CPAP on metabolic syndrome *per se* is less robust, being based largely on uncontrolled trials of short duration.

INTERPRETATION. Use of CPAP for 6 weeks, compared with sham CPAP, did not show any improvements in serum glucose, lipids, insulin resistance or the proportion of patients classified as having metabolic syndrome. However, there was a significant fall in blood pressure and an improvement in baroreceptor sensitivity. This suggests that the time course of changes in metabolic variables in OSAHS is longer than previously reported or is not as significant in a more general OSAHS population.

Comment

Of all the trials reported in the literature to date, this is the only trial that has used the randomized, placebo-controlled, blinded crossover trial method in an attempt to properly evaluate the association between treatment of OSAHS and metabolic parameters.

Thirty-four obese Caucasians (body mass index $36.1 \pm 7.6 \text{ kg/m}^2$) with severe OSAHS (respiratory disturbance index 39.7 ± 13.8) were randomized to either therapeutic CPAP or sham CPAP for a period of 6 weeks. All subjects were naive to CPAP. Subjects were excluded if there were any abnormalities on electrocardiogram (ECG), evidence of diabetes type II, renal, liver or cardiac disease or severe hypertension. The diagnosis of sleep-disordered breathing was made using polysomnography. Serum levels of insulin and fasting glucose were analysed using commercial kits according to standard hospital practice. HOMA-IR was calculated using a standard algorithm. Metabolic syndrome was defined using the National Cholesterol Education Program criteria (Table 11.1).

Compared with subjects receiving sham CPAP, those receiving therapeutic CPAP showed a decrease of 6.7 mmHg in the mean waking systolic blood pressure and a decrease of 4.9 mmHg in diastolic pressure. The difference was greatest for those using CPAP for more than 3.5 h a night.

The results overall suggest that although CPAP is sufficient to reduce sympathetic activation enough to effect change in cardiovascular variables, other factors are most likely involved in the changes observed in metabolic variables. It is possible that obesity *per se* is more intimately linked with the evolution of metabolic syndrome rather than that of sleep-disordered breathing, and that epidemiological associations are just that. The authors also postulate that there may be a threshold level of obesity at which excess body fat is the principal determinant of insulin sensitivity regardless of the degree of sleep-disordered breathing or intermittent hypoxaemia.

Conclusion

The role of sleep-disordered breathing in the development of metabolic syndrome remains inconclusive. Although there are strong epidemiological data supporting an association, treatment studies of OSAHS have proved unhelpful to date in elucidating a causal mechanism. Indices measuring insulin resistance have significant limitations and are poorly adaptable to individual cases, especially in relation to treatment effects over short time periods.

The important message is to be aware of comorbidities in OSAHS that may be amenable to lifestyle and simple pharmacological intervention, such as raised triglycerides, hypercholesterolaemia and impaired glucose tolerance.

Obstructive sleep apnoea/hypopnoea syndrome is recognized as an independent risk factor for hypertension and CPAP is a highly effective treatment [44,45]. Whether CPAP is as effective in patients without sleepiness remains to be shown [46–48].

References

1. Young T, Peppard PE, Taheri S. Excess weight and sleep-disordered breathing. *J Appl Physiol* 2005; **99**: 1592–9.

2. Marin JM, Carrizo SJ, Vicente E, Agusti AG. Long-term cardiovascular outcomes in men with obstructive sleep apnoea-hypopnoea with or without treatment with continuous positive airway pressure: an observational study. *Lancet* 2005; **365**: 1046–53.

3. Peppard PE, Young T, Palta M, Skatrud J. Prospective study of the association between sleep-disordered breathing and hypertension. *N Engl J Med* 2000; **342**: 1378–84.

4. Barcelo A, Barbe F, de la Pena M, Vila M, Perez G, Pierola J, Duran J, Agusti AG. Antioxidant status in patients with sleep apnoea and impact of continuous positive airway pressure treatment. *Eur Respir J* 2006; **27**: 756–60.

5. Lavie L, Dyugovskaya L, Lavie P. Sleep-apnea-related intermittent hypoxia and atherogenesis: adhesion molecules and monocytes/endothelial cells interactions. *Atherosclerosis* 2005; **183**: 183–4.

6. Lavie L. Sleep apnea syndrome, endothelial dysfunction, and cardiovascular morbidity. *Sleep* 2004; **27**: 1053–5.

7. Kraja AT, Hunt SC, Pankow JS, Myers RH, Heiss G, Lewis CE, Rao D, Province MA. An evaluation of the metabolic syndrome in the HyperGEN study. *Nutr Metab (Lond)* 2005; **2**: 2.

8. Haffner SM, Valdez RA, Hazuda HP, Mitchell BD, Morales PA, Stern MP. Prospective analysis of the insulin-resistance syndrome (syndrome X). *Diabetes* 1992; **41**: 715–22.

9. Isomaa B, Almgren P, Tuomi T, Forsen B, Lahti K, Nissen M, Taskinen MR, Groop L. Cardiovascular morbidity and mortality associated with the metabolic syndrome. *Diabetes Care* 2001; **24**: 683–9.

10. Lee W-J, Huang M-T, Wang W, Lin C-M, Chen T-C, Lai I-R. Effects of obesity surgery on the metabolic syndrome. *Arch Surg* 2004; **139**: 1088–92.

11. McLaughlin T, Allison G, Abbasi F, Lamendola C, Reaven G. Prevalence of insulin resistance and associated cardiovascular disease risk factors among normal weight, overweight, and obese individuals. *Metabolism* 2004; **53**: 495–9.

12. von Eyben FE, Mouritsen E, Holm J, Montvilas P, Dimcevski G, Suciu G, Helleberg I, Kristensen L, von Eyben R. Intra-abdominal obesity and metabolic risk factors: a study of young adults. *Int J Obes Relat Metab Disord* 2003; **27**: 941–9.

13. Vgontzas AN, Papanicolaou DA, Bixler EO, Hopper K, Lotsikas A, Lin HM, Kales A, Chrousos GP. Sleep apnea and daytime sleepiness and fatigue: relation to visceral obesity, insulin resistance, and hypercytokinemia. *J Clin Endocrinol Metab* 2000; **85**: 1151–8.

14. West SD, Nicoll DJ, Stradling JR. Prevalence of obstructive sleep apnoea in men with type 2 diabetes. *Thorax* 2006; **61**: 945–50.

15. Entzian P, Linnemann K, Schlaak M, Zabel P. Obstructive sleep apnea syndrome and circadian rhythms of hormones and cytokines. *Am J Respir Crit Care Med* 1996; **153**: 1080–6.

16. Mills PJ, Dimsdale JE. Sleep apnea: a model for studying cytokines, sleep, and sleep disruption. *Brain Behav Immun* 2004: **18**: 298–303.

17. Das UN. Is obesity an inflammatory condition? *Nutrition* 2001; **17**: 953–66.

18. Genuth S, Alberti KG, Bennett P, Buse J, Defronzo R, Kahn R, Kitzmiller J, Knowler WC, Lebovitz H, Lernmark A, Nathan D, Palmer J, Rizza R, Saudek C, Shaw J, Steffes M, Stern M, Tuomilehto J, Zimmet P; Expert Committee on the Diagnosis and Classification of Diabetes Mellitus. Follow-up report on the diagnosis of diabetes mellitus. *Diabetes Care* 2003; **26**: 3160–7.

19. Centers for Disease Control and Prevention. Prevalence of diabetes and impaired fasting glucose in adults–United States. 1999–2000. *MMWR Morb Mortal Wkly Rep* 2003; **52**: 833–7.

20. King H, Aubert RE, Herman WH. Global burden of diabetes, 1995–2025: prevalence, numerical estimates and projections. *Diabetes Care* 1998; **21**: 1414–31.

21. Radikova Z. Assessment of insulin sensitivity/resistance in epidemiological studies. *Endocr Regul* 2003; **37**: 189–94.

22. Matthews DR, Hosker JP, Rudenski AS, Naylor BA, Treacher DF, Turner RC. Homeostasis model assessment: insulin resistance and beta-cell function from fasting plasma glucose and insulin concentrations in man. *Diabetologia* 1985; **28**: 412–19.

23. Stumvoll M, Mitrakou A, Pimenta W, Jenssen T, Yki-Jarvinen H, Van Haeften T, Renn W, Gerich J. Use of the oral glucose tolerance test to assess insulin release and insulin sensitivity. *Diabetes Care* 2000; **23**: 295–301.

24. Rees PJ, Prior JG, Cochrane GM, Clark TJ. Sleep apnoea in diabetic patients with autonomic neuropathy. *J R Soc Med* 1981; **74**: 192–5.

25. Ip MS, Lam B, Ng MM, Lam WK, Tsang KW, Lam KS. Obstructive sleep apnea is independently associated with insulin resistance. *Am J Respir Crit Care Med* 2002; **165**: 670–6.

26. Punjabi NM, Sorkin JD, Katzel LI, Goldberg AP, Schwartz AR, Smith PL. Sleep-disordered breathing and insulin resistance in middle-aged and overweight men. *Am J Respir Crit Care Med* 2002; **165**: 677–82.

27. Brooks B, Cistulli PA, Borkman M, Ross G, McGhee S, Grunstein RR, Sullivan CE, Yue DK. Obstructive sleep apnea in obese noninsulin-dependent diabetic patients: effect of continuous positive airway pressure treatment on insulin responsiveness. *J Clin Endocrinol Metab* 1994; **79**: 1681–5.

28. Chin K, Shimizu K, Nakamura T, Narai N, Masuzaki H, Ogawa Y, Mishima M, Nakamura T, Nakao K, Ohi M. Changes in intra-abdominal visceral fat and serum leptin levels in patients with obstructive sleep apnea syndrome following nasal continuous positive airway pressure therapy. *Circulation* 1999; **100**: 706–12.

29. Cooper BG, White JE, Ashworth LA, Alberti KG, Gibson GJ. Hormonal and metabolic profiles in subjects with obstructive sleep apnea syndrome and the acute effects of nasal continuous positive airway pressure (CPAP) treatment. *Sleep* 1995; **18**: 172–9.

30. Davies RJ, Turner R, Crosby J, Stradling JR. Plasma insulin and lipid levels in untreated obstructive sleep apnoea and snoring; their comparison with matched controls and response to treatment. *J Sleep Res* 1994; **3**: 180–5.

31. Harsch IA, Schahin SP, Radespiel-Troger M, Weintz O, Jahreiss H, Fuchs FS, Wiest GH, Hahn EG, Lohmann T, Konturek PC, Ficker JH. Continuous positive airway pressure treatment rapidly improves insulin sensitivity in patients with obstructive sleep apnea syndrome. *Am J Respir Crit Care Med* 2004; **169**: 156–62.

32. Ip MS, Lam KS, Ho C, Tsang KW, Lam W. Serum leptin and vascular risk factors in obstructive sleep apnea. *Chest* 2000; **118**: 580–6.

33. Saarelainen S, Lahtela J, Kallonen E. Effect of nasal CPAP treatment on insulin sensitivity and plasma leptin. *Sleep Res* 1997; **6**: 146–7.

34. Saini J, Krieger J, Brandenberger G, Wittersheim G, Simon C, Follenius M. Continuous positive airway pressure treatment. Effects on growth hormone, insulin and glucose profiles in obstructive sleep apnea patients. *Horm Metab Res* 1993; **25**: 375–81.

35. Smurra M, Philip P, Taillard J, Guilleminault C, Bioulac B, Gin H. CPAP treatment does not affect glucose-insulin metabolism in sleep apneic patients. *Sleep Med* 2001; **2**: 207–13.

36. Stoohs RA, Facchini FS, Philip P, Valencia-Flores M, Guilleminault C. Selected cardiovascular risk factors in patients with obstructive sleep apnea: effect of nasal continuous positive airway pressure (n-CPAP). *Sleep* 1993; **16** (8 Suppl): S141–2.

37. Harsch IA, Schahin SP, Bruckner K, Radespiel-Troger M, Fuchs FS, Hahn EG, Konturek PC, Lohmann T, Ficker JH. The effect of continuous positive airway pressure treatment on insulin sensitivity in patients with obstructive sleep apnoea syndrome and type 2 diabetes. *Respiration* 2004; **71**: 252–9.

38. Hassaballa HA, Tulaimat A, Herdegen JJ, Mokhlesi B. The effect of continuous positive airway pressure on glucose control in diabetic patients with severe obstructive sleep apnea. *Sleep Breath* 2005; **9**: 176–80.

39. Bonora E, Targher G, Alberiche M, Bonadonna RC, Saggiani F, Zenere MB, Monauni T, Muggeo M. Homeostasis model assessment closely mirrors the glucose clamp technique in the assessment of insulin sensitivity: studies in subjects with various degrees of glucose tolerance and insulin sensitivity. *Diabetes Care* 2000; **23**: 57–63.

40. McLaughlin T, Abbasi F, Cheal K, Chu J, Lamendola C, Reaven G. Use of metabolic markers to identify overweight individuals who are insulin resistant. *Ann Intern Med* 2003; **139**: 802–9.

41. Netzer NC, Stoohs RA, Netzer CM, Clark K, Strohl KP. Using the Berlin questionnaire to identify patients at risk for the sleep apnea syndrome. *Ann Intern Med* 1999; **131**: 485–91.

42. Engleman HM, Martin SE, Deary IJ, Douglas NJ. Effect of continuous positive airway pressure treatment on daytime function in sleep apnoea/hypopnoea syndrome. *Lancet* 1994; **343**: 572–5.

43. Jenkinson C, Davies RJ, Mullins R, Stradling JR. Long-term benefits in self-reported health status of nasal continuous positive airway pressure therapy for obstructive sleep apnoea. *Q J Med* 2001; **94**: 95–9.

44. Faccenda JF, MacKay TW, Boon NA, Douglas NJ. Randomized placebo-controlled trial of continuous positive airway pressure on blood pressure in the sleep apnea-hypopnea syndrome. *Am J Respir Crit Care Med* 2001; **163**: 344–8.

45. Pepperell JC, Ramdassingh-Dow S, Crosthwaite N, Mullins R, Jenkinson C, Stradling JR, Davies RJ. Ambulatory blood pressure after therapeutic and subtherapeutic nasal continuous positive airway pressure for obstructive sleep apnoea: a randomised parallel trial. *Lancet* 2002; **359**: 204–10.

46. Robinson GV, Smith DM, Langford BA, Davies RJ, Stradling JR. Continuous positive airway pressure does not reduce blood pressure in nonsleepy hypertensive OSA patients. *Eur Respir J* 2006; **27**: 1229–35.

47. Hui DS, To KW, Ko FW, Fok JP, Chan MC, Ngai JC, Tung AH, Ho CW, Tong MW, Szeto CC, Yu CM. Nasal CPAP reduces systemic blood pressure in patients with obstructive sleep apnoea and mild sleepiness. *Thorax* 2006; **61**: 1083–90.

48. Barbe F, Mayoralas LR, Duran J, Masa JF, Maimo A, Montserrat JM, Monasterio C, Bosch M, Ladaria A, Rubio M, Rubio R, Medinas M, Hernandez L, Vidal S, Douglas NJ, Agusti AG. Treatment with continuous positive airway pressure is not effective in patients with sleep apnea but no daytime sleepiness. A randomized, controlled trial. *Ann Intern Med* 2001; **134**: 1015–23.

Part V

Interstitial lung disease

12

Idiopathic pulmonary fibrosis

NIK HIRANI, JOHN SIMPSON

Introduction

Idiopathic pulmonary fibrosis (IPF) is often considered an uncommon disease yet some 4000 new cases are diagnosed each year in the UK. Furthermore, the median survival time from diagnosis is 3 years. Only 40% of patients live beyond 5 years, a prognosis poorer than for cancer of the breast, colon or ovary, and for affected patients and the physicians who look after them there is an intense sense of frustration when challenged with coping with the symptoms and with managing IPF. Fortunately this frustration has driven investigators to undertake studies that have hugely advance our understanding of the disease process and may soon lead to effective therapy. The 2004 landmark study of interferon γ1b in IPF, although essentially negative, demonstrated that large multicentre, randomized trials in IPF are feasible [1]. Furthermore, the spin-off benefits of these large trials are that we now have an unprecedented insight into the natural history of IPF. Indeed, the first three papers in this chapter deal with the epidemiology and the clinical course of IPF. Clinicians will recognize from their own practice that IPF can run an unpredictable course and that some patients appear to decline rapidly after a prolonged period of apparent stability. Two of the papers discussed highlight the concept of acute exacerbation or accelerated decline in IPF, a phenomenon that has important implications for the management of IPF. Indeed, the unpredictable nature of IPF serves as a reminder that there is a need for robust, easily measured biomarkers of disease severity and progression. At present, a 10% fall in forced vital capacity (FVC) (or a 15% fall in pulmonary transfer factor for carbon monoxide [T_{LCO}]) in the first 6 months following diagnosis has emerged as the most powerful predictor of death [2–4]. In the interferon γ1b trial, a 10% decline in FVC was associated with a 2.4-fold increase in the risk of mortality, but 43% of patients still died without exhibiting any prior significant fall in FVC [5]. The roles of exercise testing, high-resolution computed tomography (HRCT) score and a serum marker of epithelial injury, all potential biomarkers of disease in IPF, are discussed below with reference to five recent key publications. Finally, four clinical trials and a meta-analysis are described and discussed in detail. In interpreting these studies, we consider various aspects of trial design and execution. It is worth contemplating two questions in particular that are highly pertinent to IPF in general and to clinical trials in IPF in particular.

Is the study population homogeneous and does it consist entirely of cases of idiopathic pulmonary fibrosis?

The 2002 joint statement of the American Thoracic Society and the European Respiratory Society (ATS/ERS) allowed a consensus view on the increasingly confusing nomenclature that has plagued the idiopathic interstitial pneumonias [6]. The committee surmised that IPF was defined by the pathological entity 'usual interstitial pneumonia' (UIP), but also established criteria for the diagnosis of IPF in the absence of a surgical lung biopsy (Table 12.1). Non-specific interstitial pneumonia (NSIP) was considered a provisional classification term. The purely cellular form of NSIP seems to be an uncommon, if not rare, disease. Fibrotic NSIP arises proportionately more often in association with connective tissue diseases than does UIP. However, it is still uncertain whether idiopathic fibrotic NSIP represents a distinct disease entirely separate from idiopathic UIP (IPF). In the absence of a highly characteristic HRCT pattern (bilateral, predominantly basal, predominantly subpleural reticular pattern with honeycomb cysts, traction bronchiectasis and minimal ground glass change), only a surgical lung biopsy will distinguish UIP (IPF) from fibrotic NSIP, and even then the histological diagnosis of NSIP is challenging, with only moderate agreement amongst expert pathologists as to what constitutes NSIP [7,8]. All recent large clinical trials of IPF have used the ATS/ERS consensus statement to define IPF, and the stringent inclusion criteria, HRCT scans and lung biopsies, where performed, have undergone rigorous assessment by expert panels. Whilst this admirably addresses the issue of a homogeneous population, it creates a genuine dilemma when attempting to extrapolate results from clinical trials back to IPF patients in everyday practice. The degree of diagnostic precision used in trial subjects is not readily attainable by most physicians seeing patients outside of speciality clinics and tertiary referral centres. On this basis it could be argued that the findings of such studies are not readily applicable to the 'average' patient. In routine clinical practice, IPF is a heterogeneous disease, in part because the clinical entity of UIP has a variable natural history but also because the diagnosis of IPF in all likelihood will encompass those with UIP and an unquantifiable proportion of patients with fibrotic NSIP. In this regard, the first paper discussed in this chapter, by Rudd *et al.*, is pertinent.

Were the appropriate end-points chosen for the study?

The aims of a clinical trial dictate the most appropriate outcome measure. For a large multicentre Phase III study of a disease with a high mortality rate, the most appropriate and robust end-point would be death. However, this requires several hundred patients if it is to be adequately powered, a formidable undertaking for an uncommon disease such as IPF. Even in the largest IPF clinical trial to date, with a total of 330 patients recruited, mortality was not used as a single end-point but rather one of a trio of 'progression-free survival' end-points [1]. Patients recruited to clinical trials in IPF tend to exhibit a more indolent course compared with IPF patients in clinical practice. This may in part be because a large number of patients

Table 12.1 ATS/ERS criteria for diagnosis of idiopathic pulmonary fibrosis in absence of surgical lung biopsy

Major criteria

Exclusion of other known causes of ILD such as certain drug toxicities, environmental exposures, and connective tissue diseases

Abnormal pulmonary function studies that include evidence of restriction (reduced VC, often with an increased FEV_1/FVC ratio) and impaired gas exchange [increased $P(A–a)O_2$, decreased PaO_2 with rest or exercise or decreased D_{LCO}]

Bibasilar reticular abnormalities with minimal ground-glass opacities on HRCT scans

Transbronchial lung biopsy or BAL showing no features to support an alternative diagnosis

Minor criteria

Age >50 yr

Insidious onset of otherwise unexplained dyspnoea on exertion

Duration of illness ≥3 mo

Bibasilar, inspiratory crackles (dry or 'Velcro'-type in quality)

In the immunocompetent adult, the presence of all of the major diagnostic criteria as well as at least three of the four minor criteria increases the likelihood of a correct clinical diagnosis of IPF. BAL, bronchoalveolar lavage; D_{LCO}, diffusing capacity of the lung for carbon monoxide; ILD, interstitial lung disease; VC, vital capacity. Source: ATS/ERS International Multidisciplinary Consensus Classification. Am J Respir Crit Care Med (2002); 165: 277–304.

recruited to IPF studies tend to be from a subgroup who have been followed up by a physician for a considerable length of time (prevalent cases) as opposed to patients who have had a new diagnosis of IPF (incident cases). In an ideal clinical trial, a high proportion of recruited patients should be incident cases of IPF.

Given that mortality is a worthy but ambitious end-point, several clinical trials in IPF, including those discussed in this chapter, have sought to employ surrogate end-points. An ideal surrogate would be one that reliably predicts subsequent mortality or at least reliably reflects a tangible benefit to the patient. This emphasizes the importance of defining physiological, radiological or molecular biomarkers of disease activity that may serve as potential end-points in clinical studies. The most robust biomarker in IPF is a >10% fall in FVC, but, as with mortality, using a >10% fall in FVC as the primary trial end-point would require a sample size of several hundred patients. The pros and cons of using alternative trial end-points are considered in the Comment sections in this chapter. An excellent detailed review of clinical trial end-points in IPF has recently been published [9].

Epidemiology and natural history of idiopathic pulmonary fibrosis

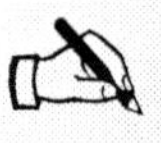

British Thoracic Society study on cryptogenic fibrosing alveolitis: response to treatment and survival.
Rudd RM, Prescott RJ, Chalmers JC, Johnston ID; British Thoracic Society.
Thorax 2007; **62**: 62–6

BACKGROUND. In 1997, the British Thoracic Society published an observational cross-sectional study of the clinical presenting features and initial treatment of 588 patients with cryptogenic fibrosing alveolitis (CFA) in the UK |10|. The term 'CFA' may be perplexing for readers outside the UK and even for younger physicians within the UK. In the ATS/ERS consensus statement of 2002, CFA was deemed to be synonymous with IPF. However, this simplistic interpretation is flawed; only a minority of CFA patients undergo surgical lung biopsy (8% in this UK cohort) and the non-biopsy criteria for diagnosing IPF are often not met because bronchoalveolar lavage (BAL) is not routinely performed in many cases. In reality, therefore, CFA should be considered a clinical syndrome rather than a disease entity, and most physicians would strive to categorize patients with CFA syndrome into those with IPF (i.e. idiopathic UIP), NSIP (fibrotic or cellular), other idiopathic interstitial pneumonias and, in some cases, hypersensitivity pneumonitis. In all likelihood, most patients with CFA syndrome have IPF but the contribution made by the other disease entities is unknown. This observational study is a follow-up of the original cohort of individuals with CFA syndrome. Whilst the relevance of the observations needs to be considered in the light of current understanding of idiopathic interstitial pneumonias, this study does provide important insights into the clinical course of a large group of patients with a uniform disease syndrome.

INTERPRETATION. This was an observational study such that the patients were treated entirely at the discretion of the participating clinicians, usually with corticosteroids with or without an immunomodulator, namely azathioprine or cyclophosphamide. One-third of the individuals started on therapy exhibited a significant improvement in lung function, defined as an increase of $\geq$10% in FVC or T_{LCO}, compared with 7% of those not receiving treatment ($P = 0.001$), and improved lung function at 3 months and at 1 year was an independent predictor of improved long-term survival. The overall 4-year survival of patients with CFA from study entry was 60.4% and the overall median survival time from entry was 2.43 years (95% confidence interval [CI] 2.17–3.18). The 445 patients who had received a specific treatment had identical survival to those who had not. CFA was the main or contributory cause in 73% of deaths and lung cancer was present in 12% of patients at death. Whilst CFA syndrome is clearly not directly analogous to IPF/UIP, the poor survival figures described here are sobering and similar to those reported in patients with IPF.

Comment

This is an observational study of 588 patients with a clinical presentation of CFA recruited between 1990 and 1992 and subsequently followed up in detail until 1996. Information regarding survival and cause of death was updated at the end of 2000. The average age at recruitment was 68 years and 63% were men. The data, therefore, were clearly being collected well before the current classification for idiopathic interstitial pneumonias as set out in the ATS/ERS consensus statement. The criteria for inclusion in this study were stated as a histological diagnosis of CFA or bilateral interstitial chest X-ray shadowing with bilateral basal inspiratory crackles together with a restrictive pattern on lung function testing. HRCT scanning, now considered a cornerstone of IPF diagnosis, was not routinely performed at the time and no data were collected subsequently.

Serial lung function data were collected but a considerable amount of data were reported missing. The results revealed that 76% of the 588 patients received some form of therapy, either just before entering the study or at some stage in the study. The majority of those who did receive therapy were started on treatment within 3 months of diagnosis (289 of 445 patients). Of the therapies given, monotherapy with prednisolone was administered in 55%, often at doses higher than 30 mg daily, and 12% received prednisolone combined with another immunomodulatory drug, usually azathioprine or cyclophosphamide. Lung function was measured 3 months after study entry and categorized into (i) improved, defined as an increase of 10% or more in either FVC or T_{LCO}; (ii) worsening, defined as a decrease in either FVC or T_{LCO} of 10%; or (iii) unchanged. One-third of the 155 patients started on treatment demonstrated improved lung function at 3 months, as defined above. Forty-four per cent remained stable and 20% had deteriorating lung function. These values compared with just 9 out of 129 patients (7%) who showed a spontaneous improvement in FVC at 3 months in the absence of treatment. The overall median survival time from entry was 2.43 years (95% CI 2.17–3.18). Younger age at entry, female sex, and higher percentage of predicted FVC and T_{LCO} were associated with greater chances of survival at 4 years. That the average age at presentation was 68 years is relevant, since this is perhaps 5–8 years older than similar case series from the USA, and may account for similar survival figures between those with CFA syndrome, which harbours some relatively benign entities, and those with IPF. The 445 patients who had received a specific treatment had identical survival to those who had not. Patients who had responded to treatment at 3 months had better lung function at 1 year and in turn better survival than those who remained stable, who in turn survived substantially longer than those who had deteriorated (Fig. 12.1). The causes of death were updated to 31 December 2000; 54% of patients had died primarily due to CFA, and 19% died partly due to CFA. Lung cancer was present in 12% of patients at death and contributed to 34 of the 398 deaths. Hence, CFA was the main or contributory cause in 292 of 398 (73%) of deaths. Smoking status did not affect survival significantly after allowing for age, sex and initial lung function.

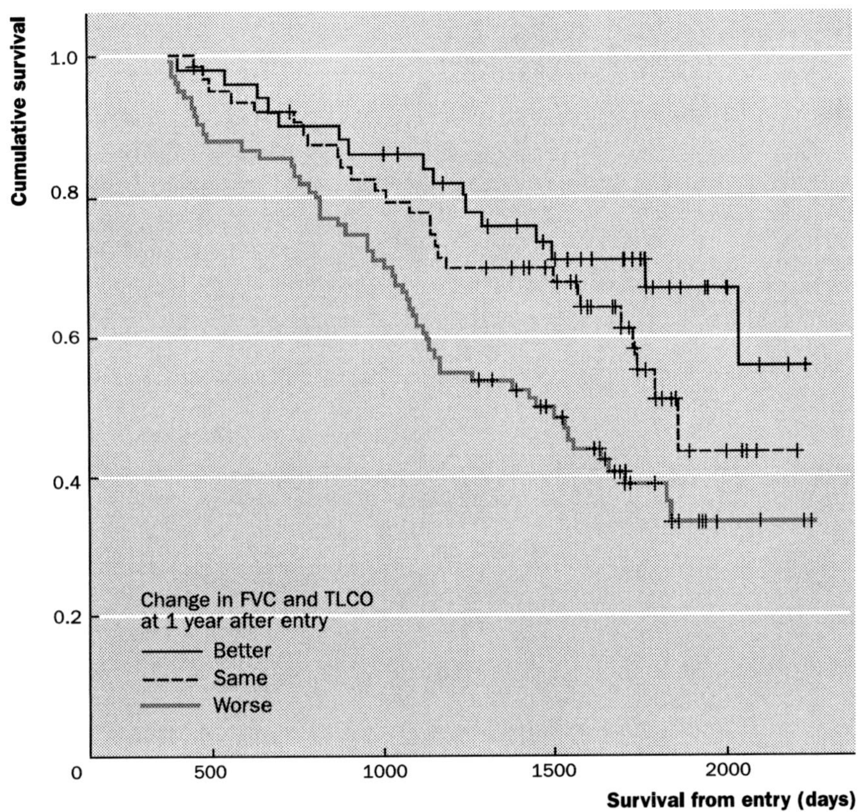

Fig. 12.1 Survival according to treatment response assessed at 1 year. Differences between groups were significant by the log-rank test ($P = 0.002$). FVC, forced vital capacity; T_{LCO}, carbon monoxide transfer factor. Source: Rudd *et al.* (2007).

The main strengths of this study were that a large number of patients were recruited in a variety of clinical settings rather than just specialist centres, and that the data on deaths were well recorded, such that survival data can be interpreted with great confidence. A median survival of only 2.43 years indicates that, despite the likely case-mix of disease entities within this group of patients, the overall clinical outcome is very similar to, if not indeed a little worse than, large case series from the USA of biopsy-proven IPF. The lung function data from this study are certainly less reliable than the survival data since a substantial number of data points were missing. For example, 3 months after study entry, lung function data were available for only 56% of eligible patients. The study hints, but by no means proves, that early treatment leads to better lung function that translates to better survival. A significant improvement in lung function following treatment is frequently reported in studies of IPF, as judged by post-ATS/ERS criteria, but this seems to occur only in approximately 10% of cases. For example, in the study by Antoniou and colleagues discussed in this chapter, only 6 of 68 patients (9%) responded to the high-dose steroids in the run-in period of the study. That 35% of patients should show a significant improvement suggests that many of these UK patients did not have IPF and may have had other idiopathic interstitial pneumonias of a predominantly inflammatory nature. Some years ago, a study by Nicholson and colleagues clearly demonstrated that in patients with a clinical diagnosis of CFA who had undergone a lung biopsy, reclassification into UIP, fibrotic NSIP and other inflammatory disorders neatly segregated the different prognoses of the three groups in addition to demonstrating that a significant response to steroid therapy was not a feature of UIP disease [11].

The clinical course of patients with idiopathic pulmonary fibrosis

Martinez FJ, Safrin S, Weycker D, Starko KM, Bradford WZ, King TE Jr, et al.
Ann Intern Med 2005; **142**: 963–7

BACKGROUND. The natural clinical course of IPF is surprisingly poorly understood and has never been studied prospectively in a large cohort of well-defined patients. The advent of international placebo-controlled, multicentre clinical trials has presented clinicians with an opportunity to study the course of the disease over time, at least in the subgroup of IPF patients deemed suitable for recruitment to clinical trials.

INTERPRETATION. In this study, the investigators took the opportunity to study the 168 participants in the placebo arm of a large multicentre, controlled study of interferon γ1b published in 2004 [1]. All patients recruited to this trial had IPF diagnosed in accordance with the ATS/ERS consensus criteria. Severity of disease ranged from mild, but showing evidence of decline, to advanced and all patients had either received or were receiving corticosteroid therapy. The main messages from the study are that patients with IPF often exhibit prolonged periods of stability that are punctuated by acute, often rapid, declines in lung function or acute exacerbation, which in turn is associated with a poor prognosis. Acute exacerbation was seen in one in ten patients, and of those who died during the 72 weeks of the study half exhibited an episode of rapid decline in the preceding 4 weeks. This insight into natural history has important clinical implications. In the subgroup of patients suitable for lung transplantation, an episode of acute exacerbation should lead to the prioritizing of that individual on the transplant list. Acute exacerbations and hospitalizations may also be potential end-points for future clinical trials.

Comment

This study of the natural history of IPF highlights aspects of the disease that many clinicians will recognize from their own practice but which had not previously been documented in a robust fashion in the literature. All patients had IPF by ATS/ERS criteria and were recruited to the placebo arm of a multicentre, controlled study of interferon γ1b [1]. The mean age of the 168 participants was 64 years and the male:female ratio was 2:1. Ninety per cent were defined as never smokers or ex-smokers. The mean time from diagnosis of IPF to recruitment into the study was 378 days. At entry, FVC ranged from 50 to 90% of predicted (median 64.5%) and T_{LCO} was required to be at least 20–25% of predicted. Hence, only those with very mild or very severe disease were excluded, and the majority had mild or moderate disease. As would be expected in a clinical trial of this type, the patients were closely monitored and various parameters were measured every 12 weeks. The paper focuses in particular on physiological variables, the number of hospitalizations and survival over the 72 weeks of the study. Each of these provides us with useful insights into the clinical course of IPF. Whereas the disease is often considered to be a relentless and progressive condition, the serial lung function data quite clearly show that many patients exhibit very little change in FVC or T_{LCO} over time (Fig. 12.2). In the 111 patients (66%) that survived to 72 weeks, the percentage of predicted FVC fell from 64.5 (SD 11.1) to 61 (SD 14.1) and the percentage of predicted T_{LCO} decreased from 37.8 (SD 11.1) to 37 (SD 19.9). Thirty-six (21.4%) patients died during the 72-week observation period and 89% of these deaths were considered to be IPF-related, as judged by the clinician investigator. Serial lung function in those who died show that, whilst there is significant variability between individuals, the overall trend is one of stable lung function followed by a rather abrupt decline in parameters, principally T_{LCO} and FVC, shortly before death (Fig. 12.3). Indeed, half of those who died exhibited an acute (4 weeks or less) deterioration just before death. Another important observation is that one-third of all recruited patients had a hospitalization on at least one occasion and in most cases this was due to a respiratory complication. Hospitalization episodes with IPF conferred a poor prognosis; of the 23% of patients who were hospitalized with a respiratory-related condition, a fifth subsequently died during the study period. In a subsequent letter to the journal, Martinez and colleagues provide further data that address a critically important question: can one predict which patients are likely to experience a sudden acute deterioration? [12] Baseline lung function variables, including the proportion of patients with a T_{LCO} of less than 40% (a cut-off shown in previous studies to identify short survival time [13]) was similar in those who did and did not exhibit acute deterioration. The baseline HRCT score also failed to distinguish those who would go on to experience acute exacerbation from those who did not.

The study does, of course, have important limitations that should curtail broad generalizations with regard to the true natural history of IPF. Firstly, and most importantly, it is well recognized that patients recruited to randomized controlled trials must by definition represent a particular subset, defined as they are by rigid inclusion/exclusion criteria. Being under the constant gaze of clinical investigators will also affect the course of disease by a magnitude that is hard to quantify. For comparison, the mortality at 48 weeks in this study was just 11%, compared with a

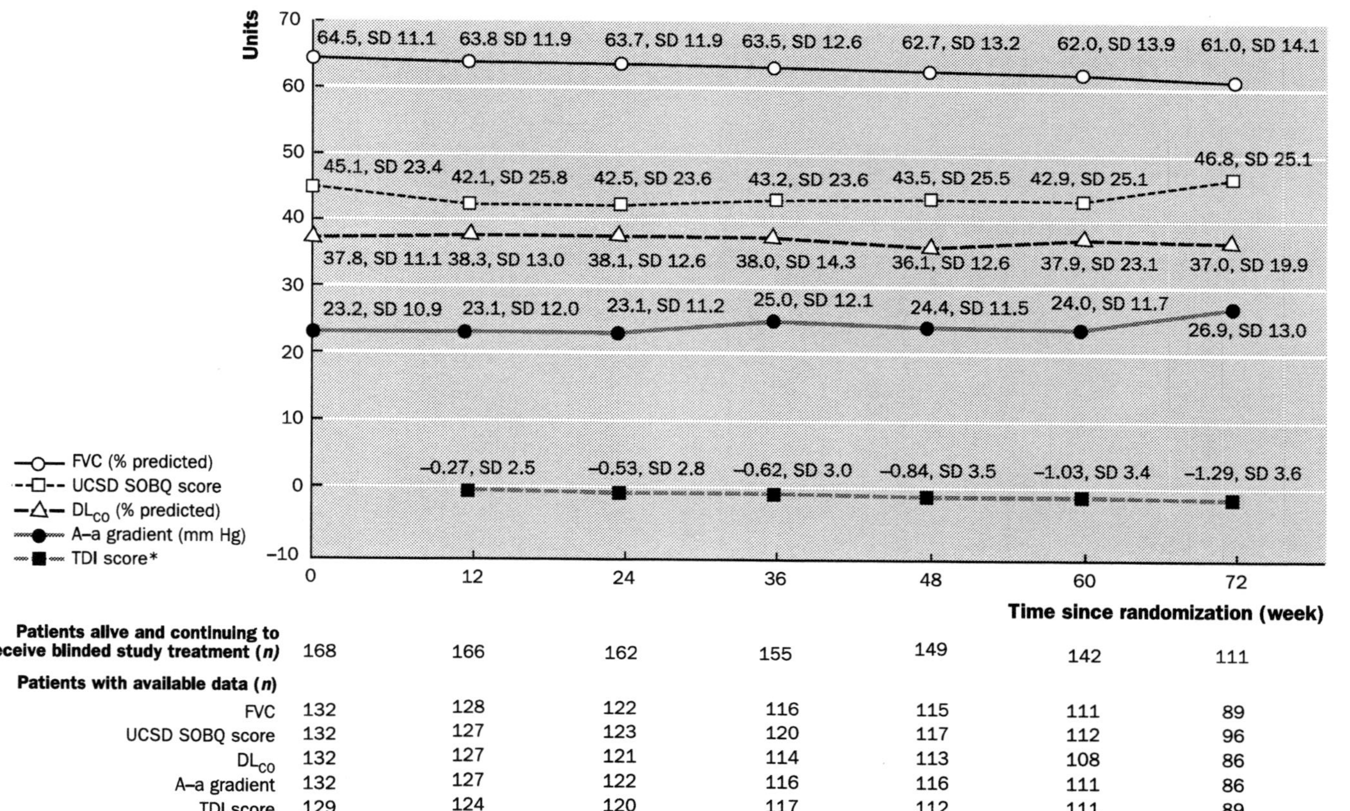

Patients alive and continuing to receive blinded study treatment (n)	168	166	162	155	149	142	111
Patients with available data (n)							
FVC	132	128	122	116	115	111	89
UCSD SOBQ score	132	127	123	120	117	112	96
DL_{CO}	132	127	121	114	113	108	86
A–a gradient	132	127	122	116	116	111	86
TDI score	129	124	120	117	112	111	89

Fig. 12.2 Measures of physiology and dyspnoea from study entry to week 72 for patients who survived throughout the trial. Values are mean and SD. A–a, alveolar–arterial gradient; $D_{L}CO$, diffusion capacity of carbon monoxide; TDI, Transition Dyspnea Index Questionnaire Score; UCSD SOBQ, score on the University of California, San Diego, Shortness of Breath Questionnaire. The TDI score denotes change from baseline. Source: Martinez et al. (2005).

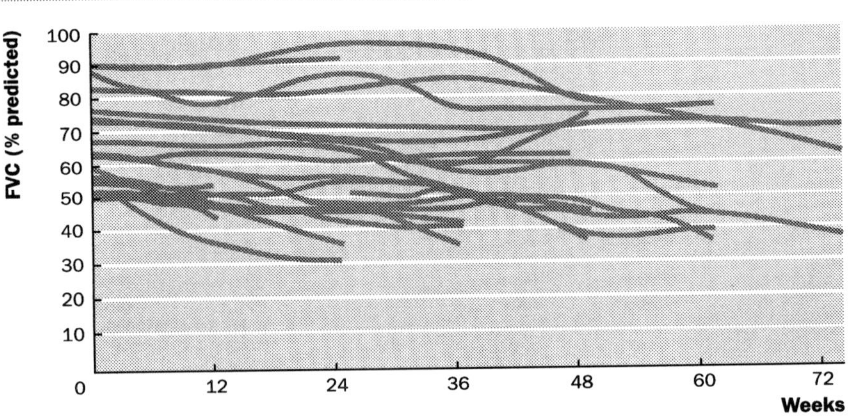

Fig. 12.3 Percentage of predicted FVC over the 72 weeks of the study period. Abrupt declines in lung function are commonly observed following periods of prolonged stability. Source: Martinez *et al.* (2005).

1-year mortality of 30% in patients with CFA syndrome under observation but outwith a clinical trial (see Rudd *et al.*). Secondly, whilst this was a placebo-controlled trial, this is not to say that participants received no treatment. Indeed, the inclusion criteria dictated that patients must have worsening of disease during the preceding 1 year despite receiving a total corticosteroid dose of 1800 mg or greater in the preceding 2 years. This is not a particularly large dose and, for example, a patient who had received a 3-month trial of prednisolone 20 mg daily would be eligible. Patients were also permitted to continue taking up to 15 mg prednisolone daily although it is not specified how many participants this applied to during the study period. A negligible number of patients received azathioprine or other immunosuppressive therapy during the study period. Thirdly, as discussed in our commentary on the paper by Kim *et al.* (below), the term 'acute exacerbation' or 'accelerated decline' does not have a readily acceptable definition. Similarly, the indications for hospitalization may be varied and were not pre-defined in this study. These issues need to be resolved before, for example, either acute exacerbation or hospitalization can be considered robust end-points for clinical studies.

From a practical point of view, the unpredictable nature of accelerated decline or acute exacerbations in IPF has a direct effect on patient care, most pressingly on the timing of lung transplantation for those who are eligible. Transplantation units should build in flexibility to allow rapid updating of their current transplant list to accommodate patients with seemingly stable IPF who exhibit sudden deterioration.

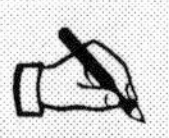

Acute exacerbation of idiopathic pulmonary fibrosis frequency and clinical features

Kim DS, Park JH, Park BK, Lee JS, Nicholson AG, Colby T. *Eur Resp J* 2006; **27**: 143–50

BACKGROUND. Many physicians who look after patients with IPF will recognize a subgroup in whom a period of stability that may continue for months or even years is punctuated by a rapid decline in lung function. Indeed, the important paper by Martinez and colleagues discussed above demonstrates this phenomenon of acute rapid deterioration, particularly in patients whose predicted diffusion capacity of carbon monoxide (T_{LCO}) is under 40%. Acute exacerbations of IPF, also termed 'accelerated decline', have been well reported in the Japanese medical literature. Sporadic descriptions have also appeared elsewhere, but the phenomenon is poorly understood and there is no universally accepted definition for acute exacerbation or accelerated decline. The original description by Kondoh defined acute exacerbation in IPF as including (i) worsening dyspnoea within 1 month; (ii) hypoxaemia with an arterial oxygen tension/inspired oxygen tension ratio of <225; (iii) newly developing chest X-ray infiltrates; and (iv) an absence of apparent infection or heart disease [14]. The present study provides further insights into the phenomenon of acute exacerbation in IPF.

INTERPRETATION. This study by Kim and colleagues reviews 147 patients from a large academic centre in Korea. All patients had a surgical lung biopsy confirming UIP. Of these 147 cases, eleven satisfied the criteria for acute exacerbation as defined by Kondoh [14]. This equated to a 1-year frequency of acute exacerbation of 8.5% and a 2-year frequency of 9.6%. All eleven patients had an HRCT scan, usually on the day of admission, and eight of the eleven patients also underwent BAL. Since these lavages were found to be sterile, these eight patients represent a well-defined subgroup of acute exacerbation in the absence of infection.

Comment

This is essentially a retrospective descriptive study but does add to our appreciation of the natural history of IPF. The 1 in 10 frequency of acute exacerbation described in this study is similar to that of acute decline in lung function described by Martinez and colleagues in North American patients in the paper discussed above. Another similarity is that predicting which patients will experience acute exacerbation remains a challenge; the authors found no obvious difference in age, sex, smoking status, the presence or absence of treatment (steroids or other cytotoxic drugs) or baseline lung function when comparing patients with acute exacerbation versus those without acute exacerbation. Two patients developed acute exacerbation shortly after surgical lung biopsy, a phenomenon that has been described previously, and other patients developed exacerbation following BAL. All eight patients displayed new diffuse bilateral ground-glass opacity on HRCT scanning, superimposed on the background fibrotic/ honeycomb changes. In addition to

BAL, culture of blood and serological testing for viruses were also negative. The differential cell count in the lavage fluid at the time of exacerbation was not significantly different from that seen in stable patients with IPF, revealing excess lymphocytes and neutrophils and, in a few cases, excess eosinophils. By definition, all patients had an HRCT scan that showed ground-glass opacification which was described as either peripheral, multifocal or diffuse. In four patients a surgical lung biopsy was performed at the time of acute exacerbation and all cases revealed UIP with superimposed diffuse alveolar damage. All patients with acute exacerbation were treated with broad-spectrum antibiotics and corticosteroids (up to 1 g methylprednisolone daily for 3 days in the case of six individuals). An important message from the study was that acute exacerbation is associated with a high mortality rate and that, despite mechanical ventilation in nine patients, the overall in-hospital mortality was 78%. The authors speculate that the phenomenon of acute exacerbation may actually be more common than they have described if one applies less rigid diagnostic criteria |**15**|. Although no clear risk factors for acute exacerbation were identified, the observation that surgical lung biopsy or possibly BAL may precipitate an acute deterioration is consistent with several previous reports |**16,17**|. From the limited literature available, diffuse alveolar damage seems to be the dominant histological finding in those who succumb to acute exacerbation. The practical implication is that, other than to exclude infection or malignancy, a surgical lung biopsy in a patient with known IPF and acute exacerbation is unlikely to provide material information that would change management. The role of corticosteroids in treating acute exacerbation of IPF is unclear. In this study all patients were given corticosteroids and the mortality rate was very high. There are numerous reports in the literature, all with small numbers, hinting that high doses of corticosteroids may be effective in this syndrome. However, several studies have now demonstrated that the outcome for patients with IPF admitted to the intensive care unit with respiratory failure is extremely poor, with a mortality of over 90% |**18–20**|.

Prognostic indicators in idiopathic pulmonary disease: lung function, HRCT and blood biomarkers

Several studies, albeit retrospective, have demonstrated the value of baseline lung function in stratifying disease severity and of changes in lung function in determining disease progression in IPF. Thus, it is accepted that lower baseline FVC and T_{LCO} generally indicate more advanced disease and early death. A baseline T_{LCO} of <40% appears to be the most robust independent cut-off for poor prognosis in multivariate analysis in patients with IPF |**13**|. Furthermore, this simple baseline measure predicts early death not just in IPF but also in fibrotic NSIP |**4**|. We now also know, from multiple retrospective studies, that 6-month changes in FVC (>10% change from baseline) and, to a lesser degree, T_{LCO} (>15% change from baseline) are powerful prognostic indicators in IPF |**2,3**|. As with baseline T_{LCO}, the 6-month changes confer prognostic significance not just in IPF but also in fibrotic NSIP, and indeed a change in physiology may be a more powerful indicator of prognosis than baseline histological diagnosis |3,21|. Intuitively, it would be reasonable to hypothesize that baseline exercise testing would provide valuable additional information with regard to the severity of disease. There are several different protocols for assessing physiology on exercise testing, but one of the most common, and indeed best studied in IPF, is the 6-min walking test. Lama and colleagues showed that desaturation to <88% was a powerful prognostic indicator in patients with fibrotic idiopathic interstitial pneumonia (UIP or NSIP) independently of other known prognostic indicators, namely age, smoking, sex, T_{LCO}, FVC or HRCT score |4,22|. In patients with IPF, the 4-year survival was 35% in those who did desaturate significantly compared with 69% in those who did not, and a fall in saturation of 4% or greater was associated with a 14-fold increase in mortality.

Thus, the baseline 6-min walking test does appear to provide important prognostic information above and beyond other measures of disease severity, and the value of this complex physiological test is further explored in the studies by Lettieri *et al.* and Lederer *et al.*, described below. With regard to changes in exercise test results over time, Eaton and colleagues |23| had demonstrated that the distance walked during the 6-min walking test, but not the amplitude of desaturation, was highly reproducible in patients with UIP and fibrotic NSIP, thus laying the foundation for the study by Flaherty and colleagues described below, in which the prognostic value of 6-month changes in exercise performance are addressed.

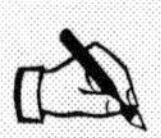

The distance-saturation product predicts mortality in idiopathic pulmonary fibrosis

Lettieri CJ, Nathan SD, Browning RF, Barnett SD, Ahmad S, Shorr AF. *Respir Med* 2006; **100**: 1734–41

BACKGROUND. This research group determined the individual prognostic accuracy of distance walked and oxygen saturation during the 6-min walking test in patients with IPF. A new composite index was defined: the distance–saturation product (DSP), which is the product of distance walked and lowest oxygen saturation during the 6-min walking test. The performance of the DSP was compared with the individual 6-min walking test parameters in predicting mortality. The group compared pulmonary function tests, 6-min walk parameters and the DSP between survivors and non-survivors. The ability of each measure to discriminate outcomes was determined by the use of receiver operating characteristic curves. Eighty-one patients (48 survivors and 33 non-survivors) were included.

INTERPRETATION. The investigators studied 81 patients with IPF who had baseline 6-min walking test results. Over 12 months, 41% died, and these individuals had walked a significantly shorter distance at baseline compared with survivors (181.3 ± 94.2 vs 407 ± 71.6 m; *P* = 0.005; summarized in Table 12.2). The DSP generated a cut-off value of ≥200 m% that was associated with greater discriminatory power (positive predictive value 87%, negative predictive value 86%) than either distance walked or degree of oxygen saturation alone (Table 12.3).

Table 12.2 Baseline patient variables

	Survivors (*n* = 48)	Non-survivors (*n* = 33)	*P*
Age (years)	59.4 ± 7.3	58.2 ± 8.7	0.31
% male	77.1	69.7	0.46
Supplemental oxygen requirement (%)	22.93	60.6	<0.001
FEV$_1$ (% predicted)	63.5 ± 14.4	62.0 ± 14.0	0.35
TLC (% predicted)	64.7 ± 15.2	66.6 ± 16.5	0.34
D$_{LCO}$ (% predicted)	41.9 ± 10.8	39.4 ± 12.6	0.22
Resting SpO$_2$ on room air (%)	97.4 ± 1.23	94.2 ± 2.6	0.007
Lowest SpO$_2$ on 6MWT (%)	89.4 ± 3.0	83.7 ± 3.3	<0.001
Desaturation during 6MWT (%)	7.9 ± 2.8	10.5 ± 3.3	0.002
Distance walked on 6MWT (m)	406.9 ± 71.6	181.3 ± 95.2	0.005
DSP (%)	364.8 ± 67.2	153.5 ± 81.5	<0.001

Abbreviations: D$_{LCO}$, diffusion capacity for carbon monoxide; DSP, distance–saturation product; FEV$_1$, forced expiratory volume in 1 s; FVC, forced vital capacity; SpO$_2$, oxygen saturation by pulse oximetry; TLC, total lung capacity; 6MWT, six-minute walk test.
Source: Lettieri *et al.* (2006).

Table 12.3 Screening characteristics of various parameters for mortality in IPF

	Sensitivity (%)	Specificity (%)	Positive predictive value (%)	Negative predictive value (%)	Accuracy (%)
DSP ≤200	78.8	91.7	86.7	86.7	86.8
Distance walked ≤300m	78.8	87.5	81.3	85.7	83.9
Lowest SpO$_2$ ≤88%	81.8	56.3	56.3	81.8	66.6
FVC 60–79% predicted	39.4	62.5	62.5	60.0	53.1

Abbreviations: DSP, distance–saturation product; FVC, forced vital capacity.
Source: Lettieri *et al.* (2006).

Comment

The value of the 6-min walking test has been further studied in this cohort of 106 patients, all fulfilling the ATS/ERS criteria for the diagnosis of IPF, from a large teaching hospital in the USA. Interestingly, the average age of these patients was just under 60 years, only slightly older than the average age of patients awaiting lung transplantation in the study by Lederer and colleagues. Of the 106 patients originally evaluated, 25 were excluded because they underwent lung transplantation, died shortly after initial evaluation or had a resting oxygen saturation of <88%, and were not able to perform the 6-min walking test on room air, as dictated in the study protocol. The primary end-point was 12-month survival following the initial 6-min walking test; of the 81 patients in the final cohort, 48 were deemed survivors and 33 non-survivors. The overall 12-month mortality of 40.7% for this seemingly unselected group of patients is certainly high and this may reflect quite advanced disease at presentation, as judged by, for example, the baseline D_{LCO}, which was just 40% of predicted. There was no difference in baseline static lung function tests between the survivors and non-survivors. Distance walked in the 6-min walking test was significantly lower in non-survivors compared with survivors (181.3 ± 94.2 vs 407 ± 71.6 m). In fact, the investigators found that a cut-off distance of 300 m or less yielded a positive predictive value of 81.3% and a negative predictive value of 85.7% for mortality.

The authors acknowledge that additional factors well known to influence survival, such as smoking history, age, comorbid conditions, HRCT appearance and lung histology, were not controlled for in their analysis. This study does, however, add to the growing body of evidence that the 6-min walking test serves as a potentially powerful baseline prognostic indicator in patients with IPF.

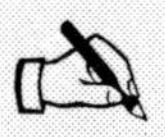

Six-minute-walk distance predicts waiting list survival in idiopathic pulmonary fibrosis

Lederer DJ, Arcasoy SM, Wilt JS, D'Ovidio F, Sonett JR, Kawut SM. *Am J Respir Crit Care Med* 2006; **174**: 659–64

BACKGROUND. The optimum time to proceed to surgery in patients with IPF suitable for lung transplantation is unknown. The investigators studied the baseline 6-min walking distance with the specific aim of determining a clinically useful cut-off distance that would reliably identify early mortality in those waiting for lung transplantation.

INTERPRETATION. Of 209 patients with IPF who were awaiting lung transplant and were followed up for 6 months after the 6-min walking test, 49 (23%) died. Using receiver operating characteristic curve analysis, an optimal cut-off distance of 207 m (683 feet) had a sensitivity of 74% (95% CI 61–86%) and a specificity of 73% (95% CI 66–79%) for death within 6 months, yielding a positive predicted value of 45% and a negative predicted value of 90%. The inability to walk more than 207 m was associated with a 5-fold increase in mortality after adjustment for age, sex, race, smoking, percentage of predicted FVC, pulmonary hypertension and other relevant factors (Fig. 12.4).

Comment

For patients with IPF who meet the required criteria, lung transplantation offers the prospect of a significantly improved prognosis and quality of life, with reported 1- and 2-year post-transplant survival rates around 80 and 65% respectively. However, around 50% of patients with pulmonary fibrosis die whilst on the waiting list for lung transplantation |24|. Lederer and colleagues have addressed a critically important question in the management of IPF: in patients suitable for transplantation, what is the optimal time to proceed to surgery? Whilst there is a body of

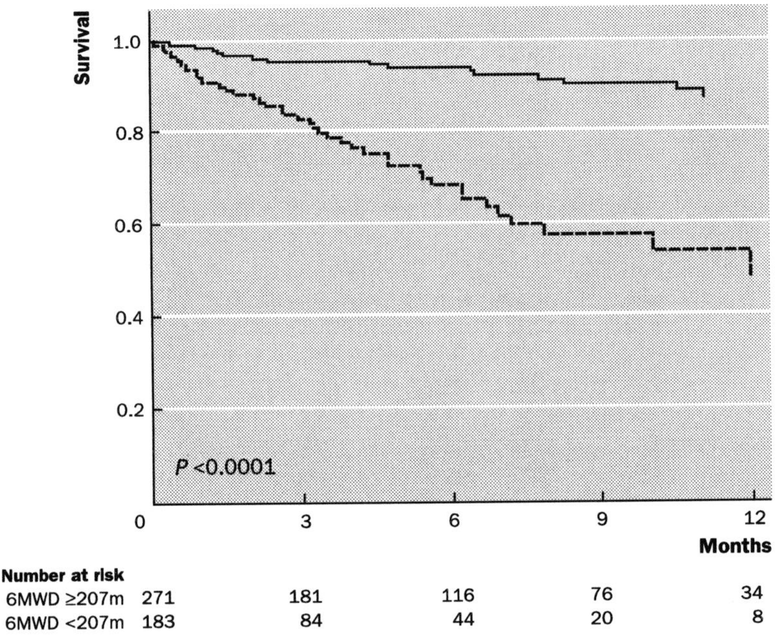

Number at risk

6MWD ≥207m	271	181	116	76	34
6MWD <207m	183	84	44	20	8

Fig. 12.4 Kaplan–Meier survival estimates for patients with idiopathic pulmonary fibrosis listed for lung transplantation. Six-minute walking distance (6MWD): *solid line* ≥207 m; *dotted line* <207 m. Source: Lederer *et al.* (2006).

data pertaining to prognostic biomarkers in IPF, by definition those listed for lung transplantation represent a distinct cohort.

In a previous study, this same group had reported that a 6-min walking distance of <350 m was associated with a shorter survival time compared with a distance of >350 m in patients with IPF evaluated for lung transplantation [25]. The present study is an extension with a specific aim of examining an optimal 6-min walking distance cut-off for mortality at 6 months. In contrast to the studies of Lettieri *et al.* and Flaherty *et al.*, patients in this study were permitted supplementary oxygen, and hence the prognostic value of desaturation <88% cannot be determined in this cohort. The United Network for Organ Sharing (UNOS) database includes 6-min walking distance as a continuous variable for candidates on a waiting list for lung transplantation. Of 454 patients classified as having IPF (not necessarily based on ATS/ERS criteria) and listed in the UNOS registry, 63 (14%) died and 191 (42%) underwent lung transplantation, roughly equally divided into single and bilateral transplants, over a 1-year period of follow-up. A total of 209 patients had a 6-month follow-up without undergoing lung transplantation, and 49 (23%) of these died during this 6-month period. Using receiver operating curve analysis, the authors found that an optimal cut-off of 207 m (683 feet) had a sensitivity of 74% (95% CI 61–86%) and a specificity of 73% (95% CI 66–79%) for death within 6 months, yielding a positive predicted value of 45% and a negative predicted value of 90%. The inability to walk more than 207 m was associated with a 5-fold increase in mortality. These figures are after adjustment for age, sex, race, height, smoking, education, percentage of predicted FVC, pulmonary hypertension, diabetes, hypertension and renal function.

Although the 6-min walking distance was a more powerful discriminator than percentage of predicted FVC, it is not necessarily clear that the 6-min walking distance is more advantageous than other simpler lung function measures, principally percentage of predicted T_{LCO}. This parameter has been shown by others to be a powerful indicator of survival in patients listed for lung transplantation |**13**|. The authors argue, however, that the 6-min walking test has advantages over T_{LCO} measurement in that it requires less specialist equipment, it may be less costly and it can be performed whilst the patient is still receiving oxygen therapy. Whilst these arguments are not entirely compelling, using the 6-min walking distance as a tool for stratifying patients on lung transplant waiting lists is attractive. Indeed, towards the end of the study period the UNOS lung allocation criteria were changed to prioritize patients to lung transplantation based on need rather than on a first come, first served basis. Under this new system the priority for lung transplantation is increased if the 6-min walking distance is <46 m (150 feet).

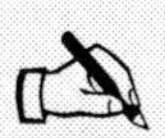

Idiopathic pulmonary fibrosis: prognostic value of changes in physiology and six-minute-walk test

Flaherty KR, Andrei AC, Murray S, *et al. Am J Respir Crit Care Med* 2006; **174**: 803–9

BACKGROUND. Full lung function tests and the 6-min walking test were performed at baseline and 6 months in 197 patients with IPF who were subsequently followed for up to 7 years.

INTERPRETATION. The investigators confirmed their earlier observations that desaturation to 88% or lower was a powerful independent predictor of subsequent mortality. Baseline distance walked provided little or no predictive value for subsequent mortality when compared with baseline desaturation. In the subgroup of patients who maintained oxygen saturation above 88% throughout the baseline 6-min walking test, the following changes at 6 months were associated with increased mortality: walking distance decreased by >61 m (200 feet); worsening of desaturation area; and a 10% relative decrease in FVC or a 15% relative decrease in T_{LCO}. In a group of patients in whom oxygen saturation fell to 88% or below during the baseline 6-min walking test, a 15% fall in T_{LCO} appeared to be the only parameter at 6 months that predicted mortality, even after multivariate analysis for age, sex and smoking.

Comment

This group of investigators have made many of the key observations that inform our understanding of progression in IPF. In this study, 197 patients with IPF (mean age 63 years) were identified using the large University of Michigan database. All the recruited patients had a confident diagnosis of IPF based on a typical HRCT pattern or a lung biopsy showing UIP. At baseline all patients underwent full lung function tests and a 6-min walking test without supplementary oxygen, with repeat investigations at 6 months. The investigators confirmed their earlier observation that desaturation of 88% or lower was a powerful independent predictor of subsequent mortality. Median survival in those with significant desaturation was 3.21 years compared with 6.83 years for those who maintained oxygen saturation above 88%. Patients who significantly desaturated were no older than those who did not desaturate but did have significantly poorer baseline lung function. The investigators also confirmed that, in the subgroup of patients who maintained an oxygen saturation of >88% on exercise, even small degrees of desaturation (as measured by desaturation area, a relatively simple calculation devised by the investigators) were associated with higher mortality. Interestingly, baseline distance walked appeared to have little or no predictive value for subsequent mortality when compared with baseline desaturation, a much more powerful predictor. This highlights the effects of supplementary oxygen, which, when permitted during a 6-min walking test, negates significant desaturation and elevates the prognostic value of distance walked.

Having established the powerful predictive value of baseline desaturation on the 6-min walking test, the investigators went on to examine the 6-month changes in lung function and 6-min walking test parameters. This is against the background that it is already known that a 10% fall in FVC and a 15% fall in T_{LCO} at 6 months are both powerful, independent predictors of mortality. Using a univariate Cox model, the investigators show that, in the subgroup of patients who maintained oxygen saturation above 88% throughout the baseline 6-min walking test, increased mortality was observed in those whose walking distance decreased by >61 m (200 feet), exhibited worsening of desaturation area, a 10% relative decrease in FVC or a 15% relative decrease in T_{LCO}. In the group of patients in whom oxygen saturation fell to 88% or below during the baseline 6-min walking test, a 15% fall in T_{LCO} appeared to be the only parameter at 6 months that predicted mortality, even after multivariate analysis for age, sex and smoking (hazard ratio [HR] 2.95; 95% CI 1.29–6.79; $P = 0.01$).

As might be expected, serial predictors outperformed baseline predictors in terms of prognostic markers for subsequent mortality. The investigators therefore suggest that, at presentation, patients with IPF should be stratified into those who do and those who do not desaturate below 88% on a 6-min walking test on air. Following stratification, those who do desaturate have a significantly poorer prognosis than those who do not. At 6 months, the most powerful predictor of subsequent mortality in those who desaturate at baseline is a 15% decline in T_{LCO}.

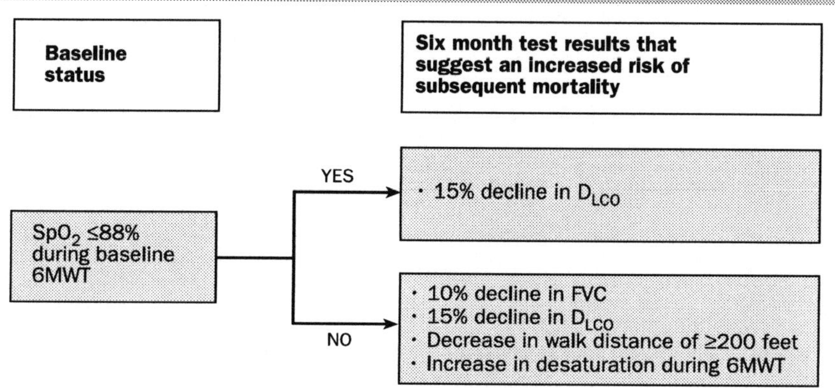

Fig. 12.5 Graphic representation of how the predictive ability of serial changes in FVC, diffusion capacity of carbon monoxide (D$_{LCO}$), change in walking distance and change in desaturation varies according to the presence/absence of desaturation to ≤88% during a baseline 6-min walking test. These data suggest that the decline in D$_{LCO}$ over 6 months is the sole predictor of increased risk of subsequent mortality and that declines in D$_{LCO}$, FVC and walking distance and worsening desaturation can be used to follow patients who do not desaturate ≤88% during a baseline 6-min walking test. SpO$_2$, oxygen saturation by pulse oximetry. Source: Flaherty *et al.* (2006).

In contrast, in those who do not desaturate at baseline, a 10% decline in FVC, a 15% decline in T$_{LCO}$, a decrease in walking distance of ≥61 m (200 feet) or worsening desaturation during a 6-min walking test are all good predictors of subsequent mortality (Fig. 12.5).

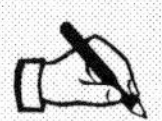

High-resolution computed tomography in idiopathic pulmonary fibrosis: diagnosis and prognosis

Lynch D, Godwin D, Safrin S, *et al. Am J Resp Crit Care Med* 2005; **172**: 488–93

BACKGROUND. The HRCT scan has become an integral part of the evaluation of interstitial lung disease and of idiopathic interstitial pneumonias in particular. Diagnostic precision in idiopathic interstitial pneumonias depends on the integration of clinical, radiological and, when available, histological evidence. An influential earlier study had shown that, when interpreted by expert radiologists, specific HRCT features, primarily the presence of bibasal peripheral honeycombing with minimal ground-glass change, have 100% specificity for UIP disease at biopsy, and therefore in the appropriate clinical setting a surgical lung biopsy is not required in order to distinguish IPF from other interstitial lung diseases, including NSIP |26|. Furthermore, among

patients with a histological diagnosis of UIP, those with a typical UIP pattern on HRCT had significantly poorer survival than those patients with a non-diagnostic HRCT pattern. These observations from specialist interstitial lung disease centres have important implications for both the diagnosis and the management of patients with IPF, if they can be extrapolated to a larger population of patients in non-specialist or community settings. Consequently, further studies of the diagnostic and prognostic roles of baseline HRCT scanning, as presented by Lynch and colleagues, are very welcome.

INTERPRETATION. The investigators reviewed 315 HRCT scans of patients with IPF recruited to a previously published randomized, controlled trial of interferon γ1b in IPF [1]. They aimed to compare the degree of agreement of interpretation of these scans between the original study site radiologists, who were from both academic and community centres, and a core group of expert radiologists not involved with the original study. Of the 263 scans that were interpreted by the study site radiologists as definite IPF, 245 (93.2%) were judged to be consistent with IPF (either typical IPF or atypical IPF) by core radiologist consensus. Core radiologists agreed between themselves on the interpretation of HRCT scans in 86% of cases. A histological diagnosis of UIP was made in 205 patients, and in 88% of these cases the baseline HRCT scan was interpreted as consistent with IPF by the core expert radiologists. However, the most important feature on HRCT scans with regard to the diagnosis of IPF is honeycombing, and the two core radiologists achieved at best only fair agreement as to the presence or absence of honeycombing ($\kappa = 0.21$; 95% CI 0.09–0.32). The core radiologists tended to report honeycombing more frequently than the original study site radiologists. On multivariate analysis the overall extent of fibrosis score was strongly associated with subsequent mortality, with a HR of 2.71 (95% CI 1.61–4.5; P <0.0001). Hence, this large study does much to consolidate the potential diagnostic role of HRCT in IPF, suggesting that robust expert HRCT interpretation, in the context of IPF, is not limited to academic institutions. It also confirms that baseline HRCT has prognostic value in IPF. However, even expert radiologists often fail to agree on a critical aspect of HRCT interpretation, namely honeycombing, and until this is resolved the diagnostic and prognostic value of HRCT scans remains uncertain when applied to widespread clinical practice.

Comment

In this study, the investigators have utilized data available from the previously published placebo-controlled Phase III study of interferon γ1b in mild to moderate IPF [1]. Virtually every one of the 330 patients randomized in this study had a baseline HRCT scan available for evaluation and Lynch and colleagues had three main aims: (i) to define the HRCT features of patients recruited to the study; (ii) to determine the extent of agreement between the study site radiologists (academic and community) involved in the original publication and a panel of three independent thoracic radiologists from an academic unit (so-called core radiologists) and also between core radiologists themselves; and (iii) to examine the association between baseline HRCT score, baseline physiological variables and subsequent mortality. Because of various exclusions, 315 baseline HRCT scans were included in the final analysis. All scans were performed using the standard high-resolution technique (1–1.5 mm thickness) at 2 cm intervals. The minimum tube exposure was 200 mA/s. In the original study the study site radiologists were asked to determine whether the baseline HRCT scan showed definite or probable IPF. A radiographic diagnosis of definite IPF required all three of the following criteria: (i) the presence of reticular abnormality and/or traction bronchiectasis with basal and peripheral predominance; (ii) the presence of honeycombing with basal and peripheral predominance; and (iii) the absence of atypical features, such as micronodules, peribronchial vascular nodules, consolidation, isolated (non-honeycomb cysts), extensive ground-glass attenuation, and extensive mediastinal adenopathy. If only the first and third of these criteria were present (i.e. if honeycombing was absent), a radiological diagnosis of probable IPF was required. All of the study site radiologists knew that IPF was a clinical consideration at the time of reporting. The core radiologists were blinded to the clinical data but of course knew that in every case the patients would have met ATS/ERS criteria for the diagnosis of IPF and had subsequently been recruited to a clinical trial of IPF. Hence, they recognized that every HRCT scan had been labelled with at least probable IPF by a study-site radiologist. The core radiologists were asked to score the baseline HRCT in a standardized manner, recording the extent of ground-glass attenuation, reticulation, honeycombing, decreased attenuation, centrilobular nodules, other nodules, consolidation, and emphysema. The extent of each of these abnormalities and the overall extent of fibrosis (measured as the extent of reticulation and honeycombing together) were determined for each entire lung using a four-point scale with 0 = no involvement and 4 = 75–100% involvement. The HRCTs were classified as typical IPF, atypical IPF or inconsistent with IPF using normal diagnostic evaluation processes and without pre-specified criteria. For subsequent data analysis, the categories of typical IPF and atypical IPF were pulled together as 'consistent' with IPF. The interpretation of this study would have been easier if the core radiologists had used the same classification as the study radiologists, namely 'definite IPF' and 'probable IPF'.

The investigators made several important observations. Firstly, the core radiologists found that 256 of the 315 baseline CT scans were consistent with IPF (81.3%). Furthermore, the two core radiologists had reasonable agreement between themselves after the interpretation of the scans ($\kappa = 0.33$; 95% CI 0.18–0.48). Of course, this means that in almost 20% of cases the core radiologists felt the CT scan to be not consistent with IPF. This does not imply that the original study by Raghu and colleagues had a large proportion of patients who did not have IPF, since most of the patients with non-diagnostic HRCT scans underwent lung biopsy.

Two hundred and five of the 315 patients had indeed undergone a surgical lung biopsy revealing the histological pattern of UIP. In 88% of cases, the baseline HRCT scan was interpreted as consistent with IPF by the core radiologist. Since the single most important feature on HRCT scans with regard to the diagnosis of IPF is honeycombing, it was notable that the two core radiologists achieved at best fair agreement as to the presence or absence of honeycombing ($\kappa = 0.21$; 95% CI 0.09–0.32). The core radiologists tended to report honeycombing more frequently

Table 12.4 High-resolution computed tomography characteristics in scans consistent with idiopathic pulmonary fibrosis versus scans inconsistent with idiopathic pulmonary fibrosis

Characteristics	Total* ($n = 313$)	Consistent with IPF ($n = 283$)	Inconsistent with IPF ($n = 30$)	P-value†
Honeycomb	287 (91.7)	270 (95.4)	17 (56.7)	<0.001
Ground-glass attenuation	94 (30.0)	66 (23.3)	28 (93.3)	<0.001
Decreased attenuation	25 (8.0)	12 (4.2)	13 (43.3)	<0.001
Centrilobular nodules	10 (3.2)	6 (2.1)	4 (13.3)	≤0.010
Reticulation	313 (100.0)	283 (95.4)	30 (100.0)	≤N/A
Emphysema	101 (32.3)	94 (33.2)	7 (23.3)	≤0.311
Nodules, not centrilobular	3 (1.0)	3 (1.1)	0 (0.0)	>0.999
Consolidation	9 (2.9)	8 (2.8)	1 (3.3)	≤0.601
Bronchiolectasis	294 (93.9)	275 (97.2)	19 (63.3)	<0.001
Mosaic attenuation	25 (8.0)	13 (4.6)	12 (40.0)	<0.001
Lower lobe volume loss	224 (71.6)	210 (74.2)	14 (46.7)	≤0.003
Traction bronchiectasis	290 (92.7)	266 (94.0)	24 (80.0)	≤0.015
Upper lobe volume loss	49 (15.7)	43 (15.2)	6 (20.0)	≤0.439
Overall extent of fibrosis, mean score ± SD	1.90 ± 0.61	1.88 ± 0.61	2.01 ± 0.65	≤0.39†

* total no. of patients with a diagnosis consistent with IPF (283) or inconsistent with IPF (30)
† p values derived by two-tailed Fisher test
Source: Lynch *et al.* (2005).

than the original study site radiologists. Ground-glass attenuation, decreased attenuation and centrilobular nodules were features that were much more likely to lead to an interpretation of being inconsistent with IPF (Table 12.4).

The baseline HRCT characteristics, in particular honeycombing, the honeycomb pattern extent score and the overall score for extent of fibrosis, correlated well with baseline lung function, in particular T_{LCO}. Finally, the investigators reported on the baseline HRCT characteristics that might predict short-term mortality: 44 (13.3%) patients died during the 600-day period of the interferon γ study. The investigators found that the overall disease extent score, reticulation pattern score and honeycomb pattern score were all strongly associated with mortality, with hazard ratios of between 2.6 and 3.1 ($P <0.0001$). These data relate to univariate analysis, but on multivariate analysis only the overall extent of fibrosis score, with a HR of 2.71 (95% CI 1.61–4.55), remained strongly associated with subsequent mortality ($P <0.0001$). This association with subsequent mortality is better than that seen with baseline percentage of predicted T_{LCO} (HR 0.94; 95% CI 0.90–0.98; $P = 0.004$). The observations are similar to those reported by Mogulkoc *et al.*, who also identified the percentage of predicted T_{LCO} and HRCT fibrosis score as the only independent predictors of 2-year mortality in 115 patients with UIP [13].

The major strength of this study is the large sample size. Furthermore, the patients were relatively uniform in having mild to moderate disease since those with severe disease were excluded in the clinical trial. The study reassures us that there is reasonable concordance between academic and community radiologists with regard to the interpretation of the HRCT in IPF. However, whilst radiologists largely agreed on whether an HRCT was consistent with IPF, there was surprisingly poor agreement amongst the core radiologists with regard to the presence or absence of honeycombing, a critical feature in the diagnosis. The investigators suggest a set of standardized CT images illustrating various HRCT features in interstitial lung disease, akin to the radiographs widely used for the International Labour Organization classification of the pneumoconiosis.

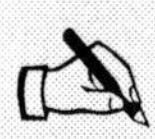

Prognostic value of circulating KL-6 in idiopathic pulmonary fibrosis

Yokoyama A, Kondo K, Nakajima M, *et al. Respirology* 2006; **11**: 164–8

BACKGROUND. A reliable, easily assayed circulating mediator that reflects disease activity, prognosis and indeed response to therapy would be a powerful clinical tool in IPF. KL-6 is a high molecular weight mucin-like glycoprotein product of alveolar type II epithelial cells and has been reported to be raised in many interstitial lung diseases, including IPF, hypersensitivity pneumonitis, sarcoidosis and connective tissue disease-associated interstitial pneumonia |27,28|. The role of serial KL-6 measurement in predicting prognosis in IPF is unknown.

INTERPRETATION. Twenty-seven patients with IPF had serum KL-6 measured by sandwich enzyme-linked immunosorbent assay (ELISA) at baseline and were followed up for at least 3 years. Investigators also measured baseline serum C-reactive protein (CRP) and serum lactate dehydrogenase. The investigators identified an optimal KL-6 cut-off level of 1000 U/ml to separate survivors from non-survivors. Following multivariate analysis, the odds ratio (OR) for subsequent mortality was 12.5 in patients with a KL-6 value of ≥1000 U/ml, with a wide 95% confidence interval (1.2–132; $P = 0.035$). This study should be seen very much as hypothesis-generating. The prognostic role of KL-6 in IPF needs to be studied prospectively in a larger cohort.

Comment

This is a retrospective study from Japan of 27 patients with IPF diagnosed by ATS/ERS criteria. The authors have been carefully building on their previous observations in order to define the prognostic role of KL-6 in disease progression. Using receiver operator curves, the investigators identified an optimal baseline KL-6 cut-off level of 1000 U/ml to separate survivors from non-survivors (Fig. 12.6). Following multivariate analysis, the odds ratio for subsequent mortality was 12.5 in patients with a KL-6 value of 1000 U/ml or greater. However, the confidence intervals are very wide (95% CI 1.2–132; $P = 0.035$). The paper does not provide the KL-6 values for each individual studied, but it is known that in patients with IPF the circulating KL-6 concentration ranges from normal to extremely high. Baseline CRP and lactate dehydrogenase did not show a relationship with

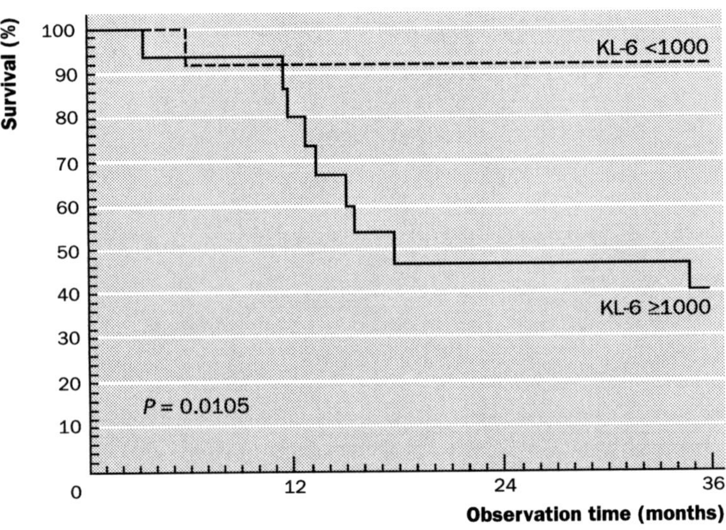

Fig. 12.6 Survival function of KL-6 at the cut-off level of 1000 U/ml was estimated using the Kaplan–Meier method. The idiopathic pulmonary fibrosis patients with KL-6 level <1000 (*n* = 12) had a significantly more favourable prognosis than those with a KL-6 level of ≥1000 U/ml. Source: Yokoyama *et al.* (2006).

subsequent mortality. The data are interesting but the numbers are small. Importantly, although baseline percentage vital capacity and age were included in the covariate analysis, other important predictors of mortality, including smoking status, percentage T_{LCO}, detailed HRCT scores and exercise physiology data were not obtained. The role of KL-6 in IPF, and indeed the roles of other putative circulating biomarkers in IPF, including surfactant protein A and surfactant protein D, need to be confirmed in a larger prospective study.

Clinical trials in idiopathic pulmonary fibrosis

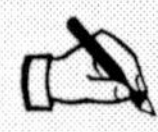

Double-blind, placebo-controlled trial of pirfenidone in patients with idiopathic pulmonary fibrosis

Azuma A, Nukiwa T, Tsuboi E, *et al. Am J Respir Crit Care Med* 2005; **171**: 1040–7

B ACKGROUND. Pirfenidone is a novel antifibrotic agent. The mechanism of action is not known, but the drug has been shown to attenuate the expression of profibrotic molecules *in vitro* and tissue fibrosis in animal models, and has shown promise in clinical studies of renal and liver fibrosis. Two previous studies in lung fibrosis were

sufficiently encouraging for Azuma and colleagues to undertake a double-blind, randomized, placebo-controlled Phase II clinical study |29,30|.

INTERPRETATION. Analysis of the primary end-point – the difference in the change in lowest oxygen saturation during a 6-min walking test between baseline and 9 months – showed no difference between pirfenidone and placebo. However, the trial was terminated early because interim analysis at 6 months revealed an excess number of deaths due to acute exacerbations of IPF in the placebo group compared with the treatment group ($n = 5$ vs $n = 0$; $P = 0.003$). This controversial decision, together with several other design aspects of the study, makes interpretation of the study difficult; this is discussed further in the Comment below. However, the study was sufficiently powerful to foster the view that pirfenidone may be efficacious in IPF and is certainly worthy of further study.

Comment

Characteristics of recruited patients

This study was performed in multiple centres in Japan and a total of 107 patients were recruited. IPF was diagnosed based on the ATS/ERS consensus criteria. In total, 23 of the 107 patients underwent a lung biopsy to confirm the presence of UIP disease. Ninety-one of the 107 patients had what is described as definite UIP by HRCT scanning, as judged by three expert chest radiologists with a reasonable degree of concurrence. Only 16 patients had HRCTs that were described as probably UIP and it is not clear what percentage of these individuals underwent a surgical lung biopsy. However, it does seem reasonable to assume that the vast majority of patients recruited to this study had IPF. Unusually for studies in IPF, 92 of the recruited individuals had not previously received corticosteroid therapy. Finally, it should be recognized that approximately half the patients recruited were diagnosed with IPF at least 3 years previously and only about one-fifth of the participants were within 1 year of diagnosis. The baseline lung function of the recruited patients suggested that, on average, the disease was by no means advanced and indeed the percentage of predicted vital capacity was approximately 80% and the percentage of predicted T_{LCO} was 57% at baseline. These values are significantly higher than those observed in patients recruited to the European multicentre study of N-acetylcysteine in IPF (discussed below). The authors point out that in Japan the national health insurance scheme promotes routine medical evaluations, including chest X-rays, in otherwise healthy individuals. This is likely to lead to earlier diagnoses of IPF, and 3 years after diagnosis lung function thus appears better preserved in patients from Japan than in patients in, say, Europe or the USA.

Study end-points

The primary end-point for the study was change in the lowest oxygen saturation during a 6-min walking test. The secondary end-points were change in lung function parameters (vital capacity, total lung capacity, T_{LCO}, arterial partial pressure of oxygen), disease progression by HRCT scanning, episodes of acute exacerbation of IPF, change in serum markers of alveolar epithelial cell injury, and change in quality of life scores. The study was planned to continue for 1 year.

Aspects of study design

Patients were administered placebo or oral pirfenidone at the highest dose tolerated, with a maximum dose of 600 mg three times a day. Upon starting this study, the investigators met an unexpected dilemma; 27 of the 107 patients recruited were unable to complete the baseline 6-min walking test required by the protocol. Normally when patients drop out of a study for any reason after recruitment, it is recommended that an intention-to-treat analysis is pursued so that all data are collected regardless of dropouts. In this study, the significant number of dropouts at such a critical stage led the investigators to perform a full analysis of the entire 107-patient data set and a separate analysis of the 87 patients who successfully completed the 6-min walking test. Whilst this appears controversial, the authors do point out that as soon as they became aware of subjects' inability to complete the test, they proactively and prospectively altered the study design. Therefore, they did not perform a retrospective subgroup analysis, which would clearly have biased the interpretation. The investigators then suffered a second unexpected event: an interim analysis of the data at 6 months revealed an excess number of deaths due to acute exacerbations of IPF in the placebo group (five) compared with the treatment group (none; $P = 0.003$). The independent Drug Safety Monitoring Board (DSMB) recommended early termination of the study based on this interim finding. All patients in fact completed a minimum of 9 months during the trial before termination but not the planned 1 year. The early termination generates a second controversial issue worthy of debate. Ending the study because of an excessive number of events in the placebo arm creates a subtext that the treatment is efficacious. The authors, however, never make this claim. A new Phase III trial is unquestionably warranted, but the decisions made in this study by an independent body will raise difficult ethical questions for the investigators and data monitoring bodies.

Drug safety

Pirfenidone appears to be reasonably well tolerated, although it should be pointed out that 15% of patients discontinued the drug during the study because of adverse side effects and only half the patients could tolerate the maximum dose of 1800 mg/day. Gastrointestinal upset with pain, heartburn and nausea, as well as fatigue, were significantly more common in patients taking pirfenidone.

Study outcome

Analysis of the primary end-point (the difference in the change in lowest oxygen saturation during a 6-min walking test between baseline and 9 months) showed no difference between pirfenidone and placebo. Analysis of the subgroup of 80 individuals who actually completed the baseline 6-min walking test does show a small but significant improvement in the extent of desaturation in the pirfenidone group compared with the placebo group at 9 months ($P = 0.03$). Of the other lung function parameters that constituted the secondary end-points, none were found to differ significantly between the treatment and placebo arms in the full data set. A further important and controversial aspect of this study is the choice of primary end-point. At the time the study was performed, there were no data to support the 6-min walking test as a valid, reproducible and prognostically useful biomarker of disease progression. Subsequently, however, there have been studies to support the use of exercise testing in IPF, as discussed in this chapter. A multicentre European Phase III study of pirfenidone is recruiting at the time of writing.

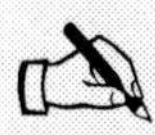

High-dose acetylcysteine in idiopathic pulmonary fibrosis
Demedts M, Behr J, Buhl R, *et al.* N Engl J Med 2005; **353**: 2229–42

BACKGROUND. Several lines of evidence suggest that oxidant–antioxidant imbalances in the lower respiratory tract play a critical role in the pathogenesis of IPF. These include the observation that patients with IPF have decreased levels of reduced glutathione in the epithelial lining fluid of their lungs |31,32|. In a small experimental medicine study, oral N-acetylcysteine (NAC) was shown to replenish deficient glutathione levels in IPF lungs |33|. This study by Demedts and colleagues of oral NAC represents the first large European multicentre clinical study in IPF.

INTERPRETATION. This is a study of prednisolone and azathioprine versus prednisolone, azathioprine and NAC. The primary end-points were absolute changes in vital capacity and T_{LCO} between baseline and month 12. The addition of NAC to prednisolone and azathioprine resulted in a significantly slower rate of decline in both vital capacity and T_{LCO} when compared with the control arm. Effectively, at the end of 12 months, lung function had fallen to a significantly lesser degree in those receiving NAC compared with those who did not. On average, vital capacity was 180 ml (9%) greater in the patients receiving antioxidant therapy ($P = 0.003$). This is the first clinical trial in IPF that has successfully met the predefined primary end-points dictated at the outset. The outcome must be reproduced in another population with IPF, ideally including a placebo arm, before the true clinical impact of NAC is known, but at present physicians who choose to treat patients with prednisolone and azathioprine should add NAC to their regimen.

Comment

Characteristics of recruited patients

The entry requirements for the diagnosis of IPF were essentially those described in the ATS/ERS diagnostic criteria. All patients were required to exhibit an HRCT that was judged very suggestive or consistent with UIP. In patients under 50 a surgical lung biopsy showing a pattern of UIP was a mandatory requirement. In older patients a lung biopsy was not a requirement but all patients were required to have a BAL that showed no features to support an alternative diagnosis at some point prior to inclusion. In the final analysis, just under 50% of patients recruited to the study had undergone a surgical lung biopsy. After randomization, 27 of the initial 182 patients were judged not to have IPF following review by an expert panel of radiologists and pathologists. Thus, the analysed data are only presented for the 155 patients (80 receiving acetylcysteine and 75 receiving placebo) who had IPF after expert review. On the one hand this is reassuring since we know the analysis is in patients with as homogeneous a disease as can be expected. On the other hand, this approach of removing patients following randomization is certainly unconventional and open to criticism from the point of view of study design. One might also say that the data may now be less applicable to the patient who is diagnosed with IPF based on the sound judgement of their physician without recourse to an expert panel.

At entry, a surprisingly large number of patients (around 50%) were recruited within 6 months of diagnosis of IPF. This proportion of incident cases is, for example, higher than in several other recent clinical trials of IPF. This might suggest that many patients will have been recruited early in the disease, but in fact the baseline lung function tests suggest that a significant proportion will have had quite advanced disease at the time of randomization. For example, one-third of patients had a vital capacity of <60% of predicted at the time of recruitment.

Study end-points

The primary end-points chosen were absolute changes in vital capacity and T_{LCO} between baseline and month 12. The pre-specified secondary end-points were changes between baseline and 12 months in vital capacity and T_{LCO} as percentages of predicted values and a number of other physiological scores together with changes in HRCT score and quality of life assessment.

Aspects of study design

This was a double-blind randomized study across multiple centres in Europe. Whilst it is described as being placebo-controlled, this is a slight misnomer since all recruited patients were given treatment with prednisolone and azathioprine according to a protocol suggested in the ATS/ERS consensus statement of 2000 [34]. Patients were then allocated to receive either NAC at 600 mg orally three times daily or placebo. A total of 182 patients were randomly assigned to the two groups (92 to acetylcysteine and 90 to placebo) but, as described above, 27 cases, equally split between the two groups, were judged not to have IPF and the final analysis was restricted to 155 randomized participants. During the 12-month course of the study, a significant number of patients were lost to follow-up or withdrawn. However, the investigators did perform an intention-to-treat analysis and used a last-observation-carried-forward strategy for missing data points. That is to say, if lung function data were available at 6 months but not 12 months, then data from the earlier time-point were carried over to the later time-point. This would seem a robust way of analysing the available data if applied, as it was in this case, with similar frequency in the two groups.

Drug tolerability and safety

Adverse effects were few and reported with equal frequency in both study groups with one exception: NAC therapy was associated with significantly fewer episodes of bone marrow toxicity (three events in acetylcysteine group versus ten events in the placebo group; $P = 0.03$). It should also be noted that the true side-effect profile of long-term steroids and azathioprine might be under-represented in this study, since patients were '. . . excluded if the standard regimen with prednisone and azathioprine was contraindicated or not justified for them'. This exclusion further detracts from the applicability of the study data to real patients.

Study outcome

The results at 12 months show that the addition of acetylcysteine to prednisolone and azathioprine results in a significantly slower rate of decline in both vital capacity and T_{LCO} when compared with the control arm. Effectively, at the end of 12 months patients receiving NAC had a vital capacity that was on average 180 ml (9%) greater and a T_{LCO} that was 0.75 mmol/min/kPa (24%) greater than that in patients receiving prednisolone and azathioprine alone ($P = 0.003$ and $P = 0.002$ respectively) (Fig. 12.7). The confidence intervals are quite large and the actual difference may be as little as 30 ml or as great as 320 ml for vital capacity, with a similarly large range for T_{LCO}. Whether this salvaging of lung function translates into real benefit is of course unknown. This is because we do not know the true relationship between the rate of decline in these lung function parameters and mortality. We do know, however, from large retrospective data sets, that a change in vital capacity of 10% between baseline and 12 months or a change in T_{LCO} of 15% between baseline and 12 months does have prognostic value. The investigators recognized this and performed a *post hoc* analysis to answer the specific question of whether NAC therapy significantly alters the number of patients whose lung function has changed by >10% in vital capacity or >15% in T_{LCO} at 12 months. This analysis showed no beneficial effect of NAC over placebo. None of the secondary end-points other than percentage change in vital capacity or T_{LCO} were statistically significant.

In the absence of a genuine placebo group, the true value of antioxidant therapy in IPF is unclear, and some have speculated that NAC simply protects tissue such as bone marrow and lung from the harmful effects of azathioprine [34,35]. Further trials that include a placebo arm are critically needed, but until that time one can draw the very reasonable conclusion that giving prednisolone and azathioprine without the addition of NAC is difficult to justify. NAC is well tolerated, inexpensive and in many countries available without prescription.

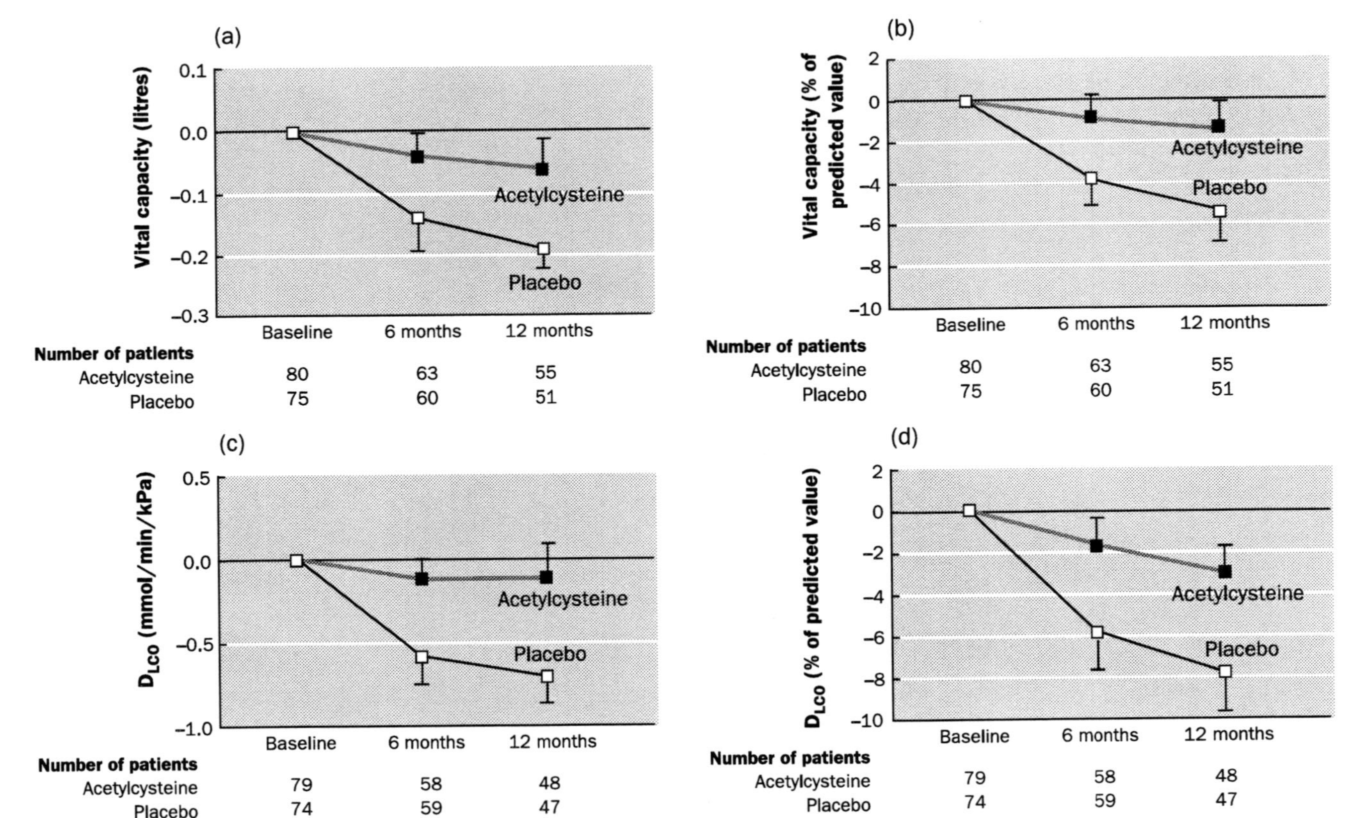

Fig. 12.7 Vital capacity and single-breath carbon monoxide diffusing capacity (T_{LCO}) at 6 and 12 months compared with baseline. Mean values for vital capacity (a, b) and D_{LCO} (c, d) are shown as absolute amounts and as percentages of the predicted value; *I bars* represent standard error of the mean. Source: Demedts *et al.* (2005).

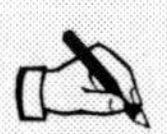

Interferon-gamma1b therapy in idiopathic pulmonary fibrosis: a metaanalysis

Bajwa EK, Ayas NT, Schulzer M, Mak E, Ryu JH, Malhotra A. *Chest* 2005; **128**: 203–6

BACKGROUND. Meta-analysis is a potentially powerful tool for pooling multiple studies of an intervention or therapy and by weighting the studies based on the quality of each trial the true magnitude of treatment effect may be determined with greater precision than in any one individual study. In this report, the authors performed a meta-analysis of studies of interferon γ1b, a promising therapy in IPF, after a systematic literature search.

INTERPRETATION. This analysis of the pooled data from three clinical trials indicates that interferon γ 1b significantly decreased the mortality rate in IPF compared with control groups at time-points of 1 year, 18 months, 650 days and 2 years. The pooled hazard ratio in the meta-analysis was 0.418, with a 95% CI of 0.253–0.690 (*P* = 0.0003), indicating that, on average, patients taking interferon γ1b were only half as likely to die as those not receiving the drug. Thus, for the first time in IPF, a truly devastating disease, a meta-analysis of randomized controlled trials has shown a significant survival benefit with therapy. Meta-analyses do, of course, have limitations, and in general they should be used for hypothesis generation and to fuel high-quality randomized controlled trials before a firm conclusion on treatment efficacy can be reached.

Comment

In this study, the authors performed a systematic literature search using appropriate terms and found four studies of interferon γ1b that fulfilled four predetermined criteria: (i) they were randomized controlled studies with an adequately controlled group; (ii) they enrolled patients who met accepted ATS/ERS clinical and pathological criteria for the diagnosis of IPF; (iii) interferon γ1b was delivered for at least 6 months; and (iv) mortality data were appropriately reported in the form of a Kaplan–Meier survival analysis. In fact, the last criterion resulted in one of the four studies being excluded because the Kaplan–Meier survival curve was not available from the lead author (this study and |45|). Of the remaining three studies, one was an unpublished study from which data had been presented at national and international meetings. The data from this paper were subsequently published and are described below in this chapter. Of the two remaining studies, one was the small but well-designed study of interferon γ1b that first brought the attention of the medical community to the potential for this agent to treat IPF |37|. The other was the first large, multicentre, randomized, placebo-controlled study in IPF |1|. Hence, the meta-analysis consists of just three studies, one of which contributed the vast majority of patients and the two others, by Ziesche *et al.* and Antoniou *et al.*, which contributed 18 and 42 patients respectively.

The analysis of the pooled data indicates that interferon γ1b significantly decreased the mortality rate in IPF compared with control groups at the time-points of 1 year, 18 months, 650 days and 2 years. The pooled HR in the meta-analysis was 0.418 with a 95% CI of 0.253–0.690; $P = 0.0003$ (Fig. 12.8).

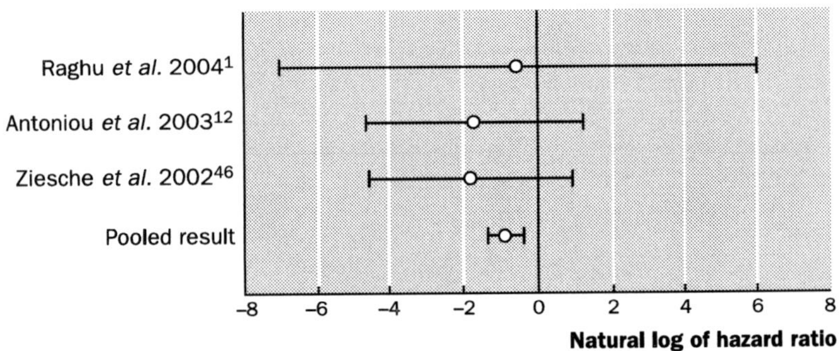

Fig. 12.8 Effect of interferon γ1b treatment on survival. A natural logarithm of 0 for the hazards ratio indicates no difference in mortality between the interferon γ1b and control groups. A negative value for the logarithm indicates a reduction in mortality rate with interferon γ1b. Source: Bajwa et al. (2005).

The authors, however, recognize that these data are not sufficient to prove efficacy. As well as being heavily skewed by one large randomized controlled trial, which in itself yielded negative results, other issues are raised. For example, the studies by Ziesche and Antoniou included steroid use as part of the treatment protocol, whilst the Raghu study [1] did not formally include corticosteroids in the protocol but allowed clinicians to use steroids at their own discretion. Although there is no proof that corticosteroids in isolation are of therapeutic value in IPF, no trial has ever been done to test this hypothesis and it is plausible that corticosteroids may modulate the natural history of the disease. The authors make the important observation that the meta-analysis is an important tool in generating hypotheses but does not in itself relieve us of the need to perform a further high-quality, randomized, placebo-controlled study of interferon γ1b. Such studies are awaited with great interest.

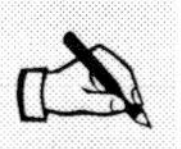

Long-term clinical effects of interferon gamma-1b and colchicine in idiopathic pulmonary fibrosis

Antoniou KM, Nicholson AG, Dimadi M, *et al. Eur Respir J* 2006; **28**: 496–504

BACKGROUND. Although this study was published in 2006, data derived from it had been in the public domain for some time following presentations at national and international meetings, and had been used in a meta-analysis of IPF by Bajwa and colleagues prior to full publication of this paper |44|. The study builds on previous observations of the promising therapeutic value of interferon γ1b and colchicine.

INTERPRETATION. In this randomized, prospective, multicentre study, subjects received either interferon γ1b plus prednisolone 10 mg daily or oral colchicine 1 mg per day plus prednisolone 10 mg daily. Pre-specified end-points were not defined and the study was continued for 24 months. Of the various parameters analysed, survival appeared to be the most striking, such that the hazard ratio of death in the interferon γ1b group compared with the colchicine group was 0.3 (95% CI 0.07–0.86; $P = 0.04$). The study has several design weaknesses but adds to the body of evidence that suggests that interferon γ1b confers a survival benefit in IPF.

Comment

Characteristics of recruited patients

Patients with IPF were identified according to the ATS/ERS consensus criteria. It should be noted that in this study around 80% of patients underwent a lung biopsy that showed a UIP histological pattern. Patients with severe IPF, as determined by FVC <55% of predicted or T_{LCO} <35% of predicted, were excluded from the study. On average, patients had experienced symptoms for around 3 years before entering the study but the time from actual diagnosis to study recruitment is not clear. It appears, however, that the proportion of incident cases of IPF was small.

Aspects of study design

This was a randomized, prospective, multicentre study, but was not blinded and not placebo-controlled. Sixty-eight patients with IPF were recruited and all had a run-in period during which prednisolone 50 mg/day was administered orally for 1 month with subsequent tapering down to 10 mg/day over a 4-week period. If during this steroid trial there was an increase of >10% in the percentage of predicted FVC and/or T_{LCO}, the individual was withdrawn from the study. This was the case in six of the 68 IPF patients and a further twelve were excluded for failing to meet other entry criteria. Hence, in the final analysis 50 subjects were randomized to receive either interferon γ1b 200 μg subcutaneously three times per week plus prednisolone 10 mg daily or oral colchicine 1 mg per day plus prednisolone 10 mg daily. The study was continued for 24 months and the analysis was performed on an intention-to-treat basis.

A significant flaw in the study design was that pre-specified end-points were not identified. The investigations evaluated changes in lung function, HRCT score, quality of life and survival.

Drug tolerability and safety

Constitutional symptoms, such as fever, myalgia, rigors, headache and flu-like syndrome, were significantly more common among patients who received interferon γ1b ($P = 0.01$), although as previously reported the symptoms did settle within 2–3 months.

Study outcome

Of the several (unspecified) end-points, mortality yielded the most striking observation. The survival curves began to diverge significantly after approximately 20 months, and by the end of the study five out of 32 (15.6%) patients receiving interferon γ1b had died compared with seven out of 18 (38.8%) patients receiving colchicine ($P = 0.028$). The hazard ratio for death in the interferon γ1b group compared with the colchicine group was 0.3 (95% CI 0.07–0.86; $P = 0.04$). The authors performed a subgroup analysis akin to that performed in the earlier large multicentre study by Raghu *et al.* |**1**| and showed that in patients with mild disease (FVC ≥71% of predicted) there was 100% survival in the 16 patients with mild IPF receiving interferon γ1b compared with four deaths in the nine patients receiving colchicine ($P = 0.008$). The impact of interferon γ1b on lung function was less impressive than on survival, although by 24 months FVC as a percentage of predicted was significantly better in the interferon γ1b group than in the groups receiving colchicine ($P = 0.04$). The change in T_{LCO} as a percentage of predicted was similar in the two groups. HRCT scores and quality of life assessments were not significantly different between groups and over the 24-month period. The authors conclude that interferon γ1b may improve survival in patients with mild to moderate IPF. The absence of pre-specified end-points and the lack of a placebo control are major limitations. However, the study does add further weight to the body of evidence that interferon γ1b may prolong survival in IPF without (for reasons that are not entirely clear) significantly affecting lung function. The outcome of the ongoing International Study of Survival Outcomes in IPF with Interferon-γ1b Early Intervention (INSPIRE) clinical trial in patients with mild to moderate IPF is eagerly anticipated.

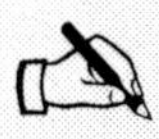

Anticoagulant therapy for idiopathic pulmonary fibrosis

Kubo H, Nakayama K, Yanai M, *et al. Chest* 2005; **128**: 1475–82

B ACKGROUND. There is a body of evidence that suggests that microvascular thrombosis and injury is an important process in the pathogenesis of IPF |47,48|. Furthermore, pulmonary embolism has been reported as an important cause of death

in IPF, although its true incidence is unclear |40|. Perhaps surprisingly, the potential therapeutic value of anticoagulation in IPF had not hitherto been studied in a clinical trial.

INTERPRETATION. This is a multicentre, randomized control study from Japan. Fifty-six patients with IPF were randomly assigned to receive oral prednisolone or prednisolone, plus oral warfarin with the aim of maintaining the international normalized ratio (INR) between 2.0 and 3.0. The primary end-points were overall survival, time to death and the hospitalization-free period during a 3-year follow-up period. Five out of 23 individuals in the anticoagulated group died compared with 20 out 33 in the non-anticoagulated group ($P = 0.006$). Kaplan–Meier survival estimates showed a statistically significant difference between survival curves of the anticoagulant and non-anticoagulant groups ($P = 0.049$). Using the Cox regression model, the hazard ratio for death in the non-anticoagulated group was 2.9 compared with the anticoagulated group after adjustment for age and baseline FVC as a percentage of predicted (95% CI 1.0–8.0; $P = 0.04$). There are several issues concerning the trial design, discussed in detail below, that preclude a conclusion that warfarin therapy reduces mortality in IPF.

Comment

This multicentre, randomized, controlled study was performed across five centres in Japan. The diagnosis of IPF was based on a combination of HRCT appearances and lung biopsy. Only nine of the 56 patients underwent open lung biopsy and for the others the diagnosis was based on HRCT scan appearances and, in some cases, a transbronchial biopsy that excluded other conditions. Whilst not strictly adhering to ATS/ERS criteria, the description given of the patients who were recruited suggests that most of them would indeed have IPF. All recruited patients received prednisolone initially at 0.5–1.0 mg/kg/day for 1 month, with subsequent tapering to a maintenance dose of between 10 and 20 mg/day. The treatment group received in addition oral warfarin with the aim of maintaining the INR between 2.0 and 3.0. Interestingly, all 56 patients had already demonstrated progressive deterioration of IPF despite having received prednisolone therapy, although the term 'progressive deterioration' is not defined.

The study was not blinded but this is understandable given the inherent difficulty of blinding warfarin studies. The mean age at the time of hospital admission was 69.4 years (range 47–89). It is not clear from the paper for how long the patients had had a diagnosis of IPF prior to study recruitment, so the proportion of incident versus prevalent cases is not known. Lung function data at baseline suggest that the majority of patients had mild disease, since the average FVC was approximately 70% of predicted and the average T_{LCO} was approximately 60% of predicted. The investigators state that there were two primary end-points over a 3-year follow-up: overall survival time to death and the hospitalization-free period. Kaplan–Meier survival estimates show a statistically significant difference between the survival curves of the anticoagulant and non-anticoagulant groups ($P = 0.049$) (Fig. 12.9). Using the Cox regression model, the hazard ratio for death in the non-anticoagulated group was 2.9 compared with the anticoagulated group after adjustment for age and baseline FVC as a percentage of predicted (95% CI 1.0–8.0; $P = 0.04$). Rehospitalization episodes and the hospitalization-free period were not significantly different between the warfarin and control groups. An interesting feature of this population of patients is the high number of reported hospitalization episodes (Table 12.5). In total there were 44 inpatient episodes amongst the 56 patients and over 70% of these were for acute exacerbation of IPF, a phenomenon described and discussed in a previous section of this chapter (see discussion of the paper by Kim *et al.*). The authors did not define acute exacerbation, but reached the diagnosis after excluding infection and heart failure using clinical assessment and transthoracic echocardiography. Pulmonary embolism was deemed not to have accounted for any of the hospital admissions in either group, although CT– pulmonary angiography was not performed routinely. Acute exacerbation was considered to be the cause of death in 17 of the 25 patients who died. More particularly, the mortality from acute exacerbation in patients in

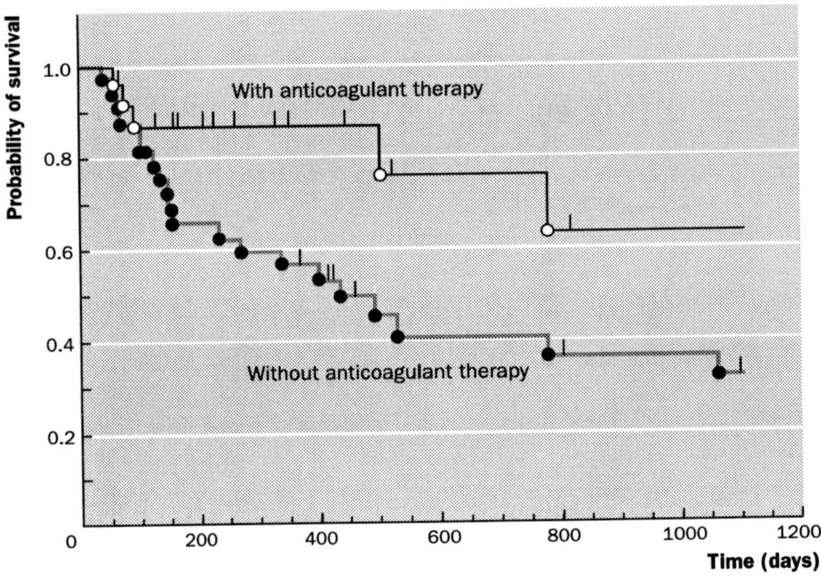

Fig. 12.9 Kaplan–Meier survival estimate with censoring ($\perp$) between the non-anticoagulated group and the anticoagulated group in regard to overall survival. *Open circles* indicate the survival curve in the anticoagulated group. *Closed circles* indicate the survival curve in the non-anticoagulated group. There was a statistically significant difference between survival curves of the anticoagulated group and the non-anticoagulated group ($P = 0.049$, log-rank test). According to the Cox regression model, the HR for death was 2.9 in the non-anticoagulated group compared with the anticoagulated group (adjusted for age and baseline FVC as percentage of predicted; 95% CI 1.0–8.0; $P = 0.04$). Source: Kubo *et al.* (2005).

Table 12.5 Clinical outcome during follow-up

Variables	Non-anticoagulant (n = 33)	Anticoagulant (n = 23)	P-value
Rehospitalization, no. of patients	22	13	0.6*
Once	17	11	
Twice	3	2	
Three times	2	0	
Causes of rehospitalization,			
total no. of hospitalizations	29	15	
Acute exacerbation	21	11	
Pneumonia	6	2	
Heart failure	1	1	
Sepsis	1	1	
Death, no. of patients	20	5	0.006†
Causes of death, total no. of patients	20	5	
Acute exacerbation	15	2	
Pneumonia	3	1	
Heart failure	1	1	
Sepsis	1	1	

* χ^2 test.
† Fisher exact test.
Source: Kubo et al. (2005).

the non-anticoagulated arm was significantly higher than that in the anticoagulated group (15 deaths in 21 acute exacerbations versus two deaths in eleven acute exacerbations; $P = 0.008$).

Can one conclude that warfarin therapy reduces the mortality of acute exacerbations in IPF? The trial design and analysis do not allow such a conclusion to be drawn. Firstly, it is apparent that 8 of 31 participants randomized to the warfarin arm of the study dropped out. The data should have been presented as an 'intention-to-treat' analysis of all 31 individuals, and analysing only the sub-group of 23 participants introduces a major bias into the study. Secondly, all patients in the anticoagulation arm were switched to intravenous low molecular weight heparin (doltaparin 75 IU/kg/day) for up to 14 days, whilst those in the steroid arm were treated with high-dose methylprednisolone (500–1000 mg/day) for 3 days. Hence, whilst the number of hospital admissions for acute exacerbation was similar between the anticoagulated and control groups, the mortality from acute exacerbation differed; this may reflect the effect of intravenous low molecular weight heparin treatment during an exacerbation rather than previous warfarin therapy. This specific hypothesis requires testing in an appropriately designed clinical trial. The investigators also studied plasma D-dimer levels during the trial period. They found that levels tended to be slightly elevated and remain elevated during the 14 days in inpatients receiving methylprednisolone, whereas they fell significantly in those receiving low molecular weight heparin (Fig. 12.10). This adds further weight to the hypothesis that the beneficial effects of anticoagulation in this study actually

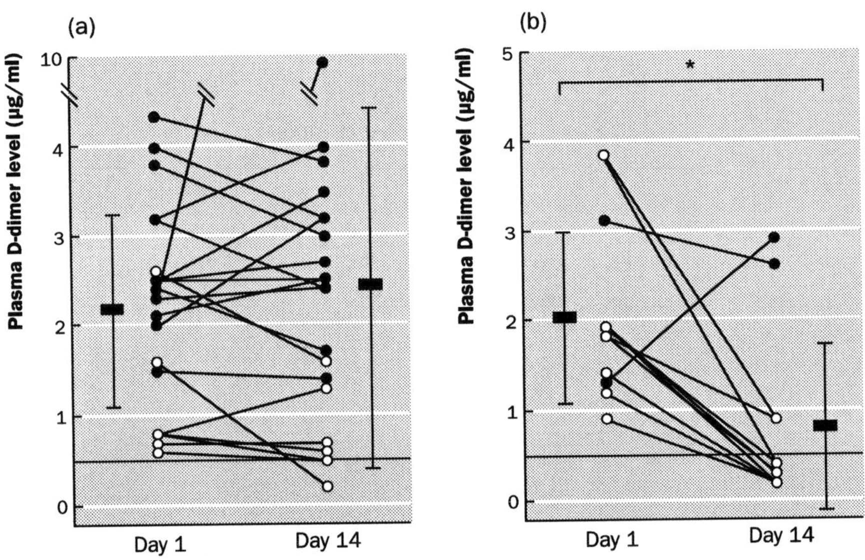

Fig. 12.10 Comparisons of plasma D-dimer levels on days 1 and 14 during hospitalization due to acute exacerbation of IPF in the non-anticoagulated group (a) and the anticoagulant group (b). *Open circles* indicate values for survivors with acute exacerbation of IPF. *Closed circles* indicate values for patients who died during hospitalization. *Bold black bars* indicate mean values of groups. *P = 0.01, paired *t*-test. The horizontal line indicates the upper limit of the plasma D-dimer level (<0.5 µg/ml). Source: Kubo *et al.* (2005).

relate to heparin treatment during an acute exacerbation rather than to long-term warfarin therapy. Post-mortem studies in those who died revealed usual interstitial pneumonia with superimposed acute lung injury (diffuse alveolar damage), the pattern of disease most commonly reported in patients with IPF and acute exacerbation.

This study provides some tantalizing data with regard to anticoagulation in IPF. It is indeed remarkable that a study of only 56 patients achieved a significant difference with mortality as a primary end-point. However, the limitations of the study preclude any firm conclusions. We have already discussed the possibility that it was therapy with intravenous low molecular weight heparin rather than warfarin therapy that conferred the survival benefit. The singular effect of anticoagulation therapy cannot be interpreted because all patients also received corticosteroid therapy. Acute exacerbation of IPF is itself a concept that is only recently being widely acknowledged. For example, in the study by Martinez *et al.* of 168 patients followed up for 72 weeks, 22 deaths might reasonably be attributed to acute exacerbation (13%). Kim and colleagues quote a 2-year frequency of acute exacerbation of 9.6%.

In the present study, the 3-year exacerbation rate is over 50%. It may be that the natural history of IPF differs significantly across ethnically diverse populations.

Conclusion

There have unquestionably been significant recent advances made in our understanding of IPF. Whilst the median survival rate of patients with IPF is poor and has been shown to be so in every population group studied, there is marked heterogeneity within the disease. This heterogeneity is apparent even within groups of patients who have a stringent diagnosis of IPF based on consensus integration of clinical, radiographic and histological features. One important manifestation of this heterogeneity is the rapid decline in function, or acute exacerbations, observed in patients with apparently stable disease. The incidence of acute exacerbation may vary with ethnicity, but these episodes uniformly herald a poor prognosis. Further studies are needed to better define acute exacerbation, to understand its pathogenesis and to treat or prevent episodes. In terms of biomarkers of disease, we know that a 10% decline in FVC (and to a lesser extent 15% decline in T_{LCO}) is associated with poorer survival in IPF, but these parameters have shortcomings. Exercise testing at baseline appears to capture an aspect of the disease that is not apparent from static lung function, but it is unclear, for example, which component of the 6-min walking test is important. Distance walked is highly reproducible but the degree of desaturation has greater prognostic significance. The extent of fibrosis on a baseline HRCT scan appears to have prognostic significance, but, perhaps worryingly, even expert radiologists have difficulty agreeing on the presence or absence of honeycombing, a key component in the IPF diagnostic process. Finally, one might consider it surprising that, at the same time as the natural history of the disease is only beginning to be fully appreciated, large-scale therapeutic trials in IPF are being undertaken. This is a reflection of the uncommon nature of the disease and its appalling prognosis, both of which have led to an understandable drive to prioritize therapeutic trials wherever possible. There is no consensus as to the best current treatment for IPF and no trial yet published can claim to radically influence current practice in the management of the disease. However, in the light of the study by Demedts and colleagues, one can make a strong claim that, in patients with IPF in whom treatment with prednisolone and azathioprine is being considered, N-acetylcysteine should be added to the regimen, based on the current evidence.

References

1. Raghu G, Brown KK, Bradford WZ, Starko K, Noble PW, Schwartz DA, King TE Jr.; Idiopathic Pulmonary Fibrosis Study Group. A placebo-controlled trial of interferon gamma-1b in patients with idiopathic pulmonary fibrosis. *N Engl J Med* 2004; **350**: 125–33.

2. Collard HR, King TE Jr, Bartelson BB, Vourlekis JS, Schwarz MI, Brown KK. Changes in clinical and physiologic variables predict survival in idiopathic pulmonary fibrosis. *Am J Respir Crit Care Med* 2003; **168**: 538–42.

3. Flaherty KR, Mumford JA, Murray S, Kazerooni EA, Gross BH, Colby TV, *et al.* Prognostic implications of physiologic and radiographic changes in idiopathic interstitial pneumonia. *Am J Respir Crit Care Med* 2003; **168**: 543–8.

4. Latsi PI, du Bois RM, Nicholson AG, Colby TV, Bisirtzoglou D, Nikolakopoulou A, *et al.* Fibrotic idiopathic interstitial pneumonia: the prognostic value of longitudinal functional trends. *Am J Respir Crit Care Med* 2003; **168**: 531–7.

5. King TE Jr, Safrin S, Starko KM, Brown KK, Noble PW, Raghu G, Schwartz DA. Analyses of efficacy end points in a controlled trial of interferon-gamma1b for idiopathic pulmonary fibrosis. *Chest* 2005; **127**: 171–7.

6. American Thoracic Society/European Respiratory Society International Multidisciplinary Consensus Classification of the Idiopathic Interstitial Pneumonias. This joint statement of the American Thoracic Society (ATS), and the European Respiratory Society (ERS) was adopted by the ATS board of directors, June 2001 and by the ERS Executive Committee, June 2001. *Am J Respir Crit Care Med* 2002; **165**: 277–304.

7. Flaherty KR, King TE Jr, Raghu G, Lynch JP III, Colby TV, Travis WD, *et al.* Idiopathic interstitial pneumonia: what is the effect of a multidisciplinary approach to diagnosis? *Am J Respir Crit Care Med* 2004; **170**: 904–10.

8. Nicholson AG, Addis BJ, Bharucha H, Clelland CA, Corrin B, Gibbs AR, *et al.* Interobserver variation between pathologists in diffuse parenchymal lung disease. *Thorax* 2004; **59**: 500–5.

9. Johnson WC, Raghu G. Clinical trials in idiopathic pulmonary fibrosis: a word of caution concerning choice of outcome measures. *Eur Respir J* 2005; **26**: 755–8.

10. Johnston ID, Prescott RJ, Chalmers JC, Rudd RM. British Thoracic Society study of cryptogenic fibrosing alveolitis: current presentation and initial management. Fibrosing Alveolitis Subcommittee of the Research Committee of the British Thoracic Society. *Thorax* 1997; **52**: 38–44.

11. Nicholson AG, Colby TV, du Bois RM, Hansell DM, Wells AU. The prognostic significance of the histologic pattern of interstitial pneumonia in patients presenting with the clinical entity of cryptogenic fibrosing alveolitis. *Am J Respir Crit Care Med* 2000; **162**: 2213–17.

12. Crowley SP, Kelly P, Egan JJ. Acute exacerbations in idiopathic pulmonary fibrosis. *Ann Intern Med* 2006; **144**: 218–19.

13. Mogulkoc N, Brutsche MH, Bishop PW, Greaves SM, Horrocks AW, Egan JJ. Pulmonary function in idiopathic pulmonary fibrosis and referral for lung transplantation. *Am J Respir Crit Care Med* 2001; **164**: 103–8.

14. Kondoh Y, Taniguchi H, Kawabata Y, Yokoi T, Suzuki K, Takagi K. Acute exacerbation in idiopathic pulmonary fibrosis. Analysis of clinical and pathologic findings in three cases. *Chest* 1993; **103**: 1808–12.

15. Akira M, Hamada H, Sakatani M, Kobayashi C, Nishioka M, Yamamoto S. CT findings during phase of accelerated deterioration in patients with idiopathic pulmonary fibrosis. *AJR Am J Roentgenol* 1997; **168**: 79–83.

16. Utz JP, Ryu JH, Douglas WW, Hartman TE, Tazelaar HD, Myers JL, *et al.* High short-term mortality following lung biopsy for usual interstitial pneumonia. *Eur Respir J* 2001; **17**: 175–9.

17. Allen MS, Deschamps C, Jones DM, Trastek VF, Pairolero PC. Video-assisted thoracic surgical procedures: the Mayo experience. *Mayo Clin Proc* 1996; **71**: 351–9.

18. Al-Hameed FM, Sharma S. Outcome of patients admitted to the intensive care unit for acute exacerbation of idiopathic pulmonary fibrosis. *Can Respir J* 2004; **11**: 117–22.

19. Saydain G, Islam A, Afessa B, Ryu JH, Scott JP, Peters SG. Outcome of patients with idiopathic pulmonary fibrosis admitted to the intensive care unit. *Am J Respir Crit Care Med* 2002; **166**: 839–42.

20. Blivet S, Philit F, Sab JM, Langevin B, Paret M, Guerin C, *et al.* Outcome of patients with idiopathic pulmonary fibrosis admitted to the ICU for respiratory failure. *Chest* 2001; **120**: 209–12.

21. Jegal Y, Kim DS, Shim TS, Lim CM, Do LS, Koh Y, *et al.* Physiology is a stronger predictor of survival than pathology in fibrotic interstitial pneumonia. *Am J Respir Crit Care Med* 2005; **171**: 639–44.

22. Lama VN, Flaherty KR, Toews GB, Colby TV, Travis WD, Long Q, *et al.* Prognostic value of desaturation during a 6-minute walk test in idiopathic interstitial pneumonia. *Am J Respir Crit Care Med* 2003; **168**: 1084–90.

23. Eaton T, Young P, Milne D, Wells AU. Six-minute walk, maximal exercise tests: reproducibility in fibrotic interstitial pneumonia. *Am J Respir Crit Care Med* 2005; **171**: 1150–7.

24. De MJ, Smits JM, Persijn GG, Haverich A. Listing for lung transplantation: life expectancy and transplant effect, stratified by type of end-stage lung disease, the Eurotransplant experience. *J Heart Lung Transplant* 2001; **20**: 518–24.

25. Kawut SM, O'Shea MK, Bartels MN, Wilt JS, Sonett JR, Arcasoy SM. Exercise testing determines survival in patients with diffuse parenchymal lung disease evaluated for lung transplantation. *Respir Med* 2005; **99**: 1431–9.

26. Flaherty KR, Thwaite EL, Kazerooni EA, Gross BH, Toews GB, Colby TV, *et al.* Radiological versus histological diagnosis in UIP and NSIP: survival implications. *Thorax* 2003; **58**: 143–8.

27. Kohno N, Awaya Y, Oyama T, Yamakido M, Akiyama M, Inoue Y, *et al.* KL-6, a mucin-like glycoprotein, in bronchoalveolar lavage fluid from patients with interstitial lung disease. *Am Rev Respir Dis* 1993; **148**: 637–42.

28. Yokoyama A, Kohno N, Hamada H, Sakatani M, Ueda E, Kondo K, *et al.* Circulating KL-6 predicts the outcome of rapidly progressive idiopathic pulmonary fibrosis. *Am J Respir Crit Care Med* 1998; **158**: 1680–4.

29. Gahl WA, Brantly M, Troendle J, Avila NA, Padua A, Montalvo C, *et al.* Effect of pirfenidone on the pulmonary fibrosis of Hermansky-Pudlak syndrome. *Mol Genet Metab* 2002; **76**: 234–42.

30. Nagai S, Hamada K, Shigematsu M, Taniyama M, Yamauchi S, Izumi T. Open-label compassionate use one year-treatment with pirfenidone to patients with chronic pulmonary fibrosis. *Intern Med* 2002; **41**: 1118–23.

31. Cantin AM, Hubbard RC, Crystal RG. Glutathione deficiency in the epithelial lining fluid of the lower respiratory tract in idiopathic pulmonary fibrosis. *Am Rev Respir Dis* 1989; **139**: 370–2.

32. Borok Z, Buhl R, Grimes GJ, Bokser AD, Hubbard RC, Holroyd KJ, *et al.* Effect of glutathione aerosol on oxidant-antioxidant imbalance in idiopathic pulmonary fibrosis. *Lancet* 1991; **338**: 215–16.

33. Meyer A, Buhl R, Magnussen H. The effect of oral N-acetylcysteine on lung glutathione levels in idiopathic pulmonary fibrosis. *Eur Respir J* 1994; **7**: 431–6.

34. American Thoracic Society. Idiopathic pulmonary fibrosis: diagnosis and treatment. International consensus statement. American Thoracic Society (ATS), and the European Respiratory Society (ERS). *Am J Respir Crit Care Med* 2000; **161**: 646–64.

35. Hunninghake GW. Antioxidant therapy for idiopathic pulmonary fibrosis. *N Engl J Med* 2005; **353**: 2285–7.

36. Strieter RM, Starko KM, Enelow RI, Noth I, Valentine VG. Effects of interferon-gamma 1b on biomarker expression in patients with idiopathic pulmonary fibrosis. *Am J Respir Crit Care Med* 2004; **170**: 133–40.

37. Ziesche R, Hofbauer E, Wittmann K, Petkov V, Block LH. A preliminary study of long-term treatment with interferon gamma-1b and low-dose prednisolone in patients with idiopathic pulmonary fibrosis. *N Engl J Med* 1999; **341**: 1264–9.

38. Magro CM, Allen J, Pope-Harman A, Waldman WJ, Moh P, Rothrauff S, Ross P Jr. The role of microvascular injury in the evolution of idiopathic pulmonary fibrosis. *Am J Clin Pathol* 2003; **119**: 556–67.

39. Imokawa S, Sato A, Hayakawa H, Kotani M, Urano T, Takada A. Tissue factor expression and fibrin deposition in the lungs of patients with idiopathic pulmonary fibrosis and systemic sclerosis. *Am J Respir Crit Care Med* 1997; **156**: 631–6.

40. Panos RJ, Mortenson RL, Niccoli SA, King TE Jr. Clinical deterioration in patients with idiopathic pulmonary fibrosis: causes and assessment. *Am J Med* 1990; **88**: 396–404.

13

Pulmonary hypertension in interstitial lung disease and systemic sclerosis

NIK HIRANI

Introduction

Pulmonary hypertension is defined as a resting mean pulmonary artery pressure (PAP) >25 mmHg or systolic PAP >35 mmHg with normal left atrial pressure. Whilst the terms 'pulmonary hypertension' and 'pulmonary arterial hypertension' (PAH) are frequently used interchangeably, the syndrome of pulmonary hypertension can be caused by underlying chronic cardiorespiratory disease causing systemic and/or regional hypoxia, pulmonary thromboembolic disease or an intrinsic disorder of the pulmonary microcirculation; only the latter is termed PAH. In a recently adopted international classification system, pulmonary hypertension associated with interstitial lung disease is categorized with hypoxic causes of pulmonary hypertension (Table 13.1 [1]). This belies the complex nature of the pulmonary hypertension associated with, for example, idiopathic pulmonary fibrosis (IPF) or sarcoidosis, in which hypoxia, microthromboembolic disease and an intrinsic vasculopathy may all play a role in the development of pulmonary hypertension. These issues are discussed in more detail within the disease-specific sections of this chapter. The clinical symptoms and signs of PAH characteristically appear late in the course of the disease and, in the case of pulmonary hypertension associated with interstitial lung disease, the symptoms will often be masked by the underlying pulmonary disorder. The gold standard method for measuring PAP, and thereby diagnosing pulmonary hypertension, is right-heart catheterization. This invasive test carries with it a small but inherent risk to the patient. There is therefore a need for reliable non-invasive indicators of pulmonary hypertension.

Transthoracic Doppler echocardiography (TTE) is a candidate tool for non-invasively detecting pulmonary hypertension, but the PAP cannot be measured directly by this technique. Instead, Doppler echocardiography is used to estimate the right ventricular systolic pressure (RVSP), which in the absence of pulmonary outflow obstruction is equivalent to the systolic PAP. In order to calculate the estimated RVSP, one is required to measure the velocity of the systolic tricuspid

Table 13.1 Clinical classification of pulmonary hypertension—Venice 2003

1. Pulmonary arterial hypertension (PAH)
    1.1. Idiopathic (IPAH)
    1.2. Familial (FPAH)
    1.3. Associated with (APAH):
        1.3.1. Connective tissue disease
        1.3.2. Congenital systemic to pulmonary shunts
        1.3.3. Portal hypertension
        1.3.4. HIV infection
        1.3.5. Drugs and toxins
        1.3.6. Other (thyroid disorders, glycogen storage disease, Gaucher's disease, hereditary haemorrhagic telangiectasia, haemoglobinopathies, meloproliferative disorders, splenectomy)
    1.4. Associated with significant venous or capillary involvement
        1.4.1. Pulmonary veno-occlusive disease (PVOD)
        1.4.2. Pulmonary capillary haemangiomatosis (PCH)
    1.5. Persistent pulmonary hypertension of the newborn (PPHN)

2. Pulmonary hypertension associated with left heart diseases
    2.1. Left-sided atrial or ventricular heart disease
    2.2. Left-sided valvular heart disease

3. Pulmonary hypertension associated with lung respiratory diseases and/or hypoxia
    3.1. Chronic obstructive pulmonary disease
    3.2. Interstitial lung disease
    3.3. Sleep-disordered breathing
    3.4. Alveolar hyperventilation disorders
    3.5. Chronic exposure to high altitude
    3.6. Developmental abnormalities

4. Pulmonary hypertension due to chronic thrombotic and/or embolic disease
    4.1. Thromboembotic obstruction of proximal pulmonary arteries
    4.2. Thromboembotic obstruction of distal pulmonary arteries
    4.3. Non-thrombotic pulmonary embolism (tumour, parasites, foreign material)

5. Miscellaneous
    Sarcoidosis, histiocytosis X, lymphangiomatosis, compression of pulmonary vessels (adenopathy, tumour, fibrosing mediastinitis)

Source: Galie *et al.* (2003) Eur Heart J 25: 2243–78

regurgitant jet (vTR) and to estimate the right atrial pressure (rAP), and then to apply the Bernoulli formula: RVSP = 4(vTR)^2 + rAP. Unfortunately, assessment of both vTR and rAP can be problematic. In skilled hands, a tricuspid regurgitant jet can be detected in at most 70–80% of cases. In one study of 347 patients with advanced interstitial lung disease, PAP could only be assessed by TTE in 44% of individuals [2], and the absence of a detectable tricuspid regurgitation jet does not rule out significant pulmonary hypertension [3]. Even when assessable, PAP measurement by TTE is susceptible to technical measurement error. Right atrial pressure can be assessed from jugular venous distension or by observing changes in the inferior vena cava diameter during respiration, but both measures are prone to subjective variation. TTE has been reported to have high sensitivity (>85%) for detecting pulmonary hypertension, but the technique tends to overestimate systolic PAP by around 10 mmHg and the overall specificity and positive predictive values are <60% in the context of fibrotic lung disease [2,4]. However, in PAH associated with systemic sclerosis the positive predictive accuracy of echocardiography compared with cardiac catheterization is 97% for values ≥45 mmHg [4]. As a final caveat, it should be borne in mind that healthy individuals exhibit RVSP values that range from 15 to 57 mmHg, the highest values being seen in the elderly and those with a high body mass index [5]. If the presence of PAH is assumed on the basis of RVSP ≥35 mmHg, as suggested in international guidelines [1], a significant number of false-positive diagnoses will be generated. The role and limitations of TTE are particularly pertinent to the article from Chang and colleagues discussed in this chapter.

A reduced pulmonary transfer factor for carbon monoxide (T_{LCO}) is of limited value in predicting pulmonary hypertension in the presence of interstitial lung disease, although it is a powerful test for predicting PAH in patients with systemic sclerosis without concomitant interstitial lung disease [6,7]. Similarly, the value of submaximal exercise testing with regard to detecting pulmonary hypertension in fibrotic lung disease is unclear (discussed in Chapter 12). Recently there has been considerable interest in the role of brain natriuretic peptide (BNP) and its role as a simple non-invasive biomarker for pulmonary hypertension. This is discussed in detail with regard to the study by Leuchte and colleagues.

Finally, there are recent international guidelines that address best practice for therapy in PAH [1,8] and an excellent review of current treatments is provided by Ghofrani and colleagues [9]. Long-term anticoagulant therapy is associated with improved survival in idiopathic PAH [10], but its risk/benefit profile has never been tested in pulmonary hypertension associated with interstitial lung disease. A growing body of evidence, including landmark clinical trials, has, however, led to three principal classes of drugs gaining approval for the treatment of PAH: the prostanoids, the endothelin antagonists and the phosphodiesterase type 5 inhibitors. When considering the use of these agents in patients specifically with pulmonary hypertension associated with interstitial lung diseases, however, there are important caveats to consider. Most large clinical trials have included a case-mix of patients with idiopathic PAH, pulmonary hypertension associated with interstitial lung disease, and systemic sclerosis-associated PAH. These forms of pulmonary hypertension may share pathobiological features, but it is a potentially fallible assumption that the therapeutic responses will be equivalent. For example, long-term intravenous prostanoid treatment improves functional capacity and survival in patients with idiopathic PAH [11], but in patients with lung fibrosis it can be detrimental by exacerbating V/Q mismatch [12]. At the time of writing, the much-anticipated Bosentan Use in Interstitial Lung Disease (BUILD) 1 study, a large, multicentre, placebo-controlled trial in patients with IPF, had only been published in abstract form and hence is not discussed in detail in this chapter. Thus, there remains a clear lack of evidence for specific vasculomodulatory therapy in interstitial lung disease-associated pulmonary hypertension.

Pulmonary hypertension in idiopathic pulmonary fibrosis

The presence of pulmonary hypertension in IPF is well recognized [13], but only recently has pulmonary hypertension been studied in large cohorts of patients with IPF, as exemplified by the articles discussed in this section. The pathogenesis of raised pulmonary artery pressure in IPF is uncertain. Hypoxia, both systemically and perhaps at a local level within fibrotic tissue, is the archetypal stimulus for pulmonary artery vasoconstriction and is likely to play some role. Thrombo-embolic and microvascular thrombosis may be relevant but to what degree thrombosis occurs during the course of disease, as opposed to a near terminal event, is unclear. Pulmonary vascular remodelling, causing PAH, is also considered to be significant and there is evidence of contemporaneous vascular ablation and neovascularization in the lungs of patients with IPF [14,15]. Whilst the pathogenesis of pulmonary hypertension is a worthy area of study, for many clinicians the key issues with regard to pulmonary hypertension and IPF are the following: How common is pulmonary hypertension in IPF? Should the presence of pulmonary hypertension be actively sought, and if so in which patients and by which method? What are the implications of developing pulmonary hypertension for the patient? In IPF patients, the presence of pulmonary hypertension at transplant assessment may be associated with early mortality after transplantation [16]. Furthermore, it is recognized that a 10% fall in forced vital capacity (FVC) within 6 months of presentation is a poor prognostic indicator in IPF, but in the interferon γ1b study of 330 patients with IPF it was notable that 43% of such patients died without a prior documented 10% fall in FVC [17]. This raises the prospect of 'hidden' factors that affect survival, one of which is speculated to be pulmonary hypertension. There is also the question of whether pulmonary hypertension in IPF requires treatment, and if so with what drug? Unfortunately, pending the outcome of the ongoing studies, there are no published trials that directly address therapy for IPF-associated pulmonary hypertension. The epidemiology and prognostic significance of pulmonary hypertension in IPF have, however, been addressed in the publications discussed in this chapter.

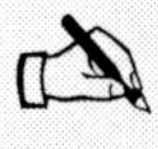

Pulmonary hypertension in patients with idiopathic pulmonary fibrosis

Nadrous HF, Pellikka PA, Krowka MJ, *et al. Chest* 2005; **128**: 2393–9

BACKGROUND. This is a retrospective study aimed at determining the incidence and prognostic significance of pulmonary hypertension, measured by TTE, in patients with IPF.

INTERPRETATION. Of 136 patients with IPF who underwent TTE at presentation, systolic PAP either could not be assessed non-invasively, or significant left ventricular or valvular disease was present, resulting in study exclusion of one-third. Of the 88 eligible subjects, 74 (84%) had pulmonary hypertension, defined as systolic PAP of >35 mmHg at rest, with mean systolic PAP of 48 ± 16 mmHg. Patients with severe pulmonary

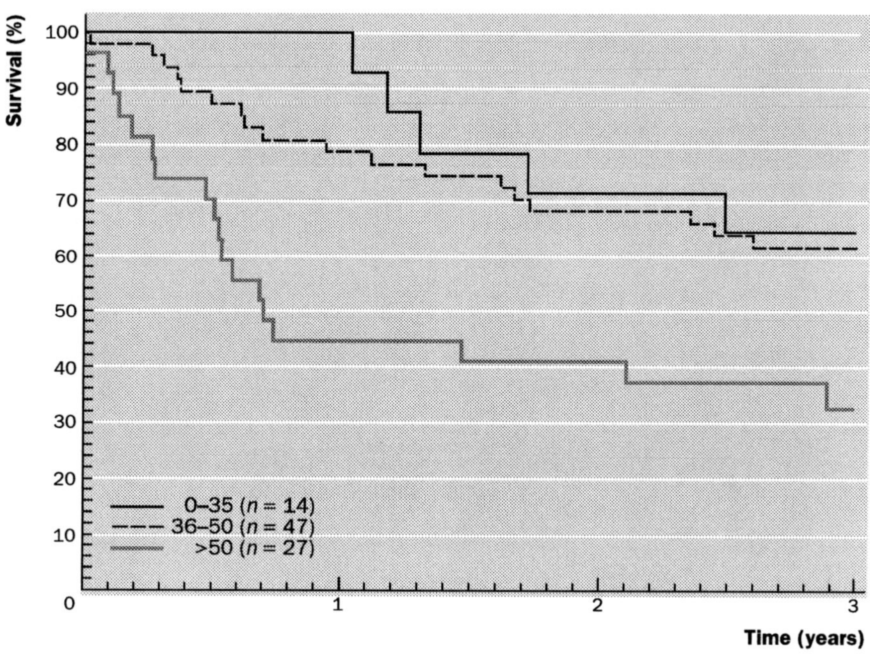

Fig. 13.1 Kaplan–Meier survival curve for 88 patients stratified by their systolic pulmonary artery pressure (mmHg). Source: Nadrous *et al.* (2005).

hypertension (systolic PAP >50 mmHg) had a 1-year mortality rate of 44%, compared with 0% in those with systolic PAP <35 mmHg (Fig. 13.1). Although the average TLCO in those with severe pulmonary hypertension was lower than that in those with normal systolic PAP, baseline lung function did not appear to be a reliable indicator of the presence or absence of pulmonary hypertension. Hence, high systolic PAP predicted in particular for early (1-year) mortality. The retrospective nature of this study introduces the likelihood of significant bias and the data should be interpreted in this light.

Comment

The authors identified 487 patients with IPF who had attended the Mayo Clinic over a 2-year period. Of these, 136 patients (28%) had undergone transthoracic TTE evaluation within 3 months of their first visit and 88 patients from within this group met the required inclusion criteria, namely PAP accessible by TTE, normal left ventricular function and absence of valvular heart disease. These 88 individuals were considered to have IPF by the consensus criteria of the American Thoracic Society and the European Respiratory Society (ATS/ERS). Pulmonary artery hypertension was defined as a systolic PAP of >35 mmHg at rest, calculated by the modified Bernoulli equation. The investigators found that 74 (84%) patients had evidence of pulmonary hypertension, with a mean systolic PAP of 48 ± 16 mmHg (range 28–116 mmHg). The investigators divided patients into three groups: those with normal pulmonary artery pressure (≤35 mmHg, $n = 14$); those with mild pulmonary hypertension (36–50 mmHg, $n = 47$); and those with severe pulmonary hypertension (>50 mmHg, $n = 27$). The Kaplan–Meier survival curves for the three groups showed that those with systolic PAP >50 mmHg had the poorest overall survival, with a 1-year mortality of 44% compared with 0% in those with systolic PAP ≤35 mmHg and 20% in those with systolic PAP 36–50 mmHg (Fig. 13.1). The mean percentage of predicted T_{LCO} in those with PAP >50 mmHg was 39 ± 12.3 (range 18–60%), significantly lower than in those with normal PAP (53.9 ± 16.5; range 27–79%). However, given the wide range in both groups, the severity of lung dysfunction at presentation was not a reliable indicator of the presence or absence of pulmonary hypertension.

In this study, high systolic PAP predicted in particular for early (1-year) mortality. It is not clear whether high PAP is an independent predictor of poor prognosis when corrected for other parameters known to be associated with poor survival, such as male gender and lower T_{LCO}. The retrospective nature of this study does introduce the likelihood of significant bias in the data. For example, the 136 patients with IPF studied using TTE represented a subgroup of the total IPF population seen in this centre, selected for assessment of PAP at the discretion of the attending physician without pre-specified criteria. The prevalence of pulmonary hypertension in an unselected population of patients with IPF is almost certainly considerably lower than the 84% cited in this study. The limitation of TTE in assessing pulmonary hypertension is discussed in the Introduction of this chapter, and, since TTE tends to overestimate PAP by around 10 mmHg, it possible that as many as 50% of individuals in this study may not in fact have had pulmonary hypertension if assessed by right heart catheter measurement.

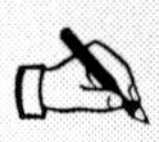

Prevalence and outcomes of pulmonary arterial hypertension in advanced idiopathic pulmonary fibrosis
Lettieri CJ, Nathan SD, Barnett SD, Ahmad S, Shorr AF. *Chest* 2006; **129**: 746–52

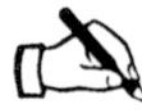

Pulmonary hypertension and pulmonary function testing in idiopathic pulmonary fibrosis
Nathan SD, Shlobin OA, Ahmad S, Urbanek S, Barnett SD. *Chest* 2007; **131**: 657–63

BACKGROUND. These two retrospective studies emanate from the same specialist IPF clinic and lung transplant referral centre in North America. The aims were to

assess the prevalence of pulmonary hypertension in patients with IPF and to determine the relationship between underlying pulmonary hypertension and lung function parameters.

INTERPRETATION. All patients underwent right heart catheterization, and 48 of 118 patients (40.7%) were found to have pulmonary hypertension, as defined by mean PAP >25 mmHg. The presence of pulmonary hypertension was associated with a 1-year mortality of 28% compared with 5.5% in those with normal pulmonary artery pressure ($P = 0.002$). Subjects with T_{LCO} <40% of predicted and resting oxygen saturation <88% were 10 times more likely to have underlying pulmonary hypertension than those with T_{LCO} >40% of predicted and a resting oxygen saturation of 88% or greater. Percentage of predicted FVC was not a reliable indicator of the presence of pulmonary hypertension and there were proportionately at least as many patients with pulmonary hypertension in the group with preserved lung volume (FVC >70% of predicted) compared with the group with severe restrictive disease (FVC <40% of predicted). This observation hints that the development of pulmonary hypertension in IPF is not entirely attributable to progressive parenchymal fibrosis.

Comment

All recruited patients had IPF as defined by ATS/ERS consensus criteria and had undergone right-sided cardiac catheterization as part of the initial evaluation prior to being considered for transplantation. Consequently, all but twelve of the patients were ≤65 years of age and in general had moderate to severe disease. The prevalence of pulmonary hypertension, as defined by a mean PAP of >25 mmHg, was 40.7%, substantially lower than the figure reported by Nadrous *et al.* The presence of pulmonary hypertension was clearly associated with a significantly poorer prognosis. The Kaplan–Meier curve (Fig. 13.2) reveals that patients with pulmonary hypertension suffer a high early mortality rate, 28% of patients dying within 1 year compared with 5.5% in those with normal pulmonary artery pressure ($P = 0.002$). It is also noteworthy that left ventricular dysfunction, one of the commonest causes of mild pulmonary hypertension, was not a potential confounding factor in these studies and left ventricular dysfunction did not independently predict survival. Patients who had both a T_{LCO} of <40% of predicted and significant resting hypoxaemia, as defined above, were 10 times more likely to have underlying PAH than those with T_{LCO} >40% of predicted and a resting oxygen saturation of ≥88%. However, individual lung function parameters were found to be a poor guide to the presence or absence of PAH (Table 13.2). In fact, rather paradoxically, there was a higher proportion of patients with PAH in those with FVC >70% of predicted, compared with the group with FVC <40% of predicted (P <0.008), although the statistical significance was lost when individuals with elevated pulmonary capillary wedge pressure (present in 16% of subjects) were excluded. As might be predicted, performance on a 6-min walking test was a useful predictor of underlying pulmonary hypertension, such that those with elevated PAP walked significantly shorter distances and experienced significantly greater desaturation than those with normal PAP.

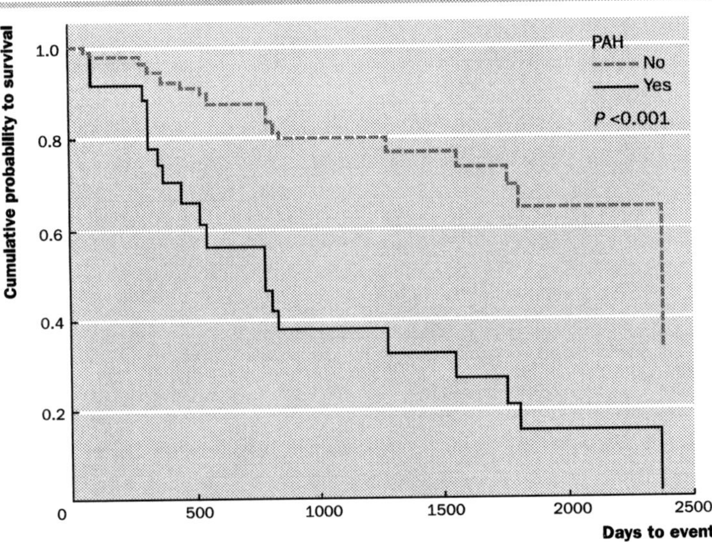

Fig. 13.2 Pulmonary hypertension (mean PAP >25 mmHg) as a predictor of survival in patients with idiopathic pulmonary fibrosis. Source: Lettieri *et al.* (2006).

The observation that pulmonary hypertension was observed in 16 patients in whom FVC was >70% of predicted is interesting. The authors speculate that this reinforces the hypothesis that parenchymal fibrosis is not directly responsible for pulmonary hypertension. However, there is no comment on the prevalence of emphysema in this population of patients that could account for the relatively well-

Table 13.2 Patient characteristics and baseline physiological parameters (*n* = 118)

Parameters	mPAP <25 mmHg (*n* = 70)	mPAP ≥25 mmHg (*n* = 48)	P-value
Male gender	45 (64.3)	29 (60.4)	0.558
Age, yr	59.7 ± 7.0	58.4 ± 7.0	0.923
FVC%	52.4 ± 14.7	54.6 ± 17.3	0.469
D_{LCO}%	36.3 ± 14.1	33.2 ± 18.0	0.331
FVC%/D_{LCO}% ratio	2.8 ± 5.9	2.0 ± 0.8	0.420
FEV_1%	55.8 ± 15.7	56.0 ± 15.3	0.575
TLC%	54.4 ± 13.5	58.6 ± 15.9	0.196
PCWP, mmHg	8.2 ± 4.6	12.2 ± 5.8	0.001
Interval between RHC and PFT, d	70.5 ± 60.7	83.2 ± 68.6	0.298

Data are presented as no. (%) or mean ± SD.
D_{LCO}, diffusing capacity for carbon monoxide; PCWP, pulmonary capillary wedge pressure; PFT, pulmonary function test; RHC, right heart catheterization TLC, total lung capacity.
Source: Nathan *et al.* (2007).

maintained lung volumes and low T_{LCO}. Indeed, the authors acknowledge that FVC may not be the best parameter to define the extent of underlying parenchymal lung disease in a cohort of patients who are often current or ex-smokers. The investigators did evaluate the composite physiological index (CPI), a previously described tool for assessment in IPF in relation to pulmonary hypertension. To some extent, this is an index that corrects for associated emphysema, and the observation that the CPI did not correlate with mean PAP does hint that pulmonary hypertension may occur as a specific entity within IPF and not necessarily as a direct consequence of progressive fibrosis.

A significant strength of these studies is that all patients underwent right heart catheterization rather than TTE alone. A limitation is the retrospective nature of the report, which concerns a rather select group of patients with advanced disease and relatively young age. However, selection bias is offset to some extent since in this particular institution it is a policy to evaluate all patients under the age of 65 for transplantation at the time of initial presentation, regardless of the severity of disease.

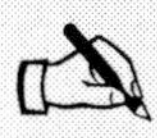

Significance of pulmonary arterial pressure and diffusion capacity of the lung as prognosticators in patients with idiopathic pulmonary fibrosis

Hamada K, Nagai S, Tanaka S, *et al. Chest* 2007; **131**: 650–6

BACKGROUND. This prospective study aimed to define the incidence and clinical course of pulmonary hypertension in 70 patients with IPF. Pulmonary hypertension was assessed by right heart catheterization and was defined as a mean PAP >25 mmHg.

INTERPRETATION. In this study, the incidence of pulmonary hypertension was 8%. The investigators identified a critical cut-off of 17 mmHg, such that mean PAP below this value was associated with a 5-year survival of 62.2% compared with 16.7% in those with mean PAP >17 mmHg. The implication is that even pulmonary artery pressures within the normal range may have a prognostic implication in patients with IPF.

Comment

This is the first long-term longitudinal study of the incidence and clinical course of pulmonary hypertension in IPF. Seventy-eight patients with a diagnosis of IPF (usual interstitial pneumonia pattern histologically [$n = 59$] or unspecified criteria [$n = 19$]) underwent right heart catheterization, in addition to routine clinical work-up at presentation. A number of patients were excluded because of early post-operative deaths, a re-evaluation of the diagnosis of IPF or loss to follow-up, such that 61 individuals were available for 5-year survival analysis. Pulmonary hypertension was defined as mean PAP >25 mmHg. On this basis, six out of 70 patients (8%) had pulmonary hypertension at initial work-up. This value is markedly lower than the values of around 40–80% reported by Nadrous *et al.* and Lettieri *et al.*, albeit in different populations and, in the case of Nadrous *et al.*, using transthoracic echocardiography as opposed to right heart catheterization. These differences may reflect differences in the stage of disease at which PAP was assessed or may perhaps reflect differences between populations of different ethnicity. Rather than comparing the long-term survival of patients with and without pulmonary hypertension, the authors chose to perform a receiver operating characteristic curve analysis to determine an optimal cut-off value of mean PAP for predicting 5-year mortality. Although the analysis is not shown in the paper, a value of 17 mmHg was judged to be critical, presumably suggesting that this value had the highest sensitivity and specificity for predicting death. The investigators found that 23 of the 37 patients (62.2%) with mean PAP <17 mmHg survived for 5 years compared with only 4 of only 24 patients (16.7%) with PAP ≥7mmHg (*P* <0.001; relative risk of mortality 2.2; 95% confidence interval [CI] 1.4–3.45) (Fig. 13.3). The predicted vital capacities of those with high and low PAP were not significantly different, but those with a PAP of ≥17 mmHg did have a significantly lower percentage of predicted T_{LCO} (36 ± 10 vs 51 ± 15%; *P* <0.001). Also consistent with several previous studies was the observation that T_{LCO} <40% of predicted confers a poor prognosis. The message from this paper is that even mean PAP values that by definition fall within the normal range (17–25 mmHg) may have prognostic significance, and that T_{LCO} is a useful but not entirely reliable way of predicting which patients have PAH or PAP of >17 mmHg on baseline resting physiology

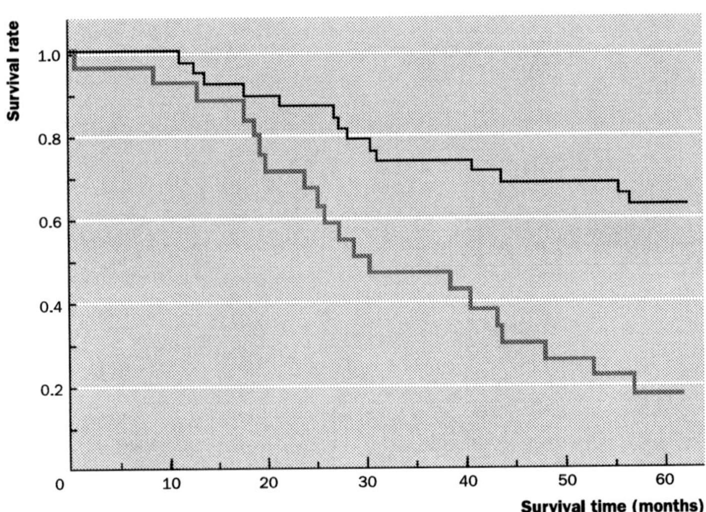

Fig. 13.3 Five-year survival rates of patients grouped according to pulmonary artery pressure (PAP). *Thin line*, normal PAP group (mean PAP [mPAP] <17 mmHg; *n* = 37); *bold line*, high PAP group (mean PAP ≥17 mmHg; *n* = 24). Source: Hamada *et al.* (2007).

testing alone. The role of exercise testing in identifying pulmonary hypertension was not explored in this study. The incidence of true pulmonary hypertension (>25 mmHg) was less than 1 in 10 in this relatively unselected group of patients.

Pulmonary hypertension in sarcoidosis

Pulmonary hypertension has long been recognized as an uncommon complication of sarcoidosis, but it is only with the publication of recent studies, discussed in this chapter, that a clear description of the epidemiology and natural history of sarcoidosis-associated pulmonary hypertension has begun to emerge. What are the implications of developing pulmonary hypertension for the patient with sarcoidosis? In individuals listed for lung transplantation, the presence of pulmonary hypertension is associated with an adverse prognosis [18,19]. Shorr *et al.* detail the characteristics of over 300 patients with sarcoidosis awaiting lung transplantation with the aim of defining clinical and radiological features that might predict the presence of pulmonary hypertension. Although pulmonary hypertension in sarcoidosis is generally associated with parenchymal lung disease, it can occur in Stage 0 and Stage 1 sarcoidosis, as described in a recently reported retrospective study in which 10% of cases of sarcoidosis-associated pulmonary hypertension occurred in subjects with Stage 0 or Stage 1 disease [20], and this observation is reinforced in the prospective study by Handa *et al.* This raises intriguing questions about the pathogenesis of pulmonary hypertension in sarcoidosis. In addition to hypoxia secondary to lung disease, the mechanisms for generating pulmonary hypertension in sarcoidosis include compression of large pulmonary arteries by mediastinal/hilar adenopathy, granulomatous vasculitis, secondary pulmonary veno-occlusive disease and heightened sensitivity to vasoactive factors; in these respects the report by Nunes and colleagues is enlightening.

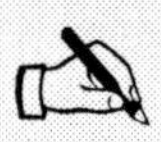

Pulmonary hypertension in advanced sarcoidosis: epidemiology and clinical characteristics

Shorr AF, Helman DL, Davies DB, Nathan SD. *Eur Respir J* 2005; **25**: 783–8

BACKGROUND. The investigators reviewed the United Network of Organ Sharing (UNOS) Registry and identified all patients with sarcoidosis listed for lung transplantation over a 7-year period with the aim of determining the prevalence of pulmonary hypertension in this population.

INTERPRETATION. Pulmonary hypertension (mean PAP >25 mmHg) was reported in 75% of the 363 patients, and 36% exhibited severe pulmonary hypertension (mean PAP ≥40 mmHg). The requirement for supplementary oxygen, but not spirometry or 6-min walking distance, proved to be a useful parameter for distinguishing those with pulmonary hypertension from those with normal PAP.

Comment

The UNOS registry is a comprehensive database of all patients listed for organ transplantation in North America. The investigators identified all patients listed for single lung, double lung and heart–lung transplantation for sarcoidosis over a 7-year period up to December 2002. Registered patients had recorded data for resting spirometry, 6-min walk distance, the need for supplementary oxygen and right heart catheterization with measures of cardiac performance. Pulmonary hypertension was defined as a mean PAP of >25 mmHg and severe pulmonary hypertension defined as a mean PAP of ≥40 mmHg. The UNOS registry does not, however, record T_{LCO} or arterial oxygen tension or, at least until 1999, the ratio of forced expiratory volume in 1 second (FEV_1) to FVC, and there were no high-resolution computed tomography (HRCT) data for these patients. Three hundred and sixty-three individuals listed for lung transplantation and with complete right heart catheter data, representing 72.5% of all sarcoidosis patients listed, were reported in the data analysis. The mean age of this cohort was 46 years, 70% were African-American and two-thirds were female. Only 25% of patients had normal PAP and 131 patients (36%) had severe pulmonary hypertension. Pulmonary function based on spirometry indicated at least moderately severe disease, as might be expected of patients listed for lung transplantation. However, the only parameter that distinguished patients with pulmonary hypertension from those with normal PAP was a documented need for supplementary oxygen, which was required in 91.8% of patients with pulmonary hypertension compared with 67.3% of patients with normal PAP (P <0.001). Neither spirometry nor 6-min walking distance was a useful clinical marker for pulmonary hypertension. Interestingly, the authors also found that patients with pulmonary hypertension had higher pulmonary capillary wedge pressure and were significantly more likely to be suffering from systemic hypertension compared with those with normal PAP. This raises the distinct possibility that the pulmonary hypertension in sarcoidosis may in part be a consequence of left ventricular systolic or diastolic dysfunction.

The main limitations of this study are its retrospective nature and the lack of complete lung function data, itself a consequence of the way UNOS registry data are recorded. However, at the time of writing, this study is by far the most comprehensive report of the prevalence of pulmonary hypertension in sarcoidosis.

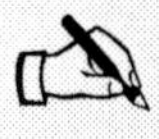

Incidence of pulmonary hypertension and its clinical relevance in patients with sarcoidosis

Handa T, Nagai S, Miki S, Fushimi Y, Ohta K, Mishima M, Izumi T. *Chest* 2006; **129**: 1246–52

BACKGROUND. This is a large prospective study of sarcoidosis from Japan. The aim was to determine the incidence of pulmonary hypertension and determine the clinical and radiological characteristics of patients with elevated PAP. The investigators used

TTE to determine the systolic PAP, and pulmonary hypertension was defined as a systolic PAP of ≥40 mmHg.

INTERPRETATION. In this prospective observational study the investigators report that 5.7% of 246 patients with Stage 0–4 sarcoidosis screened by TTE had pulmonary hypertension, defined as a systolic PAP of ≥40 mmHg. Almost 75% of patients had Stage 0 or Stage 1 disease at assessment. In addition to non-invasive estimation of PAP, all patients underwent HRCT scanning and static lung function testing. Measurement of systolic PAP by TTE was possible in 212 (86%) of the 246 screened patients, a higher proportion than is often cited in clinical studies. Although parenchymal lung disease was proportionately more common in those with pulmonary hypertension and there were statistically significant differences in lung function between patients with and without pulmonary hypertension, there were no clinically useful parameters that could reliably be used to predict the presence of pulmonary hypertension. The incidence of pulmonary hypertension in this unselected group of patients is consistent with previous reports.

Comment

The investigators compared clinical, lung function and radiographic findings between the 200 patients with normal PAP and the twelve patients with pulmonary hypertension. Five of the twelve individuals with pulmonary hypertension had Stage 0 or Stage 1 disease. The comparison of lung function tests between those with and without pulmonary hypertension does show some statistically significant differences in spirometry between the two groups, but on univariate analysis there was no single clinical lung function or radiological parameter that could be usefully used to predict the presence of PAH. This study is helpful in that it shows that, in an unselected group of patients with sarcoidosis and generally mild lung dysfunction, the prevalence of pulmonary hypertension is under 6%, a finding similar to those of previous studies of similar groups of patients in which right heart catheterization had been used to determine PAP |21|. There are well-described differences in the clinical features of sarcoidosis between ethnic groups. For example, in contrast to sarcoidosis in North America, lung disease due to sarcoidosis in Japan is relatively mild and most sarcoidosis-associated deaths are due to cardiac involvement.

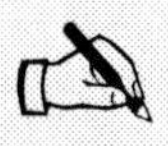

Pulmonary hypertension associated with sarcoidosis: mechanisms, haemodynamics and prognosis

Nunes H, Humbert M, Capron F, *et al. Thorax* 2006; **61**: 68–74

BACKGROUND. This retrospective case–control study sought to investigate the clinical significance of pulmonary hypertension in sarcoidosis, and more specifically to explore the pathogenesis of pulmonary hypertension in patients with sarcoidosis but without significant pulmonary fibrosis.

INTERPRETATION. The investigators confirmed that the presence of pulmonary hypertension was associated with poor prognosis in sarcoidosis, with a 5-year survival of under 60%. Detailed histopathological studies in a small subgroup of patients with sarcoidosis-associated pulmonary hypertension revealed the presence of vascular wall granulomata, specifically an occlusive venopathy, which may account for pulmonary hypertension even in the absence of parenchymal fibrosis.

Comment

This small but detailed retrospective study reports on 22 consecutive patients with sarcoidosis and pulmonary hypertension seen at a highly specialized tertiary referral centre in France. All patients had undergone right heart catheterization, and pulmonary hypertension was defined as mean PAP $\geq$25 mmHg with normal pulmonary capillary wedge pressure. Each study patient was matched with two demographically, physiologically and radiologically matched control patients with sarcoidosis. The patients with pulmonary hypertension were divided into those with and without pulmonary fibrosis based on HRCT scanning. Two patients with pulmonary hypertension had Stage 0 sarcoidosis at the time of assessment and 30% had pulmonary hypertension in the absence of lung fibrosis. Survival follow-up of the patients confirmed that the presence of pulmonary hypertension in sarcoidosis is a poor prognostic indicator. The 1-, 2- and 5-year survival rates were 84.8, 73.5 and 59% respectively compared with 100, 96.4 and 96.4% in the carefully matched controls without PAH ($P = 0.003$). Mortality was therefore not associated with patient demographical features, resting lung function, the 6-min walking test or other haemodynamic parameters measured at right heart catheterization.

The investigators sought to determine the causes of pulmonary hypertension in patients with sarcoidosis, but were hampered by the inevitable lack of lung biopsies available for study. They speculate that granulomatous pulmonary vascular occlusive disease (PVOD) may account for some cases of pulmonary hypertension in Stage 0–3 sarcoidosis, since a larger proportion of these patients had significant ground-glass change on HRCT scanning compared with controls without pulmonary hypertension (85.7 vs 14.3%; P <0.01). However, whilst ground-glass change is a feature of PVOD, it is by no means pathognomic. CT scanning also identified extrinsic compression of large pulmonary arteries by mediastinal or hilar glands in 21.4% of the patients, which may have accounted for a degree of pulmonary hypertension. The investigators were able to study native lungs obtained from patients with fibrotic sarcoidosis who had undergone lung transplantation. A number of histological findings were reported, but most striking was the presence of sarcoidosis granulomas predominantly in the veins, and occlusive venopathy with very little in the way of arterial lesions. Previous studies have found that vascular involvement at all levels from large pulmonary arteries to venous structures is very common in pulmonary sarcoidosis [22,23], but the finding of an intrinsic venopathy with marked lesions of intimal fibrosis is a novel observation that might account for the subgroup of patients with sarcoidosis, pulmonary hypertension and minimal parenchymal fibrosis. This form of granulomatous occlusive venopathy may not be responsive to corticosteroids, and the authors cite two previous studies in which corticosteroids were shown to clearly improve physiological and radiological parameters in sarcoidosis, but only reduced PAP in under half of the 24 patients studied |24,25|.

The limitations of the study are that it is retrospective and by necessity performed in a highly specialized centre with an interest in sarcoidosis and pulmonary vascular disease. However, this is a careful evaluation of pulmonary hypertension in sarcoidosis and offers new insights into the pathogenesis of this disease.

Pulmonary hypertension in systemic sclerosis

Pulmonary disease is a major cause of mortality in patients with systemic sclerosis, and amongst the pulmonary complications pulmonary hypertension is the most frequent. Pulmonary hypertension frequently occurs in the absence of significant interstitial lung disease, i.e. isolated PAH. Most studies indicate that between 10 and 20% of patients with systemic sclerosis exhibit significant pulmonary hypertension |26–28|. Moreover, patients with systemic sclerosis-associated PH are at higher risk of death than patients with idiopathic PAH, despite similar haemodynamic patterns and treatments |29|. The value of screening for PH in systemic sclerosis remains uncertain, however, and, once detected, the natural history of the disease and the value of therapeutic intervention are also poorly understood. In this regard the recent studies discussed in this section have significantly improved our understanding of pulmonary hypertension in systemic sclerosis.

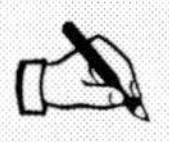

Early detection of pulmonary arterial hypertension in systemic sclerosis: a French nationwide prospective multicenter study

Hachulla E, Gressin V, Guillevin L, et al. Arthritis Rheum 2005; **52**: 3792–800

BACKGROUND. This was a large prospective study conducted with the aim of developing an algorithm for the assessment of pulmonary hypertension in systemic sclerosis. Patients with significant interstitial lung disease were largely excluded, so this is principally a study of isolated systemic sclerosis-associated PAH in the absence of parenchymal lung disease.

INTERPRETATION. Screening of 570 patients with systemic sclerosis using TTE identified 33 with suspected PAH, of whom 18 (55%) were confirmed at right heart catheterization. The mean PAP in the 18 confirmed cases of PAH was 30 ± 9 mmHg, indicating mild disease. Patients found to have PAH following screening were significantly older and more likely to be breathless and had significantly lower T_{LCO} than the 548 individuals without PAH. The authors conclude that screening with TTE and performing right heart catheterization in patients who have mildly elevated peak velocity of tricuspid regurgitation (vTR) and who are breathless for no other cause will detect a significant number of patients with PAH. However, the natural history and implications for the patient of detecting mild 'early' PAH are not known.

Comment

This was a prospective study conducted at 21 referral centres in France over a 10-month period. The authors sought to develop an algorithm based on clinical symptoms, TTE and right heart catheterization that would allow screening for PAH in patients with systemic sclerosis. Patients with systemic sclerosis who had significant pulmonary function abnormalities, defined as FVC, total lung capacity or FEV_1 <60% of predicted, were excluded in an attempt to study a relatively homogeneous population of patients with isolated systemic sclerosis-associated PAP in the absence of significant parenchymal lung disease. However, the report does not include a description of chest radiology and so it is hard to determine how many patients may have had mild or even moderately severe interstitial lung disease. Of 709 consecutive patients with systemic sclerosis, 110 were excluded because of the presence of significant heart disease, and 29 of the remaining 599 individuals had known PAH. Thus, 570 individuals were screened by TTE. In 20% of those screened, PAP could not be estimated because of the absence of tricuspid regurgitation or because of poor views. Pulmonary hypertension was suspected in patients with vTR >3 m/s or, if associated with unexplained breathlessness, between 2.5 and 3 m/s. The investigators made the assumption that pulmonary artery hypertension was not present in patients in whom the vTR could not be quantified, provided the right ventricle was normal |30|. The use of vTR to estimate systolic PAP requires the use of the modified Bernoulli equation and this technique has been shown to correlate well with systolic PAP recorded at right heart catheterization, as discussed in the Introduction. The authors chose a threshold vTR level of >2.5 m/s based on their own previous experience and that of others in the literature, and, using this cut-off, pulmonary hypertension was suspected in 33 patients. Subsequent right heart catheter studies confirmed pulmonary hypertension in 18 (55%); the remaining individuals either had evidence of left ventricular dysfunction or exhibited normal pulmonary arterial pressure. The mean PAP in the 18 confirmed cases of PAH was 30 ± 9 mmHg, indicating mild disease, although one individual had a mean PAP >45 mmHg. When the authors went back to study the characteristics of the 18 patients with newly diagnosed PAH compared with the 548 without pulmonary hypertension, they found that patients with PAH were significantly older, more likely to be breathless and had significantly lower T_{LCO} (Table 13.3). Patient breathlessness was evaluated using the New York Heart Association (NYHA) functional class, which is commonly used for the assessment of PAH. A quarter of individuals with pulmonary hypertension had T_{LCO} values >60% of predicted. Interestingly, the investigators found no difference in the incidence of PAH in patients with limited versus diffuse systemic sclerosis, whereas several other studies have suggested that PAH is more common in the limited form of the disease.

With an estimated 7000 adult patients with systemic sclerosis in France, these investigators successfully enrolled close to 10% of the affected population, an admirable achievement. The authors conclude that screening with TTE and performing right heart catheterization in patients who have mildly elevated vTR and who are breathless for no other cause will detect a significant number of patients

Table 13.3 Clinical characteristics, signs, symptoms and pulmonary function test results in patients with newly diagnosed pulmonary arterial hypertension (PAH) and those with no PAH (n = 566)

Parameter	Newly diagnosed PAH (n = 18)	No PAH (n = 548)	P
Age, years	65.0 ± 11.7	54.1 ± 12.9	<0.001
Female, no. (%)	16 (88.9)	46 (84.9)	≤1.00
Body mass index, kg/m²	26.6 ± 5.9	23.9 ± 4.5	≤0.014
SSc subtype, no. (%) limited	10 (55.6)	409 (74.6)	≤0.10
Age at first non-RP SSc symptom, years	52.0 ± 14.7	45.7 ± 13.8	≤0.07
Age at SSc diagnosis, years	57.4 ± 13.4	47.3 ± 13.6	≤0.003
Time since first non-RP symptom, years	11.9 ± 12.6	8.5 ± 7.8	≤0.29
Rodnan score	13.8 ± 8.6	13.0 ± 10.7	≤0.77
Dyspnoea, no. (%)	15 (83.3)	147 (26.8)	<0.0001
Fatigue, no. (%)	11 (61.1)	182 (33.2)	≤0.014
Palpitations, no. (%)	6 (33.3)	78 (14.2)	≤0.037
Syncope or presyncope during exercise, no. (%)	3 (16.7)	15 (2.7)	≤0.016
Chest pain, no. (%)	1 (5.6)	17 (3.1)	≤0.45
Lower limb oedema, no. (%)	6 (33.3)	37 (6.8)	<0.001
Hepatojugular reflux, no. (%)	4 (22.2)	4 (0.7)	<0.0001
Jugular venous distention, no. (%)	4 (22.2)	6 (1.1)	<0.0001
D_{LCO}, % of predicted	56.2 ± 23.3	72.6 ± 18.0	<0.0004
Patients with D_{LCO} <60%, no. (%)	13 (72.2)	149 (27.2)	<0.0001
$PaO_2 + PaCO_2$, mm Hg	111.3 ± 12.6	127.5 ± 15.1	<0.0001

Four patients with left heart disease were excluded. Except where indicated otherwise, values are mean ± SD. P-values were determined by analysis of variance or Student's t-test. D_{LCO}, diffusing capacity for carbon monoxide; RP, Raynaud's phenomenon; SSc, systemic sclerosis.
Source: Hachulla *et al.* (2005)

with pulmonary hypertension. The suggested algorithm used by the investigators is shown in Fig. 13.4. Clearly, the expertise of the echocardiographer is critical to the success of this screening protocol. This study did not include patients with moderate to severe pulmonary function abnormalities and therefore the screening algorithm may not be applicable to all patients with systemic sclerosis. Furthermore, the implications of early detection of PAP will need to be assessed in long-term follow-up to determine the natural history of mild PAH detected in this way.

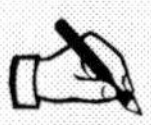

Natural history of mild–moderate pulmonary hypertension and the risk factors for severe pulmonary hypertension in scleroderma

Chang B, Schachna L, White B, Wigley FM, Wise RA. *J Rheumatol* 2006; **33**: 269–74

BACKGROUND. Recent clinical studies have shown that patients with severe symptomatic isolated PAH, principally individuals who have NYHA class III or IV

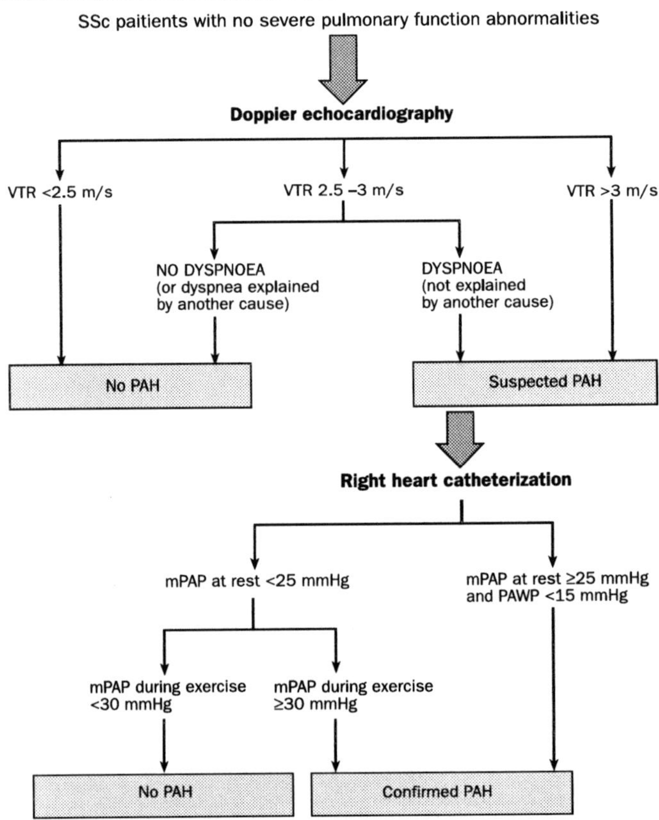

Fig. 13.4 Screening algorithm for the diagnosis of pulmonary arterial hypertension (PAH) in patients with systemic sclerosis. VTR, peak velocity of tricuspid regurgitation; mPAP, mean pulmonary artery pressure; PAWP, pulmonary artery wedge pressure. Right heart catheterization was performed except when Doppler echocardiography provided evidence of left heart disease. Source: Hachulla *et al.* (2005).

functional status, may be candidates for one of the several therapeutic options now available. What is less certain is whether early intervention in patients with mild to moderate pulmonary hypertension is of clinical benefit. A better understanding of the natural history of mild to moderate pulmonary hypertension and establishment of the risk factors that identify the subgroup who progress to severe pulmonary hypertension would have significant clinical value. Previous studies have shown that there is a direct relationship between pulmonary hypertension and survival. In a prospective study over 4 years, patients with a mean PAP of <32 mmHg at the time of right heart catheterization had a 1-year survival rate of 93% compared with 61% in those with a mean PAP of >45 mmHg |27|.

INTERPRETATION.   This was a retrospective study of 820 patients with systemic sclerosis who had undergone TTE for the assessment of pulmonary hypertension and a subgroup of 457 individuals who had undergone serial TTE. The study included patients with significant interstitial lung disease. Of the 361 individuals who did not have evidence of pulmonary hypertension at initial screening, 38% developed pulmonary hypertension over a mean period of 3.2 years. Serial TTE in the 96 individuals who did have pulmonary hypertension at first assessment revealed that, in most individuals, the severity of pulmonary hypertension did not change significantly over the period of follow-up, but that in 17.7% of individuals PAP increased significantly and in 15.6% PAP fell to within the normal range. The extent to which these observations reflect the true natural history of pulmonary hypertension in systemic sclerosis, as opposed to variations in the measurement of PAH by TTE, is uncertain.

Comment

This is a large retrospective study from a major scleroderma centre in North America. Of 1136 patients with systemic sclerosis (limited cutaneous and diffuse forms of the disease) 820 (72.1%) had undergone echocardiography suitable for the evaluation of pulmonary hypertension and a smaller subgroup of 457 (40.2%) had undergone serial echocardiography. Of the 361 individuals who did not have evidence of pulmonary hypertension at initial screening, 38% developed raised PAP over a 3.2-year period, and in more than one-third this was considered to be severe pulmonary hypertension (Fig. 13.5). Serial TTE in the 96 patients who did have pulmonary hypertension on an initial echocardiogram, yielded intriguing data. In those with mild to moderate PAH initially, 17.7% progressed to severe pulmonary hypertension and 15.6% actually regressed to having no evidence of pulmonary hypertension. Indeed, even in those with severe pulmonary hypertension on first echocardiogram, the PAP appeared to fall significantly on subsequent scans and in a handful of patients it returned to normal. It is unclear whether changes in PAP were reflected in the symptom score since the authors were unable to measure and report on the NYHA functional status at around the time of each echocardiogram. In identifying risk factors that might predict the development of severe pulmonary hypertension, the investigators observed that male sex ($P = 0.02$), fulfilment of the American College of Rheumatology criteria for scleroderma at presentation ($P = 0.04$) and older age at disease onset ($P = 0.04$) all predicted the development of severe pulmonary hypertension. Other factors, including smoking status and the disease subtype (limited versus diffuse), did not predict the development of severe pulmonary hypertension. In contrast to the French study by Hachulla *et al.*, this study did not seek to exclude patients with significant interstitial lung disease. Indeed, individuals with more severely impaired lung function, particularly reduced T_{LCO}, were also at higher risk of developing pulmonary hypertension. The authors do not report on the presence or absence of interstitial lung disease based on radiology so it is difficult to be certain what proportion of these patients had isolated pulmonary artery hypertension associated with systemic sclerosis and how many had pulmonary hypertension in conjunction with fibrotic lung disease. The authors do state that the risk of developing pulmonary hypertension increased significantly when the initial T_{LCO} was <50% of predicted, a finding in keeping with several other studies [31].

A possible interpretation of this study is that the natural history of pulmonary hypertension in systemic sclerosis is quite variable and can show improvement as well as progression. However, before drawing this conclusion one has to consider the potential variability in measuring PAP by TTE. The investigators used Doppler echocardiography to estimate RVSP, a surrogate for systolic PAP. There is a reasonably high correlation (0.57–0.93) between transthoracic echocardiography estimation of RVSP and systolic PAP measured by right heart catheterization [32]. The limitations of using TTE to estimate PAP have been discussed in the Introduction. The measurement of pulmonary hypertension by TTE is dependent on the expertise of the performer and little is known about intra- and inter-observer variability over time. Hence, the changes reported by Chang and colleagues may represent genuine changes in the natural history of pulmonary hypertension over time, observer variation or a combination of the two.

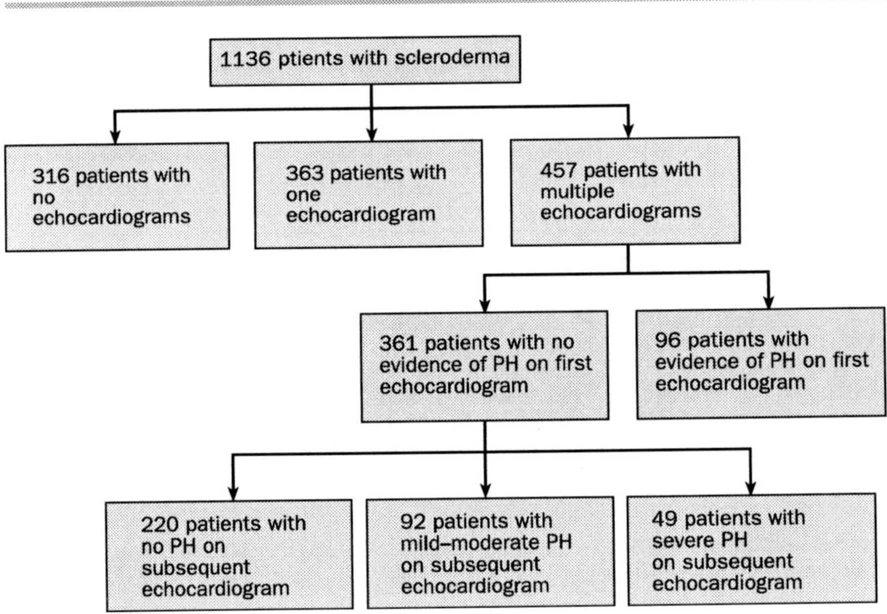

Fig. 13.5 Classification of patients with and without echocardiograms, including serial echocardiograms. PH, pulmonary hypertension. Source: Chang *et al.* (2006).

Novel screening tools for pulmonary hypertension in lung disease

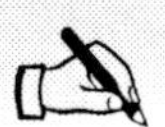

Brain natriuretic peptide is a prognostic parameter in chronic lung disease

Leuchte HH, Baumgartner RA, Nounou ME, *et al. Am J Respir Crit Care Med* 2006; **173**: 744–50

BACKGROUND. A common theme that has emerged from a number of the studies is the need for a safe and robust non-invasive method of identifying patients with clinically significant pulmonary hypertension. TTE has technical limitations and T_{LCO} and oxygen desaturation on exercise have high sensitivity for detecting pulmonary hypertension but low specificity in a setting of interstitial lung disease. A novel robust tool would be of great value if it also served as a biomarker, indicating the mortality risk and the response to therapy. BNP is predominantly secreted by cardiac ventricles under stress |33|. The value of BNP measurements in identifying pulmonary hypertension in patients with interstitial lung disease is unclear.

INTERPRETATION. This is a prospective study of 176 patients with a variety of obstructive and interstitial lung diseases, although almost one-third had IPF. All patients underwent right heart catheterization and had undergone baseline investigations including a 6-min walking test and plasma BNP assay. Over a mean follow-up of 1 year, 31 individuals died and the investigators report that mean PAP $\geq$35 mmHg, present in a quarter of patients, was associated with a 3.67-fold increased risk of death. Elevated BNP concentration identified significant pulmonary hypertension with a sensitivity of 0.85 and specificity of 0.88 and was itself associated with an almost 3-fold increased risk of death on univariate analysis. In a stepwise multivariate analysis, an elevated BNP ratio (see Comment below) predicted increased mortality independent of lung function impairment.

Comment

This is an important, well-designed, prospective study primarily designed to evaluate the value of circulating BNP levels in detecting pulmonary hypertension in patients with chronic lung disease, but also yields interesting insights into the prognostic implications of pulmonary hypertension in this setting. Of the 176 consecutive patients recruited, a quarter had chronic obstructive pulmonary disease, 55 patients were diagnosed with IPF, 17 with connective tissue disease and ten patients had sarcoidosis. All patients underwent right heart catheterization and a mean PAP of >35 mmHg was considered significant pulmonary hypertension. None of the patients had received specific vasodilator therapy at initial evaluation. Other baseline tests included lung function tests, a 6-min walking test, and normalized BNP ratio, calculated as measured BNP divided by age- and sex-corrected normal values (range 18–75 pg/ml). Elevated BNP is therefore considered to be present when the BNP ratio is >1. Impressively, for a study of this size performed over a period of just over 4 years, no patients were lost to follow-up.

Of the 176 patients with chronic lung disease, 47 (26.7%) were diagnosed with pulmonary hypertension based on right heart catheterization; 18 of these 47 patients (38.3%) died after a mean survival time of 22.36 ± 3.1 months, compared with 13 deaths in the remaining 129 patients (10.08%), who experienced a mean survival time of 34.23 ± 1.84 months (P <0.001). An elevated mean PAP of ≥35 mmHg was associated with a 3.67-fold increase in the risk of death. The poor survival in the study population as a whole emphasizes that this cohort of patients had advanced chronic lung disease. The authors report on the characteristics of the 31 patients who died during the study compared with the 145 survivors. Using univariate analysis, the investigators identified a number of variables that were significantly more frequent in non-survivors compared with survivors and that independently predicted increased mortality (Table 13.4).

Use of receiver operator characteristic analysis showed that a normalized BNP ratio of >1 had a sensitivity of 0.85 and specificity of 0.88 and the positive and negative predicted values were 0.73 and 0.92 respectively for the presence of pulmonary hypertension. An elevated BNP ratio conferred an almost 3-fold increase in the risk of death (risk ratio 2.94; 95% CI 1.45–5.99; P <0.01), a prognostic indicator that compares favourably with that of PAP assessment by right heart catheterization (Fig. 13.6). Subgroup analysis revealed that the association between elevated BNP and mortality applied equally well to patients with interstitial lung disease and chronic obstructive pulmonary disease. Among patients with interstitial lung disease, 31 out of 88 (35.2%) had elevated BNP levels, and 11 (35.5%) of these died compared with 10 (17.5%) of those with normal BNP (P <0.05).

So is BNP measurement a robust biomarker for pulmonary hypertension in chronic lung disease? It has recently been shown that patients with elevated BNP levels are at overall increased risk of cardiovascular events and death, in part because BNP levels rise with left ventricular dysfunction [34]. Hence, elevated BNP levels may be a surrogate marker of underlying left heart failure rather than PAH. In the present study, however, the investigators sought to exclude patients with left ventricular failure on clinical and haemodynamic grounds and so the association between BNP and pulmonary hypertension does appear to be independent of left heart disease. The population of patients studied clearly had advanced lung disease, as indicated both by the baseline lung function tests (mean FVC was <50% of the predicted value and mean T_{LCO} was <30% of predicted) and by the overall poor survival of only 2–3 years. Yet, even within this group, the presence of pulmonary hypertension was associated with an even further reduction in survival. Echocardiography data were not reported in this study, but the sensitivity and specificity of BNP for predicting pulmonary hypertension is at least as good, if not better, than that seen in other studies that have used TTE to predict pulmonary hypertension.

Studies of this type need to be repeated in other centres and in patients with less severe lung disease, and ideally should incorporate serial BNP measurement. However, if the highly promising role of BNP were confirmed, there would be a good case for integrating this test into routine clinical practice as a screening tool

Table 13.4 Parameters predictive of survival after univariate analysis

Variable	Risk ratio estimates	95% confidence interval	P Value
Mean PAP, $\leq$35 mmHg	3.67	1.79–7.51	<0.001
PVR, $\geq$320 dyne $\cdot$ s $\cdot$ cm^{-5}	4.24	1.89–9.5	<0.01
CO, $\leq$4.4 l/min	2.4	1.16–4.95	<0.05
CI, $\leq$2.55 l $\cdot$ min^{-1} $\cdot$ m^{-2}	2.45	1.2–5	<0.05
Cap. Po_2, $\leq$50 mmHg	3.04	1.36–6.81	<0.01
TLC, $\leq$3.72 l	3.05	1.38–6.75	<0.01
FVC, <1.52 l	2.1	1.02–4.33	<0.05
BNP, normalized ratio $\geq$1	2.94	1.45–5.99	<0.01

CI, cardiac index; CO, cardiac output; Cap. Po_2, capillary partial pressure of oxygen; PVR, pulmonary vascular resistance.
Source: Leuchte et al. (2006).

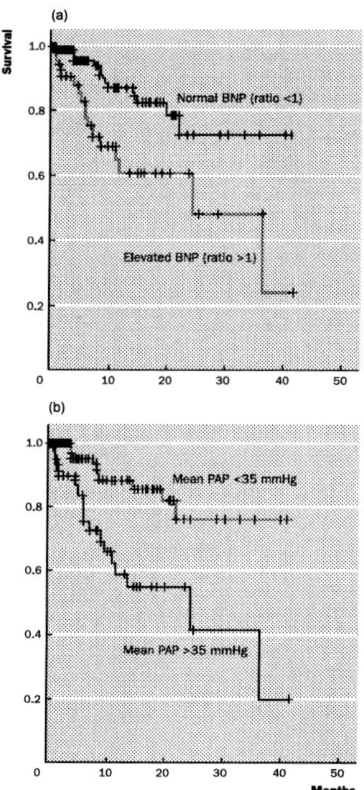

Fig. 13.6 (a) Parameters predictive of survival after univariate analysis. The brain natriuretic peptide (BNP) ratio was calculated as measured BNP concentration/individual normal BNP concentration. (b) Survival estimates based on the presence of significant pulmonary hypertension. PAP, pulmonary artery pressure. Source: Leuchte et al. (2006).

for the presence of pulmonary hypertension. Further studies are also required to determine whether therapeutic intervention can influence BNP levels.

Treatment of interstitial lung disease-associated pulmonary hypertension

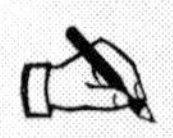

Bosentan in pulmonary arterial hypertension secondary to scleroderma

Joglekar A, Tsai FS, McCloskey DA, Wilson JE, Seibold JR, Riley DJ.
Rheumatology 2006; **33**: 61–8

BACKGROUND. Endothelin 1 (ET-1) is a powerful vasoconstrictor with mitogenic properties that has been implicated in the pathogenesis of pulmonary hypertension. Inhibition of ET-1 activity can be achieved by the blockade of two endothelin receptors, ETA and ETB. Bosentan is the first orally bioavailable, non-selective endothelin antagonist and is approved for the treatment of PAH. Bosentan therapy has been shown to improve exercise capacity and haemodynamics and to slow the time to symptomatic deterioration in two clinical trials of patients with PAH |35,36|. However, patients with pulmonary hypertension associated with systemic sclerosis made up only a small proportion of recruits to these studies and patients with significant interstitial lung disease in addition to pulmonary hypertension were excluded.

INTERPRETATION. In this retrospective study, 23 patients with systemic sclerosis-associated pulmonary hypertension were treated with oral bosentan, initially a twice-daily dose of 62.5 mg for 1 month followed by a twice-daily dose of 125 mg. Clinical benefit, assessed by World Health Organization (WHO) functional class status, was observed by 3 months, maintained to 9 months, and subsequently declined to below baseline values. The mean systolic PAP was 54 ± 2 mmHg at baseline and remained stable throughout the period of therapy, as did lung function. Hence, bosentan therapy resulted in clinical benefit for up to 9 months after therapy but did not influence pulmonary haemodynamics or lung function.

Comment

All patients in this retrospective observational study were diagnosed with systemic sclerosis based on the American College of Rheumatology Criteria and had WHO class II, III or IV functional status. A third of the patients had restrictive lung disease (total lung capacity <70% of predicted) although no radiology data are presented so the prevalence of associated interstitial lung disease in the study population is not known. Pulmonary hypertension was defined as PAP ≥45 mmHg based on TTE. Bosentan was given at a dose of 62.5 mg twice daily for 1 month followed by 125 mg twice daily. Although there was no control group, the investigators cite two seminal earlier randomized control trials of bosentan therapy (Bosentan Randomized Trial of Endothelin Antagonist Therapy for Pulmonary Hypertension 1 [BREATHE-1] |36| and Channik *et al.* |35|), using the data therein as a comparator.

In both the comparator studies, the 6-min walking test was the primary outcome measure and haemodynamic measurements and WHO functional class were secondary outcome measures. However, a 6-min walking test was not used consistently in the present study. The data show improvement in functional class during the first 3 months after bosentan therapy followed by stabilization between 3 and 6 months and a trend towards worsening after 12 months (Table 13.5). The use of the WHO functional classification is perhaps confusing since many other studies use the NYHA functional class, from which the former is derived. Serial echocardiography revealed that systolic PAP during the treatment period improved in one-third of patients, remained stable in one-third and rose in the remainder, thus remaining stable in the group overall (Fig. 13.7). Similarly, lung function remained stable or showed a downward trend overall. The degree of functional improvement observed was very similar to that seen in BREATHE-1 |36|, and the observation that bosentan does not consistently lower PAP but may tend to stabilize it is also consistent with previous observations in a placebo-controlled trial |35|. Indeed, it does appear that improved functional status is a better predictor of survival in PAH than improved haemodynamics |37|.

So what is the role of bosentan in systemic sclerosis-associated pulmonary hypertension? In the published pivotal studies, systemic sclerosis-associated PAH represents only a small subgroup of patients |35,36|. A recent subgroup analysis of these studies does, however, suggest functional benefit from bosentan treatment and it does appear that the survival of systemic sclerosis patients with pulmonary hypertension is significantly better now than it was in the previous era when treatment consisted only of oxygen, diuretics, warfarin and prostanoids |37–39|. Bosentan is approved by the FDA (U.S. Food and Drug Administration) for the treatment of PAH and it would be ethically contentious to embark on a placebo-controlled study in patients with class III or IV disease. The BUILD 2 trial (unpublished at the time of writing) is a randomized placebo-controlled study of bosentan therapy in patients with systemic sclerosis-associated interstitial lung

Table 13.5 Changes in World Health Organization classification

Change in WHO class	Baseline vs 3 mo (*n* = 12)*	3 mo vs 6 mo (*n* = 21)*	6 mo vs 9 mo (*n* = 21)*	9 mo vs 12 mo (*n* = 19)*	12 mo vs 15 mo (*n* = 15)*	15 mo vs 18 mo (*n* = 14)*
+2	14	0	0	0	0	0
+1	43	14	0	5	5	7
−1	0	14	5	16	5	21
−2	0	0	0	0	5	0

Numbers indicate the percentage of patients with baseline WHO functional class III or IV who changed class compared with the previous period. Positive numbers indicate improvement by one or two classes; negative numbers indicate worsening by one or two classes. 'Baseline' refers to data collected before study entry; 'mo' refers to 30-month periods during which data were combined. *Number of data pairs from consecutive time periods; this number may differ from the number of WHO class observations for individual time periods. Source: Joglekar *et al.* (2006).

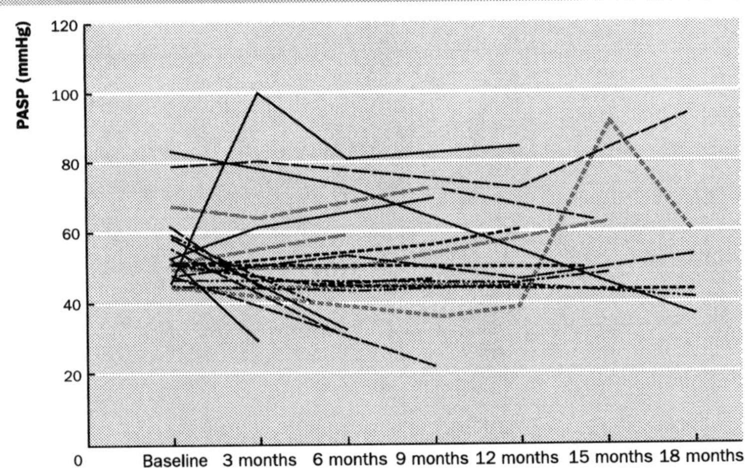

Fig. 13.7 Pulmonary artery systolic pressure (mmHg) over time (months) in individual patients. Source: Joglekar *et al.* (2006).

disease but specifically excludes those with pulmonary hypertension. Thus observational reports such as this study by Joglekar and colleagues are important and provide insight into the role of therapy in routine clinical practice.

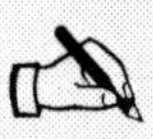

Immunosuppressive therapy and connective tissue diseases-associated pulmonary arterial hypertension

Sanchez O, Sitbon O, Jais X, Simonneau G, Humbert M. *Chest* 2006; **130**: 182–9

BACKGROUND. The role of specific vasculomodulatory drugs in pulmonary hypertension associated with connective tissue disease is receiving considerable attention. However, many such patients will receive standard immunosuppressive therapy as routine management of their systemic disease. Anecdotal evidence suggests that treatment with corticosteroids and/or immunosuppressive therapy may attenuate PAH in this setting |40,41|. The pathogenesis of pulmonary hypertension in association with connective tissue diseases and in the absence of significant parenchymal lung disease is incompletely understood, but there is evidence of an inflammatory process with elevated serum pro-inflammatory cytokines, an inflammatory cell infiltrate within plexiform lesions and an imbalance of growth factors and chemokines in diseased pulmonary arteries |42–44|.

INTERPRETATION. In this single-centre retrospective study, the clinical and haemodynamic effects of first-line immunosuppressant therapy alone on PAH was assessed in 28 consecutive patients with connective tissue disease. All patients received intravenous cyclophosphamide 600 mg/m^2 monthly for at least 3 months and 22 of the 28 patients received systemic corticosteroids in addition. Eight of the 28 patients were considered responders, as defined by stable or improved NYHA functional class, with sustained haemodynamic improvement after at least 1 year of therapy and without the addition of prostanoids, phosphodiesterase type 5 inhibitors or endothelin receptor antagonists. Of these eight responders, five had systemic lupus erythematosus (SLE) and three had mixed connective tissue disease. No patient with systemic sclerosis-associated PAH responded to the therapeutic regime.

Comment

The authors identified 28 patients with connective tissue disease and PAH who had not received prior treatment with prostacyclin derivatives, endothelin receptor antagonists or phosphodiesterase type 5 inhibitors and who had not previously received immunosuppressants or corticosteroids. The patients were classified as having SLE ($n = 13$), mixed connective tissue disease ($n = 8$), systemic sclerosis (limited disease, $n = 5$; diffuse disease, $n = 1$) or rheumatoid arthritis ($n = 1$). The diagnosis of PAH was established by right heart catheterization. The majority of patients had NYHA class III or IV disease with a mean ($\pm$ SD) PAP of 50 $\pm$ 13 mmHg. No patient had significant parenchymal lung disease, as demonstrated by detailed pulmonary function tests and an HRCT scan showing, at most, mild interstitial disease. All patients received conventional therapy, including oral anticoagulation, diuretics, supplementary oxygen and in addition a monthly intravenous bolus of cyclophosphamide 600 mg/m^2 for at least 3 months. Twenty-two of the 28 patients also received corticosteroid therapy, principally prednisolone.

Eleven of the 20 patients (55%) who did not respond to immunosuppressive therapy died within 5 years of initiation of the immunosuppressive therapy. In contrast, in patients who responded to immunosuppressive therapy, the survival rates at 1, 3 and 5 years were 100, 65 and 38% respectively ($P = 0.007$ compared with non-responders). Most patients on immunosuppressive therapy experienced the minor complications commonly seen with cyclophosphamide therapy. None of the patients with systemic sclerosis benefited from immunosuppressive therapy, whereas the response rate in those with SLE was 38% and in those with mixed connective tissue disease it was 37%. Patients who responded also tended to have less severe disease than non-responders.

The main limitations of the study are its retrospective nature and the inevitably biased selection of patients who are referred to a specialist centre of this type. Clearly definitive conclusions on the value of immunosuppressive therapy in connective tissue disease-associated pulmonary artery hypertension cannot be drawn. However, the feasibility of performing large controlled studies in which patients are given immunosuppressive therapy alone, without specific vasculo-modulatory drugs, is remote. It is likely, therefore, that future data will largely be retrospective or case-controlled. The limited evidence available does suggest that therapy with cyclophosphamide and corticosteroids may be beneficial when PAH occurs with SLE or mixed connective tissue disease.

Conclusion

The papers discussed in this chapter have shed new light on the diagnosis and epidemiology of pulmonary hypertension and pulmonary artery hypertension associated with interstitial lung disease and systemic sclerosis. The true incidence of pulmonary hypertension in unselected patients with IPF is still unknown, and in all likelihood depends upon the stage of fibrotic disease at which PAP is measured, but in advanced IPF up to 80% of individuals may have significantly elevated PAP. There is an association between elevated PAP and mortality in IPF and an unproven but tantalizing suggestion that significant pulmonary hypertension (systolic PAP >50 mmHg) may be particularly important in predicting very early mortality. In sarcoidosis, pulmonary hypertension may occur in 5–10% of patients and may be present in Stage 0 or 1 disease. The pathogenesis is likely to be complex but includes a granulomatous occlusive venopathy that may not be responsive to steroids. The current panel of drugs for treating pulmonary hypertension, including prostanoids, endothelin antagonists and phosphodiesterase type 5 inhibitors, have an established role in Stage 3 and 4 idiopathic PAH and systemic sclerosis-associated PAH. The roles of these agents in interstitial lung disease-associated pulmonary hypertension, however, remain unknown and until further trial data with mortality end-points are available, routine screening for pulmonary hypertension in patients with interstitial lung disease with TTE or promising new tools such as plasma BNP assay, is difficult to justify.

References

1. Galie N, Torbicki A, Barst R, Dartevelle P, Haworth S, Higenbottam T, Olschewski H, Peacock A, Pietra G, Rubin LJ, Simonneau G, Priori SG, Garcia MA, Blanc JJ, Budaj A, Cowie M, Dean V, Deckers J, Burgos EF, Lekakis J, Lindahl B, Mazzotta G, McGregor K, Morais J, Oto A, Smiseth OA, Barbera JA, Gibbs S, Hoeper M, Humbert M, Naeije R, Pepke-Zaba J. Guidelines on diagnosis and treatment of pulmonary arterial hypertension. The Task Force on Diagnosis and Treatment of Pulmonary Arterial Hypertension of the European Society of Cardiology. *Eur Heart J* 2004; **25**: 2243–78.

2. Arcasoy SM, Christie JD, Ferrari VA, Sutton MS, Zisman DA, Blumenthal NP, Pochettino A, Kotloff RM. Echocardiographic assessment of pulmonary hypertension in patients with advanced lung disease. *Am J Respir Crit Care Med* 2003; **167**: 735–40.

3. Borgeson DD, Seward JB, Miller FA Jr, Oh JK, Tajik AJ. Frequency of Doppler measurable pulmonary artery pressures. *J Am Soc Echocardiogr* 1996; **9**: 832–7.

4. Mukerjee D, St George D, Knight C, Davar J, Wells AU, du Bois RM, Black CM, Coghlan JG. Echocardiography and pulmonary function as screening tests for

pulmonary arterial hypertension in systemic sclerosis. *Rheumatology (Oxford)* 2004; **43**: 461–6.

5. McQuillan BM, Picard MH, Leavitt M, Weyman AE. Clinical correlates and reference intervals for pulmonary artery systolic pressure among echocardiographically normal subjects. *Circulation* 2001; **104**: 2797–802.

6. Kawut SM, Taichman DB, Archer-Chicko CL, Palevsky HI, Kimmel SE. Hemodynamics and survival in patients with pulmonary arterial hypertension related to systemic sclerosis. *Chest* 2003; **123**: 344–50.

7. Steen V, Medsger TA Jr. Predictors of isolated pulmonary hypertension in patients with systemic sclerosis and limited cutaneous involvement. *Arthritis Rheum* 2003; **48**: 516–22.

8. Rubin, LJ. Diagnosis and management of pulmonary arterial hypertension: ACCP evidence-based clinical practice guidelines. *Chest* 2004; **126**: 7S–10S.

9. Ghofrani HA, Voswinckel R, Reichenberger F, Weissmann N, Schermuly RT, Seeger W, Grimminger F. Hypoxia- and non-hypoxia-related pulmonary hypertension—established and new therapies. *Cardiovasc Res* 2006; **72**: 30–40.

10. Fuster V, Steele PM, Edwards WD, Gersh BJ, McGoon MD, Frye RL. Primary pulmonary hypertension: natural history and the importance of thrombosis. *Circulation* 1984; **70**: 580–7.

11. Barst RJ, Rubin LJ, Long WA, McGoon MD, Rich S, Badesch DB, Groves BM, Tapson VF, Bourge RC, Brundage BH. A comparison of continuous intravenous epoprostenol (prostacyclin) with conventional therapy for primary pulmonary hypertension. The Primary Pulmonary Hypertension Study Group. *N Engl J Med* 1996; **334**: 296–302.

12. Olschewski H, Ghofrani HA, Walmrath D, Schermuly R, Temmesfeld-Wollbruck B, Grimminger F, Seeger W. Inhaled prostacyclin and iloprost in severe pulmonary hypertension secondary to lung fibrosis. *Am J Respir Crit Care Med* 1999; **160**: 600–7.

13. King TE Jr, Tooze JA, Schwarz MI, Brown KR, Cherniack RM. Predicting survival in idiopathic pulmonary fibrosis: scoring system and survival model. *Am J Respir Crit Care Med* 2001; **164**: 1171–81.

14. Ebina M, Shimizukawa M, Shibata N, Kimura Y, Suzuki T, Endo M, Sasano H, Kondo T, Nukiwa T. Heterogeneous increase in CD34-positive alveolar capillaries in idiopathic pulmonary fibrosis. *Am J Respir Crit Care Med* 2004; **169**: 1203–8.

15. Renzoni EA, Walsh DA, Salmon M, Wells AU, Sestini P, Nicholson AG, Veeraraghavan S, Bishop AE, Romanska HM, Pantelidis P, Black CM, du Bois RM. Interstitial vascularity in fibrosing alveolitis. *Am J Respir Crit Care Med* 2003; **167**: 438–43.

16. Whelan TP, Dunitz JM, Kelly RF, Edwards LB, Herrington CS, Hertz MI, Dahlberg PS. Effect of preoperative pulmonary artery pressure on early survival after lung transplantation for idiopathic pulmonary fibrosis. *J Heart Lung Transplant* 2005; **24**: 1269–74.

17. King TE Jr, Safrin S, Starko KM, Brown KK, Noble PW, Raghu G, Schwartz DA. Analyses of efficacy end points in a controlled trial of interferen-gamma1b for idiopathic pulmonary fibrosis. *Chest* 2005; **127**: 171–7.

18. Arcasoy SM, Christie JD, Pochettino A, Rosengard BR, Blumenthal NP, Bavaria JE, Kotloff RM. Characteristics and outcomes of patients with sarcoidosis listed for lung transplantation. *Chest* 2001; **120**: 873–80.

19. Shorr AF, Davies DB, Nathan SD. Predicting mortality in patients with sarcoidosis awaiting lung transplantation. *Chest* 2003; **124**: 922–8.

20. Sulica R, Teirstein AS, Kakarla S, Nemani N, Behnegar A, Padilla ML. Distinctive clinical, radiographic, and functional characteristics of patients with sarcoidosis-related pulmonary hypertension. *Chest* 2005; **128**: 1483–9.

21. Rizzato G, Pezzano A, Sala G, Merlini R, Ladelli L, Tansini G, Montanari G, Bertoli L. Right heart impairment in sarcoidosis: haemodynamic and echocardiographic study. *Eur J Respir Dis* 1983; **64**: 121–8.

22. Rosen Y, Moon S, Huang CT, Gourin A, Lyons HA. Granulomatous pulmonary angiitis in sarcoidosis. *Arch Pathol Lab Med* 1977; **101**: 170–4.

23. Takemura T, Matsui Y, Saiki S, Mikami R. Pulmonary vascular involvement in sarcoidosis: a report of 40 autopsy cases. *Hum Pathol* 1992; **23**: 1216–23.

24. Gluskowski J, Hawrylkiewicz I, Zych D, Wojtczak A, Zielinski J. Pulmonary haemodynamics at rest and during exercise in patients with sarcoidosis. *Respiration* 1984; **46**: 26–32.

25. Gluskowski J, Hawrylkiewicz I, Zych D, Zielinski J. Effects of corticosteroid treatment on pulmonary haemodynamics in patients with sarcoidosis. *Eur Respir J* 1990; **3**: 403–7.

26. MacGregor AJ, Canavan R, Knight C, Denton CP, Davar J, Coghlan J, Black CM. Pulmonary hypertension in systemic sclerosis: risk factors for progression and consequences for survival. *Rheumatology (Oxford)* 2001; **40**: 453–9.

27. Mukerjee D, St George D, Coleiro B, Knight C, Denton CP, Davar J, Black CM, Coghlan JG. Prevalence and outcome in systemic sclerosis associated pulmonary arterial hypertension: application of a registry approach. *Ann Rheum Dis* 2003; **62**: 1088–93.

28. Ungerer RG, Tashkin DP, Furst D, Clements PJ, Gong H Jr, Bein M, Smith JW, Roberts N, Cabeen W. Prevalence and clinical correlates of pulmonary arterial hypertension in progressive systemic sclerosis. *Am J Med* 1983; **75**: 65–74.

29. Kawut SM, Taichman DB, Archer-Chicko CL, Palevsky HI, Kimmel SE. Hemodynamics and survival in patients with pulmonary arterial hypertension related to systemic sclerosis. *Chest* 2003; **123**: 344–50.

30. Berger M, Haimowitz A, Van Tosh A, Berdoff RL, Goldberg E. Quantitative assessment of pulmonary hypertension in patients with tricuspid regurgitation using continuous wave Doppler ultrasound. *J Am Coll Cardiol* 1985; **6**: 359–65.

31. Steen VD, Graham G, Conte C, Owens G, Medsger TA. Isolated diffusing capacity reduction in systemic sclerosis. *Arthritis Rheum* 1992; **35**: 765–70.

32. Denton CP, Cailes JB, Phillips GD, Wells AU, Black CM, Bois RM. Comparison of Doppler echocardiography and right heart catheterization to assess pulmonary hypertension in systemic sclerosis. *Br J Rheumatol* 1997; **36**: 239–43.

33. Mukoyama M, Nakao K, Hosoda K, Suga S, Saito Y, Ogawa Y, Shirakami G, Jougasaki M, Obata K, Yasue H. Brain natriuretic peptide as a novel cardiac hormone in humans. Evidence for an exquisite dual natriuretic peptide system, atrial natriuretic peptide and brain natriuretic peptide. *J Clin Invest* 1991; **87**: 1402–12.

34. Wang TJ, Larson MG, Levy D, Benjamin EJ, Leip EP, Omland T, Wolf PA, Vasan RS. Plasma natriuretic peptide levels and the risk of cardiovascular events and death. *N Engl J Med* 2004; **350**: 655–63.

35. Channick RN, Simonneau G, Sitbon O, Robbins IM, Frost A, Tapson VF, Badesch DB, Roux S, Rainisio M, Bodin F, Rubin LJ. Effects of the dual endothelin-receptor antagonist bosentan in patients with pulmonary hypertension: a randomised placebo-controlled study. *Lancet* 2001; **358**: 1119–23.

36. Rubin LJ, Badesch DB, Barst RJ, Galie N, Black CM, Keogh A, Pulido T, Frost A, Roux S, Leconte I, Landzberg M, Simonneau G. Bosentan therapy for pulmonary arterial hypertension. *N Engl J Med* 2002; **346**: 896–903.

37. McLaughlin VV, Sitbon O, Badesch DB, Barst RJ, Black C, Galie N, Rainisio M, Simonneau G, Rubin LJ. Survival with first-line bosentan in patients with primary pulmonary hypertension. *Eur Respir J* 2005; **25**: 244–9.

38. Denton CP, Humbert M, Rubin L, Black CM. Bosentan treatment for pulmonary arterial hypertension related to connective tissue disease: a subgroup analysis of the pivotal clinical trials and their open-label extensions. *Ann Rheum Dis* 2006; **65**: 1336–40.

39. Williams MH, Das C, Handler CE, Akram MR, Davar J, Denton CP, Smith CJ, Black CM, Coghlan JG. Systemic sclerosis associated pulmonary hypertension: improved survival in the current era. *Heart* 2006; **92**: 926–32.

40. Dahl M, Chalmers A, Wade J, Calverley D, Munt B. Ten year survival of a patient with advanced pulmonary hypertension and mixed connective tissue disease treated with immunosuppressive therapy. *J Rheumatol* 1992; **19**: 1807–9.

41. Groen H, Bootsma H, Postma DS, Kallenberg CG. Primary pulmonary hypertension in a patient with systemic lupus erythematosus: partial improvement with cyclophosphamide. *J Rheumatol* 1993; **20**: 1055–7.

42. Balabanian K, Foussat A, Dorfmuller P, Durand-Gasselin I, Capel F, Bouchet-Delbos L, Portier A, Marfaing-Koka A, Krzysiek R, Rimaniol AC, Simonneau G, Emilie D, Humbert M. CX(3)C chemokine fractalkine in pulmonary arterial hypertension. *Am J Respir Crit Care Med* 2002; **165**: 1419–25.

43. Humbert M, Monti G, Brenot F, Sitbon O, Portier A, Grangeot-Keros L, Duroux P, Galanaud P, Simonneau G, Emilie D. Increased interleukin-1 and interleukin-6 serum concentrations in severe primary pulmonary hypertension. *Am J Respir Crit Care Med* 1995; **151**: 1628–31.

44. Tuder R. Groves MB, Badesch DB, Voelkel NF. Exuberant endothelial cell growth and elements of inflammation are present in plexiform lesions of pulmonary hypertension. *Am J Pathol* 1994; **144**: 275–85.

Abbreviations

5-HT2A	5 hydroxytryptamine [serotonin] receptor 2A
ABCS	Active Bacterial Core Surveillance
AHI	apnoea/hypopnoea index
AHR	airway hyper-reactivity
ALT	alanine aminotransferase
ApoE	apoliprotein E
ASL	aspartate aminotransferase
ASM	airway smooth muscle
ASV	adaptive servoventilation
ATS	American Thoracic Society
BAL	bronchoalveolar lavage
BCG	Bacillus Calmette-Guérin
BNP	brain natriuretic peptide
BODE	(index based on) body mass index, airflow obstruction, dyspnoea and exercise capacity
BREATHE-1	Bosentan Randomized Trial of Endothelin Antagonist Therapy for Pulmonary Hypertension 1
BRONCUS	Bronchitis Randomized on N-acetylcysteine Cost-Utility Study
BTS	British Thoracic Society
BUILD	Bosentan Use in Interstitial Lung Disease
c.f.u.	colony-forming unit
cAMP	cyclic nucleotide adenosine 3'5'-monophosphate
CANPAP	Canadian Continuous Positive Airway Pressure for Patients with Central Sleep Apnea and Heart Failure
CAP	community-acquired pneumonia
CCHS	Copenhagen City Heart Study
CDC	Centres for Disease Control and Prevention
CFA	cytogenic fibrosing alveolitis
CFP	culture filtrate protein
cGMP	cyclic nucleotide guanosine 3'5'-monophosphate
CGMS	continuous glucose monitoring system
CI	confidence interval
COPD	chronic obstructive pulmonary disease
COSMIC	COPD and Seretide: a Multi-Center Intervention and Characterization
CPAP	continuous positive airway pressure
CPI	composite physiological index
CPMP	(European Union) Committee on Proprietary Medicinal Compounds
CRP	C-reactive protein
CSA-CSR	central sleep apnoea, Cheyne-Stokes respiration
CT	computed tomography
des-CIC	desisobutyryl-ciclesonide
DL_{CO}	diffusion capacity of carbon monoxide
DOTS	Directly Observed Treatment
DSMB	Drug Safety Monitoring Board
DSP	distance–saturation product
EBUS	endobronchial ultrasonography

ECG	electrocardiogram
EEVcw	change in Vcw at end of expiration
EGFR	epidermal growth factor receptor
ELISA	enzyme-linked immunosobent assay
EMG	??electromyography
ERS	European Respiratory Society
ESAT	early secretory antigenic target
ESS	Epworth Sleepiness Score
ET-1	endothelin 1
EUS	endoscopic ultrasono-graphy
FDA	Federal Drug Administration (or Food and Drug Administration?)
FDG	18-flurodeoxyglucose
FE_{NO}	fraction of exhaled nitric oxide
FEV_1	forced expiratory volume in 1 second
FFMI	fat-free mass/height^2
FiO_2	fraction of inspired oxygen
FRC	functional residual capacity
FVC	forced vital capacity
GINA	Global Initiative for Asthma
GLUCOLD	Groningen Leiden Universities and Corticosteroids in Obstructive Lung Disease
GOAL	Gaining Optimal Asthma Control
GOLD	Global Initiative for Chronic Obstructive Lung Disease
GPRD	General Practice Research Database
$HbA1_c$	glycosylated haemoglobin
HEC	hyperinsulinaemic–euglycaemic clamp
HIF	hypoxia-inducible factor
HIV	human immunodeficiency virus
HOMA-IR	homeostasis model assessment of insulin resistance
HR	hazard ratio
HRCT	high-resolution computed tomography
IC/TLC	inspiratory capacity to total lung capacity ratio
ICS	inhaled corticosteroids
ICU	intensive care unit
IDF	International Diabetes Federation
Ig	immunoglobulin
IGF	insulin-like growth factor
IL	interleukin
IMV	invasive mechanical support
INR	international normalized ratio
INSPIRE	International Study of Survival Outcomes in IPF with Interferon-γ1b Early Intervention
INTEREST	Iressa™ NSCLC Trial Evaluating Response and Survival against Taxotere
INVITE	Iressa™ versus vinorelbine
IPF	idiopathic pulmonary fibrosis
ITT	intention-to-treat
LABA	long-acting β-2 agonist
LOS	length of stay
LVEF	left ventricular ejection fraction
MDA	malondialdehyde
MDI	metered-dose inhaler
MDRTB	Multidrug-resistant tuberculosis
MEF_{50}	maximal expiratory flow at 50% of FVC
MMP-9	matrix metalloproteinase 9
MRC	Medical Research Council
MRI	magnetic resonance imaging

MRSA	methicillin-resistant *Staphylococcus aureus*
NAC	N-acetylcysteine
NFκB	nuclear factor κB
NHANES	National Health and Nutrition Examination Survey
NICE	National Institute for Clinical Excellence
NIV	non-invasive positive pressure ventilation
NLST	national lung screening trial
NSIP	non-specific interstitial pneumonia
NYHA	New York Heart Association
OGTT	oral glucose tolerance test
OR	odds ratio
OSAHS	obstructive sleep apnoea/hypopnoea
PAC	Prevention of Asthma in Childhood
$PaCO_2$	arterial partial pressure of carbon dioxide
PAH	pulmonary arterial hypertension
PaO_2	arterial partial pressure of oxygen
PAP	pulmonary artery pressure
PC_{20}	20% fall in FEV in response to methacholine challenge
$PDFEV_1$	post-bronchodilator FEV_1
PEAK	Prevention of Early Asthma in Kids
PEF	peak expiratory flow
PET	positron emission tomography
PITT	primary intention-to-treat
Ppa	pulmonary artery mean pressure
PPB	potentially pathogenic bacteria
PPP	per protocol population
PPV	pneumococcal vaccine
PSI	pneumonia severity index
PVOD	pulmonary vascular occlusive disease
rAP	right atrial pressure
rATS	revised American Thoracic Society (score)
REM	rapid eye-movement
ROS	reactive oxygen species
RR	risk ratio
RVSP	right ventricular systolic pressure
SEER	Surveillance, Epidemiology and End Results
SF-36	Short Form 36-item questionnaire
SGRQ	St George's Respiratory Questionnaire
SLE	systemic lupus erythematosus
SSRI	selective serotonin reuptake inhibitor
SVM	support vector machine
TBNA	transbronchial needle aspiration
TELICAST	Telithromycin, Chlamydophila, and Asthma Trial
TennCare	Tennessee Medicaid programme
TIMP-1	tissue inhibitor of metalloproteinase 1
TLCO	transfer factor for carbon monoxide
TNF	tumour necrosis factor
TRISTAN	Trial of Inhaled Steroids and Long-acting β_2 Agonists
TTE	transthoracic Doppler echocardiography
UIP	usual interstitial pneumonia
UNOS	United Network for Organ Sharing
VAP	ventilator-associated pneumonia
Vco_2	carbon dioxide production

Vcw	volume of entire chest wall	vTR	velocity of systolic triscupid regurgitation
VE	minute ventilation		
VNTR	variable number tandem repeat	WHO	World Health Organization

Index of papers reviewed

Imperatori A, Harrison RN, Leitch DN, *et al.* Lung cancer in Teeside (UK) and Varese (Italy): a comparison of management and survival. *Thorax* 2006; 61: 232–9. **148**

Joglekar A, Tsai FS, McCloskey DA, Wilson JE, Seibold JR, Riley DJ. Bosentan in pulmonary arterial hypertension secondary to scleroderma. *Rheumatology* 2006; 33: 61–8. **282**

Johnston SL, Blasi F, Black PN, Martin RJ, Farrell DJ, Nieman RB. The effect of telithromycin in acute exacerbations of asthma. *New Engl J Med* 2006; 354: 1589–600. **26**

Kim DS, Park JH, Park BK, Lee JS, Nicholson AG, Colby T. Acute exacerbation of idiopathic pulmonary fibrosis frequency and clinical features. *Eur Resp J* 2006; 27: 143–50. **227**

Kiri VA, Pride NB, Soriano JB, Vestbo J. Inhaled corticosteroids in chronic obstructive pulmonary disease: results from two observational designs free of immortal time bias. *Am J Respir Crit Care Med* 2005; 172: 460–4. **42**

Koeman M, van der Ven AJ, Hak E, *et al.* Oral decontamination with chlorhexidine reduces the incidence of ventilator-associated pneumonia. *Am J Respir Crit Care Med* 2006; 173: 1348–55. **100**

Koopmans JG, Lutter R, Jansen HM, van der Zee JS. Adding salmeterol to an inhaled corticosteroid: long term effects on bronchial inflammation in asthma. *Thorax* 2006; 61: 306–12. **15**

Kubo H, Nakayama K, Yanai M, *et al.* Anticoagulant therapy for idiopathic pulmonary fibrosis. *Chest* 2005; 128: 1475–82. **250**

Kumaran M, Benamore RE, Vaidhyanath R, *et al.* Ultrasound guided cytological aspiration of supraclavicular lymph nodes in patients with suspected lung cancer. *Thorax* 2005; 60: 229–33. **140**

Lapperre TS, Postma DS, Gosman MME, *et al.* Relation between duration of smoking cessation and bronchial inflammation in COPD. *Thorax* 2006; 61: 115–21. **37**

Lardinois D, Weder W, Roudas M, *et al.* Etiology of solitary extrapulmonary positron emission tomography and computed tomography findings in patients with lung cancer. *J Clin Oncol* 2005; 23: 6846–53. **143**

Lardizabal A, Passannante M, Kojakali F, Hayden C, Reichman LB. Enhancement of treatment completion for latent tuberculosis infection with 4 months of rifampicin. *Chest* 2006; 130: 1712–7. **72**

Larkin EK, Patel SR, Redline S, Mignot E, Elston RC, Hallmayer J. Apolipoprotein E and obstructive sleep apnea: evaluating whether a candidate gene explains a linkage peak. *Genet Epidemiol* 2006; 30: 101–10. **173**

Le Blanc JK, Devereaux BM, Imperiale TR *et al.* Endoscopic ultrasound in non-small cell lung cancer and negative mediastinum or computed tomography. *Am J Respir Crit Care Med* 2005; 171: 177–82. **137**

Lederer DJ, Arcasoy SM, Wilt JS, D'Ovidio F, Sonett JR, Kawut SM. Six-minute-walk distance predicts waiting

Martinez FJ, Safrin S, Weycker D, Starko KM, Bradford WZ, King TE Jr, *et al.* The clinical course of patients with idiopathic pulmonary fibrosis. *Ann Intern Med* 2005; 142: 963–7.   **223**

Maskell NA, Davies CW, Nunn AJ, *et al.* U.K. Controlled trial of intrapleural streptokinase for pleural infection. *N Engl J Med* 2005; 352: 865–74. Erratum in: *N Engl J Med* 2005; 352: 2146.   **104**

Masoli M, Weatherall M, Holt S, Beasley R. Moderate dose inhaled corticosteroid plus salmeterol versus higher doses of inhaled corticosteroids in symptomatic asthma. *Thorax* 2005; 60: 730–34.   **13**

Mercken EM, Hageman GJ, Scols AM, Akkermans MA, Bast A, Wouters EF. Rehabilitation decreases exercise-induced oxidative stress in chronic obstructive pulmonary disease. *Am J Respir Crit Care Med* 2005; 172: 994–1001.   **51**

Meyers BF, Haddad F, Siegel BA. Cost effectiveness of routine mediastinoscopy in computed tomography and positron emission tomography – screened patients with Stage I lung cancer. *J Thorac Cardiovasc Surg* 2006; 131: 822–9.   **141**

Michalopoulos A, Kasiakou SK, Mastora Z, Rellos K, Kapaskelis AM, Falagas ME. Aerosolized colistin for the treatment of nosocomial pneumonia due to multidrug-resistant Gram-negative bacteria in patients without cystic fibrosis. *Crit Care* 2005; 9: R53–9.   **101**

Misthos P, Sepsas E, Konstantinou M, Athanassiadi K, Skottis I, Lioulias A. Early use of intrapleural fibrinolytics in the management of postpneumonic empyema. A prospective study. *Eur J Cardiothorac Surg* 2005; 28: 599–603.   **103**

Murray CS, Woodcock A, Langley SJ, Morris J, Custovic A. Secondary prevention of asthma by the use of inhaled fluticasone propionate in wheezy infants (IFWIN): double-blind, randomised, controlled study. *Lancet* 2006; 368: 754–62.   **7**

Nadrous HF, Pellikka PA, Krowka MJ, *et al.* Pulmonary hypertension in patients with idiopathic pulmonary fibrosis. *Chest* 2005; 128: 2393–9.   **262**

Nakamura H, Kawasaki N, Taguchi M, *et al.* Survival impact of epidermal growth factor receptor overexpression in patients with non-small lung cancer: a meta-analysis. *Thorax* 2006; 61: 140–5.   **157**

Nathan SD, Shlobin OA, Ahmad S, Urbanek S, Barnett SD. Pulmonary hypertension and pulmonary function testing in idiopathic pulmonary fibrosis. *Chest* 2007; 131: 657–63.   **264**

Newell JN, Baral SC, Pande SB, Bam DS, Malla P. Family-member DOTS and community DOTS for tuberculosis control in Nepal: cluster-randomised controlled trial. *Lancet* 2006; 367: 903–9.   **78**

Nunes H, Humbert M, Capron F, *et al.* Pulmonary hypertension associated with sarcoidosis: mechanisms, haemodynamics and prognosis. *Thorax* 2006; 61: 68–74.   **271**

Oosterheert JJ, Bonten MJ, Schneider MM, *et al.* Effectiveness of early switch

Effectiveness Evaluation Unit (CEEu). UK National COPD Audit 2003: impact of hospital resources and organisation of care on patient outcome following admission for acute COPD exacerbation. *Thorax* 2006; 61: 837–42. **62**

Puhan MA, Schüemann, Frey M, Scharplatz M, Bachmann LM. How should COPD patients exercise during respiratory rehabilitation? Comparison of exercise modalities and intensities to treat skeletal muscle dysfunction. *Thorax* 2005; 60: 367–75. **52**

Rabe KF, Atienza T, Magyar P, Larsson P, Jorup C, Lalloo UG. Effect of budesonide in combination with formoterol for reliever therapy in asthma exacerbations: a randomised controlled, double-blind study. *Lancet* 2006; 368: 744–53. **14**

Rabe KF, Bateman ED, O'Donnell D, Witte S, Bredenbröker D, Bethke TD. Roflumilast – an oral anti-inflammatory treatment for chronic obstructive pulmonary disease: a randomised controlled trial. *Lancet* 2005; 366: 563–71. **48**

Ramírez-Venegas A, Sansores RH, Pérez-Padilla R, *et al*. Survival of patients with chronic obstructive pulmonary disease due to biomass smoke and tobacco. *Am J Respir Crit Care Med* 2006; 173: 393–7. **61**

Riha RL, Brander P, Vennelle M, Douglas NJ. A cephalometric comparison of patients with the sleep apnea/hypopnea syndrome and their siblings. *Sleep* 2005; 28: 315–20. **170**

Rintoul RC, Skwarski KM, Murchison JT, *et al*. Endobronchial and endoscopic ultrasound-guided real time fine-needle aspiration for mediastinal staging. *Eur Respir J* 2005; 25: 416–21. **139**

Rodrigo GJ. Comparison of inhaled fluticasone with intravenous hydrocortisone in the treatment of adult acute asthma. *Am J Respir Crit Care Med* 2005; 171: 1231–36. **25**

Rudd RM, Prescott RJ, Chalmers JC, Johnston ID; British Thoracic Society. Study on cryptogenic fibrosing alveolitis: response to treatment and survival. *Thorax* 2007; 62: 62–6. **220**

Ryan S, Taylor CT, McNicholas WT. Predictors of elevated nuclear factor-kappaB-dependent genes in obstructive sleep apnea syndrome. *Am J Respir Crit Care Med* 2006; 174: 824–30. **172**

Sanchez O, Sitbon O, Jais X, Simonneau G, Humbert M. Immunosuppressive therapy and connective tissue diseases-associated pulmonary arterial hypertension. *Chest* 2006; 130: 182–9. **284**

Schechter M, Zajdenverg R, Falco G, *et al*. Weekly rifapentine/isoniazid or daily rifampin/pyrazinamide for latent tuberculosis in household contacts. *Am J Respir Crit Care Med* 2006; 173: 922–6. **74**

Scheinberg P, Shore E. A pilot study of the safety and efficacy of tobramycin solution for inhalation in patients with severe bronchiectasis. *Chest* 2005; 127: 1420–6. **112**

Schoch OD, Rieder P, Tueller C, *et al*. Diagnostic yield of sputum, induced sputum, and bronchoscopy after radiologic tuberculosis screening. *Am J*

Respir Crit Care Med 2007; 175: 80–6. **77**

Schwab RJ, Pasirstein M, Kaplan L, *et al.* Family aggregation of upper airway soft tissue structures in normal subjects and patients with sleep apnea. *Am J Resp Crit Care Med* 2006; 173: 453–63. **170**

Sethi S, Maloney J, Grove L, Wrona C, Berenson CS. Airway inflammation and bronchial bacterial colonisation in chronic obstructive pulmonary disease. *Am J Respir Crit Care Med* 2006; 173: 991–98. **35**

Shepherd FA Rodrigues Pereira J, Cinleanu T, *et al.* Erlotinib in previously treated non-small-cell lung cancer. *N Engl J Med* 2005; 353: 123–32. **151**

Shieh FK, Snyder G, Horsburgh CR, Bernardo J, Murphy C, Saukkonen JJ. Predicting non-completion of treatment for latent tuberculous infection: a prospective survey. *Am J Respir Crit Care Med* 2006; 174: 717–21. **71**

Shorr AF, Helman DL, Davies DB, Nathan SD. Pulmonary hypertension in advanced sarcoidosis: epidemiology and clinical characteristics. *Eur Respir J* 2005; 25: 783–8. **269**

Sin DD, Wu L, Anderson JA, Anthonisen NR, *et al.* Inhaled corticosteroids and mortality in chronic obstructive pulmonary disease. *Thorax* 2005; 60: 992–7. **43**

Smith AD, Cowan JO, Brassett KP, Herbison GP, Taylor DR. Monitoring exhaled nitric oxide to guide inhaled steroid dosage in asthma. *N Engl J Med* 2005; 352: 263–73. **11**

Smith JR, Mildenhall S, Noble MJ, Shepstone L, Koutantji M, Mugford M, Harrison BDW. The Coping with Asthma Study: a randomised controlled trial of a home-based, nurse-led pschoeducational intervention for adults at risk of adverse asthma outcomes. *Thorax* 2005: 60; 1003–11. **23**

Soler-Cataluua JJ, Martínez-García, Román-Sánchez P, Salcedo E, Navarro M, Ochando R. Severe acute exacerbations and mortality in patients with chronic obstructive pulmonary disease. *Thorax* 2005; 60: 925–31. **57**

Soriano T, Alegre J, Aleman C, *et al.* Factors influencing length of hospital stay in patients with bacterial pleural effusion. *Respiration* 2005; 72: 587–93. **102**

Steentoft J, Konradsen HB, Hilskov J, Gislason G, Andersen JR. Response to pneumococcal vaccine in chronic obstructive lung disease – the effect of ongoing, systemic steroid treatment. *Vaccine* 2006; 24: 1408–12. **115**

Stockley RA, Chopra N, Rice L, on behalf of the SMS40026 Investigator Group. Addition of salmeterol to existing treatment in patients with COPD: a 12 month study. *Thorax* 2006; 61: 122–28. **40**

Swensen SJ, Jett JR, Hartman TE, *et al.* CT Screening for lung cancer: five-year prospective experience. *Radiology* 2005; 235: 259–65. **133**

Szefler SJ, Phillips BR, Martinez FD, *et al.* Characterization of within-subject responses to fluticasone and montelukast in childhood asthma. *J Allergy Clin Immunol* 2005; 115: 233–42. **17**

Index